Adverse Effects of Herbal Drugs

Volume 1

Editors

P.A.G.M. De Smet (Managing Editor)   K. Keller

R. Hänsel   R.F. Chandler

Adverse Effects of Herbal Drugs 1

Edited by
P.A.G.M. De Smet (Managing Editor)
K. Keller   R. Hänsel   R.F. Chandler

Contributors
I.H. Bowen   E.L. Boyd   D. Corrigan   I.J. Cubbin
P.A.G.M. De Smet   D. Frohne   R. Hänsel   B.M. Hausen
K. Keller   K.F. Lampe   C.-P. Siegers   U. Sonnenborn
J. Westendorf

In collaboration with the Pharmaceuticals Programme
of the World Health Organization, Regional Office for Europe

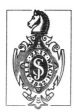

Springer-Verlag

Berlin Heidelberg New York
London Paris Tokyo
Hong Kong Barcelona
Budapest

Dr. PETER A.G.M. DE SMET
Drug Information Center
Royal Dutch Association for the Advancement of Pharmacy
Alexanderstraat 11, NL-2514 The Hague
The Netherlands

Dr. KONSTANTIN KELLER
Institut für Arzneimittel des Bundesgesundheitsamtes
Seestraße 10, W-1000 Berlin 65
Germany

Prof. DR. RUDOLF HÄNSEL
Westpreußenstraße 71, W-8000 München 81
früher: Fachbereich Pharmazie der Freien Universität Berlin
Germany

Prof. DR. R.FRANK CHANDLER
College of Pharmacy, Dalhousie University, Halifax B3H 3J5
Canada

ISBN 3-540-53100-9 Springer-Verlag Berlin Heidelberg New York
ISBN 0-387-53100-9 Springer-Verlag New York Berlin Heidelberg

Production Editor: B. Reichenthaler
Typesetting: International Typesetters Inc. Makati, Metro Manila, Philippines
13/3145-543210 − Printed on acid-free paper

To Katelijne
A Boisterous Barong

Preface

This book is the first volume of a series on the adverse effects of herbal drugs. We begin this series not because we are opposed to phytotherapy, or because we want to share our ammunition with adversaries of herbal drug treatments. We realize that several remedies of natural origin (e.g., senna, ipecac) have retained a prominent place in the conventional drug armamentarium. We also recognize that the general public appreciates so-called mildly acting herbs for self-medication purposes. We acknowledge that even when such herbs have no pronounced pharmacological activity, their psychosocial effect remains an asset that should not be ignored. Moreover, we do not hold the often heard opinion that traditional remedies are nothing but a collection of worthless relics from the remote past which cannot possibly be relevant for modern medicine. We consider this an erroneous assumption thas has been refuted repeatedly by experimental research on traditional botanicals. The encouraging results with the herbal remedy feverfew as a prophylactic antimigraine agent is a recent illustration that botanical medicine can still provide exciting therapeutic discoveries.

For these reasons it is not our intention to place botanical remedies indiscriminately in an unfavorable light. We do not seek to dam up the "green" wave that is sweeping over our society. We do consider it important, however, that this wave be appropriately chanelled, and with this basic attitude we have assumed editorial responsibility. One of the major reasons cited for the current revival of natural medicines is a widespread fear of side effects of synthetic drugs. This fear is often associated with an intuitive feeling that naturalness is a guarantee of harmlessness. However, it is a serious error to assume that anything deriving from is necessarily beneficial and benign. The genus *Aristolochia* is natural, but it contains one of the most potent animal carcinogens yet identified. It is also a grave mistake to assume that a long tradition of empiricism is an adequate safeguard against any kind of botanical health risk. At least 67 different species of *Aristolo-chia* have been used medicinally all over the world, and yet no one suspected that these plants contained a potent carcinogen until this was accidentally discovered a few years ago in laboratory animals.

Since the herbal wave sweeping over our health market may thus do harm as well as good, there is a compelling need for reliable and detailed information on the adverse effects of botanical medicines. We personally feel that such information is urgently needed in drug information centers, governmental offices, and academic institutes. It is also our experience that retrieving the full adverse reaction profile of a herbal drug is often difficult. The usual textbooks on drug information pay insufficient attention to botanical remedies, and pharmacognostic sources tend to focus on nonclinical aspects or on the beneficial side of medicinal plants. Searching computerized bibliographic files may also not provide ready answers, as botanicals are often less well indexed than chemical entities. Moreover, many herbal remedies were long ago replaced by synthetic medicines and were only recently reintroduced to the market. As a result, valuable data on these agents may be hidden in references that were published before the first database went online.

We have ourselves the task of filling this informational vacuum with a scientific series in which the adverse effects of herbal medicines are evaluated critically and comprehensively. This plant-oriented approach is supplemented by adding introductory chapters on more general topics.

November 1991   THE EDITORS

Contents

Contributors

Dr. IAN H. BOWEN
School of Pharmaceutical and Chemical Sciences,
Sunderland Polytechnic, Langham Tower, Ryhope Road,
Sunderland SR2 7EE
United Kingdom

Dr. EDDIE L. BOYD
College of Pharmacy, Xaiver University of Louisiana,
7325 Palmetto Street, New Orleans LA 70125
United States

Dr. DESMOND CORRIGAN
Department of Pharmacognosy, School of Pharmacy,
Trinity College, 18 Shrewsbury Road, Dublin 4
Ireland

Mr. Ian J. CUBBIN
School of Pharmaceutical and Chemical Sciences,
Sunderland Polytechnic, Langham Tower, Ryhope Road,
Sunderland SR2 7EE
United Kingdom

Dr. PETER A.G.M. DE SMET
Drug Information Center,
Royal Dutch Association for the Advancement of Pharmacy,
Alexanderstraat 11, 2514 JL The Hague
The Netherlands

Prof. Dr. DIETRICH FROHNE
Institut für Pharmazeutische Biologie,
Christian-Albrechts-Universität, Grasweg 9, 2300 Kiel
Germany

Prof. DR. RUDOLF HÄNSEL
Westpreußenstraße 71, W-8000 München 81
früher: Fachbereich Pharmazie der Freien Universität Berlin
Germany

Prof. Dr. B.M. HAUSEN
Universitäts-Hautklinik, Martinistraße 52, W-2000 Hamburg 20
Germany

Dr. KONSTANTIN KELLER
Institut für Arzneimittel des Bundesgesundheitsamtes,
Seestraße 10, W-1000 Berlin 65
Germany

Dr. KENNETH F. LAMPE †

Prof. Dr. C.-P. SIEGERS
Institut für Toxikologie, Medizinische Universität zu Lübeck
Ratzeburger Allee 160, W-2400 Lübeck 1
Germany

Dr. ULRICH SONNENBORN
Fa. Dr. Poehlmann & Co., Loerfeldstraße 20, W-5804 Herdecke
Germany

Prof. Dr. JOHANNES WESTENDORF
Institut für Pharmakologie, Universität Hamburg,
Grindelallee 117, W-2000 Hamburg 13
Germany

Toxicological Outlook on the Quality Assurance of Herbal Remedies

Peter A.G.M. De Smet

Introduction

The use of natural medicines is a persistent aspect of present-day health care. According to the American firm Frost & Sullivan, Europeans spent 560 million dollars on natural remedies and food supplements in 1986, and this market is expected to show substantial growth in the years to come [1]. A remarkable feature of this development is the belief of many consumers that naturalness is a guarantee of harmlessness. Yet there can be no doubt that some of the botanicals that have been traditionally used as medicines can produce dangerous and sometimes even lethal poisoning [2-12]. It is not surprising then that the professional medical literature regularly contains case reports about toxic reactions to herbal medicines. An example recently published in the *British Medical Journal* involved a 13-year-old boy who developed a veno-occlusive disease of the liver after the regular ingestion of a herbal tea prepared from comfrey leaves (*Symphytum officinale*) for two to three years. Although the patient was tolerably well at the time of writing, his prognosis remained uncertain [13]. This case history is just one of various reports that show beyond doubt that botanical medicines may produce serious side effects. Numerous reviews have therefore expressed concern about the safety of herbal medicines [1,14-38].

When the original reports on the subject are carefully screened, it becomes obvious that many of the cases where herbal products have been associated with actual human poisoning were not in fact caused by the herbs mentioned on the product label, but resulted from substitution or contamination of the declared ingredients, intentionally or by accident, with a more toxic botanical, a poisonous metal, or a potent nonherbal drug substance. In other words, the present dangers of herbal drug therapy are all too often due to a lack of stringent quality assurance rather than to the pharmacological activity of the herbal ingredients themselves. This volume therefore opens with a general introductory chapter on the quality control of botanical medicines.

In its recent "Note for Guidance on the Quality of Herbal Remedies," the influential Committee for Proprietary Medicinal Products of the European Community (EC) has described the need to control the purity of herbal remedies as follows: "As a general rule, vegetable drugs must be tested for microbiological quality and for residues of pesticides and fumigation agents, radioactivity, toxic metals, likely contaminants and adulterants, etc., unless otherwise justified" [39].

In the light of this guideline, the following types of potential contaminants will be considered in this chapter:

— Toxic botanicals
— Micro-organisms and microbial toxins
— Pesticides and fumigation agents
— Radioactivity
— Toxic metals
— Synthetic and animal drug substances

A more detailed overview furnished with examples is presented in Table 1. It should be noted that this chapter concentrates on information that is toxicologically relevant, such as safe levels of contamination and clinical findings. Analytical results are discussed in this context only, and data about analytical methodology (e.g., [40,41]) are completely outside the scope of this survey.

Besides the risk of contamination, reports on adverse reactions to botanical medicines reveal another important aspect of herbal poisoning that also needs to be dealt with by improving the quality control on herbal remedies. It is far from uncommon that the toxic effects of a herbal drug are the result of the inappropriate use of that drug by an uneducated user. For this reason, a separate section

Table 1. Potential contaminants that should be taken into account in the quality control of herbal medicines

Type of contaminant	Examples
Botanicals	*Atropa belladonna, Digitalis, Colchicum, Rauwolfia serpentina*, pyrrolizidine-containing plants
Micro-organisms	*Staphylococcus aureus, Escherichia coli* (certain strains), *Salmonella, Shigella, Pseudomonas aeruginosa*
Microbial toxins	Bacterial endotoxins, aflatoxins
Pesticides	Chlorinated pesticides (e.g., DDT, DDE, HCH isomers, HCB, aldrin, dieldrin, heptachlor), organic phosphates, carbamate insecticides and herbicides, dithiocarbamate fungicides, triazin herbicides
Fumigation agents	Ethylene oxide, methyl bromide, phosphine
Radioactivity	Cs-134, Cs-137, Ru-103, I-131, Sr-90
Metals	Lead, cadmium, mercury, arsenic
Synthetic drugs	Analgesic and anti-inflammatory agents (e.g., aminophenazone, phenylbutazone, indomethacin), corticosteroids, hydrochlorothiazide, diazepam
Animal drugs	Thyroid hormones

is devoted to the need to provide herbal medicinal products with accurate and comprehensible consumer information on how to use the products correctly and safely.

Toxic Botanicals

Introduction

The most basic requirement in the quality assurance of herbal drug products is, of course, that the correct botanical ingredients be used. This essential rule may be broken by the adulteration of commercially available botanical remedies as well as by the inexpert self-collection of medicinal plants growing wild. Case reports in the literature show that both types of breaches occasionally lead to serious poisoning due to the unexpected presence of toxic botanicals in herbal medicines.

Adulteration of Commercial Products

Potential Causes

Herbal drug dealers may deviate from pharmacopoeial or other authoritative specifications of botanical identity for various reasons:

— A justifiable motive can be that the officinal plant species is not available but may be replaced by an equivalent related species. For instance, it has become difficult to obtain real golden rod (*Solidago virgaurea*), but this species can be justifiably substituted with the related *S. gigantea* or *S. canadensis* [42]. It is obvious that such changes are only acceptable when the replacing herb is properly labeled with its correct identity.
— A less honorable practice is the deliberate, undeclared substitution of medicinal herbs by inferior and/or cheaper species. Some years ago, a Belgian consumer organization reported that the majority of locally purchased peppermint herbs and capsules did not contain *Mentha piperita* at all, but the much cheaper species *M. crispa*. Likewise, most samples of lime-tree flower did not originate from *Tilia cordata* or *T. platyphyllos*, but from the inferior species *T. argentea* [43]. Another eloquent example is the recent widespread availability of roots marketed as *Echinacea* but in reality coming from the less expensive composite *Parthenium integrifolium* [44,45].
— It is also conceivable that the careless gathering, storage, or distribution of medicinal plant material results in accidental substitution or contamination with another botanical. Inexpert or negligent herbal drug dealers may fail to recognize such a problem in time.

Toxicological Consequences

In many cases of botanical adulteration, direct toxicological implications for the user are unlikely or remain unknown. As the following examples show, however, every now and then a report appears in the literature about increased health hazards of a herbal medicine due to substitution or contamination with a toxic botanical:

— Ginseng preparations on the US market were reported to be adulterated with *Rauwolfia serpentina* and *Mandragora officinarum* species [46]. These contaminants yield the well-known toxic compounds reserpine and belladonna alkaloids, respectively [47].
— In Arizona, two cases of liver injury (one fatal) were observed in infants who had taken large quantities of a locally purchased tea called gordolobo yerba. This tea is a popular gargle and cough medicine among the Hispanic population to which the children belonged. It should be made from *Gnaphalium* leaves, but analysis showed that both materials fed to the children contained *Senecio longilobus*, a herb with hepatotoxic pyrrolizidine alkaloids [48–51].
— Seeds of the poison hemlock (*Conium maculatum*) have occasionally been found in anise seed, and roots of *Veratrum album* are sometimes mislabeled as *Primula* roots [52]. *Conium* seeds have well-known nicotine-like toxicity due to the presence of coniine and related alkaloids, and *Veratrum* alkaloids can produce severe toxic symptoms, such as bradycardia and hypotension [8].
— Fruits of the star anise tree (*Illicium verum*) may be adulterated with those of the related shikimi tree (*I. anisatum*). The latter are more dangerous than the former due to the presence of the toxic sesquiterpene dilactones anisatin and neoanisatin [42,53].
— A young female resident of Great Britain developed fatal hepatic veno-occlusive disease following the consumption of large quantities of mate tea (*Ilex* sp.) over a period of years. A sample recovered from the patient was shown to contain trace amounts of pyrrolizidine alkaloids [54]. Their presence must have been due to contamination, because the occurrence of pyrrolizidine alkaloids in *Ilex* has never been reported [55,56].
— Belladonna root (*Atropa belladonna*) has been identified as a substitute for marshmallow root, an admixture to elfdock root, and as an adulterant of burdock root [42]. Burdock root tea preparations and other commercial herbal products that normally do not contain atropine-like substances have been regularly associated over the past years with delirium and the vegetative symptoms of anticholinergic poisoning (see Table 2 for details).

Negative Markers

The detection of intentional and unintentional adulterants in herbal medicines is the domain of classical pharmacognosy and falls outside the scope of this review. For detailed information on the subject, the reader is referred to the pharmacognostical literature, in particular to German textbooks (e.g., [42,66]) and

Table 2. Anticholinergic poisoning due to the unexpected presence of atropine or atropine-like substances in commercially available herbal products

Botanical drug	Country	Victim(s)	Preparation and contents	Reference
Burdock root (*Arctium* sp.)	United States	26-year-old female	Packaged tea with 30 mg/g atropine	Bryson et al. 1978 [57,58]
	France	No details	Commercial tea contaminated with belladonna root	Anonymous 1984 [59]
	United States	59-year-old female	Packaged tea with 0.76 mg/g atropine	Rhoads et al. 1984-85 [60]
Nettle (*Urtica* sp.)	Austria	57-year-old female	Commercial tea with leaf fragments of *Atropa belladonna*	Scholz et al. 1980 [61]
Comfrey (*Symphytum officinale*)	United Kingdom	Elderly couple	No analytical details[a]	Galizia 1983 [63]
	United Kingdom	30-year-old male	Tea from health food store with ≥0.14 mg/g atropine	Routledge and Spriggs 1989 [64]
Mallow (*Malva* sp.)	Canada	Two patients	Packaged tea with berries of *Atropa belladonna* and a hyoscyamine/atropine content of > 3 mg/g	Awang and Kindack 1989 [65]

[a] Earlier that year, the UK Department of Health and Social Security had issued a warning about a commercial comfrey leaf tea because a batch of this product was contaminated with belladonna [62].

journal articles (e.g., [45,52,67–69]). The *Deutsche Apotheker Zeitung*, for instance, recently started a useful series on present-day adulterations of herbal drugs [70-72]. There is one particular point about pharmacognostic quality control, however, which deserves to be outlined here because of its toxicological significance, namely, the usefulness of negative markers.

Chemically defined constituents of medicinal plants can play an important role in the quality control of herbal products. Some constituents may serve a qualitative purpose; their presence in a herbal product assures that the product has been prepared from the correct botanical ingredient. For example, a TLC check on the presence of menthofurane in a peppermint drug may verify that it comes from *Mentha piperita* and not from *M. arvensis* var. *piperascens* [42]. Other constituents are used in a more quantitative way, that is to say, a certain level in a herbal remedy is taken as a measure of the amount of the herbal ingredient in that product. For instance, in an evaluation of commercial ginseng products on the US market, ginsenosides (= panaxosides) were determined to assess the amount of *Panax* root in each product. Capsules containing powdered root or slurries of ground root showed a total ginsenoside level comparable to dried root samples, but teas for infusion yielded only low concentrations, and tablets did not contain detectable ginsenosides [73].

If possible, one should monitor the constituents which are held responsible for the pharmacological activity of a herbal drug. When the active constituents are uncertain or unknown, however, quality control may be based on so-called chemical markers, i.e., constituents which are considered characteristic for the herbal ingredient. The usefulness of markers in the quality assurance of herbal remedies has been explicitly recognized by the Committee for Proprietary Medicinal Products of the EC. This Committee specifies in its recent "Note for Guidance on the Quality of Herbal Remedies" that a marker may serve to calculate the quantity of vegetable drug or preparation in a finished product if that marker has been quantitatively determined in the vegetable drug or preparation when the starting materials were tested [39].

From the point of view of drug safety, the quantitative determination of constituents is particularly useful when they are pharmacologically active compounds with a relatively small therapeutic window. In the case of aloe, for instance, the European Pharmacopoeia prescribes that the dry extract should be standardized to contain 19.0%–21.0% of hydroxyanthracene derivatives, calculated as anhydrous barbaloin [74]. Sometimes it can also be rewarding, however, to ensure the *absence* of a herbal constituent. Certain medicinal plants are known to have constituents which do not contribute in any known way to the established or alleged beneficial effects of the plant, but which are capable of producing adverse reactions. On the analogy of such a concept of positive markers, it would be prudent to denote such superfluous and harmful compounds as negative markers which should not reach unsafe levels in the finished herbal product.

As is made clear by the examples in Table 3, the principle of negative marking may serve not only to distinguish between safe and less safe plant species and varieties, but it can also be used to monitor whether superfluous toxic constituents of a source plant are still present in the finished product.

Self-Collection of Medicinal Plants

The risk that a poisonous plant is used instead of the required medicinal herb may become particularly high when people without botanical expertise start to collect their own plant material. Every now and then, a case report in the literature makes it abundantly clear that the erroneous identification of self-selected plant material can result in serious or even lethal poisoning:

Table 3. Examples of superfluous and toxic constituents of medicinal plants that should not reach unsafe levels in finished herbal products (so-called negative markers)

Negative marker	Details
Anthecotulid	Topical pharmaceutical and cosmetic chamomile products should be free of this sesquiterpene lactone as it has well-established sensitizing properties and can cross-react with other allergenic sesquiterpene lactones.[a] Concentrations up to 7.3% have been isolated from the chamomile substitute *Anthemis cotula* (dog fennel). It is also detectable in one of the four chemical strains of genuine chamomile (*Chamomilla recutita*) in lower levels up to 0.23% [76].
β-Asarone	Calamus products should contain no or negligible amounts of β-asarone since this compound has a chromosome-damaging effect on human lymphocytes [77], mutagenic properties in bacteria [78], and carcinogenic activity in rats [79]. The source plant (*Acorus calamus*) has several varieties with different levels of β-asarone in the rhizome. The diploid variety does not contain detectable amounts, the triploid variety provides 0.3%, and the tetraploid variety yields two races with 2% and 4%–8% of β-asarone, respectively [80]. Measurements in isolated guinea pig ileum have shown that the spasmolytic activity of β-asarone-free calamus oil is superior to that of calamus oil with a low content of β-asarone, and that β-asarone-rich oil does not show any spasmolytic activity at all [81].
Estragole	It is prudent to avoid estragole-rich chemotypes of fennel, particularly in small children (for a detailed discussion, see the chapter on *Foeniculum vulgare* elsewhere in this volume).
Pyrrolizidine alkaloids	As pyrrolizidine alkaloids have well-established hepatotoxic and hepatocarcinogenic potential [56], their occurrence in certain medicinal herbs entails a serious health risk. This risk is unnecessary since the beneficial effects of such plants are usually attributed to non-pyrrolizidine constituents [36,44]. Research has been started to develop special extraction techniques [82,83] and pyrrolizidine-free varieties [84].

[a] It should be noted that anthecotulid may not be responsible for immediate-type reactions to chamomile [75]

— An elderly American woman with limited knowledge of plants mistook foxglove for comfrey when picking material for a herbal tea. The tea killed both her and her husband [48].
— Another case of serious *Digitalis* poisoning due to the accidental substitution of foxglove for comfrey has been reported from Great Britain. The patient was an elderly man, and he needed intensive care treatment to recover [85].
— Five people in Spain took by mistake an infusion of the roots of *Atractylis gummifera* (birdlime thistle), thinking that it was another root often used as a herbal home remedy. Severe hepatocellular damage and acute renal failure developed, and one patient died because of hepatic failure and massive gastrointestinal hemorrhage. The other four patients recovered, but all of them needed one or more hemodialysis sessions [86].

— Some years ago, *Colchicum* was mistaken for ramson herb (*Allium ursinum*) by a man gathering leaves for a salad. The initial effects of the salad (vomiting, diarrhea) were not recognized as symptoms of *Colchicum* poisoning, and the patient died after a few days because of multiple organ dysfunction, including circulatory collapse [10].

Micro-organisms and Microbial Toxins

Introduction

The microbiological quality of medicinal products has attracted much attention ever since a Swedish report in the 1960s made clear that microbial contamination of medicines can lead to clinical infection [87]. Among the various aspects which have been investigated in detail so far is the microbial status of crude medicinal herbs and their finished products. From the data which have become available it is apparent that vegetal materials entail the same types of microbial health risks for the user as other pharmaceuticals, namely:

— Infection by pathogenic micro-organisms, such as *Salmonella*
— Microbial transformation of botanical constituents into more toxic compounds
— Production of microbial toxins, such as bacterial endotoxins and mycotoxins

Before these three aspects are discussed here, this section first provides some general information on the microbial status of crude herbal materials and the effects of processing.

Microbial Contamination

Levels of Contamination
Until recently, there were no special pharmacopoeial or other official regulations providing concrete upper limits for the microbial contamination of phytotherapeutical materials. For lack of something better, most investigators compared their results to the so-called FIP requirements for the microbial purity of non-sterile medicines which were proposed in the 1970s by the Committee of Official Laboratories and Control Services of the Fédération Internationale Pharmaceutique (Table 4). However, these requirements offered general limits for the microbiological quality of medicines without taking into account that drug materials of vegetal origin tend to show much higher levels of contamination than synthetic materials (Table 5). Representative figures for the microbial status of dried herbal materials are [90,92–94]:

— An *aerobic bacterial count* between 10^2 and 10^8 CFU/g (= colony forming units per g), mostly $> 10^4$ CFU/g

Table 4. FIP requirements for the microbial purity of nonsterile medicines not intended for topical use [40,88]

Micro-organism	Limit	
Aerobic bacteria	$\leq 10^3 - 10^4$	per g or ml
Yeasts and molds	$\leq 10^2$	per g or ml
Escherichia coli	n.d.	in 1 g or ml
and in certain cases:		
Salmonella	n.d.	in 1 g or ml
Other enterobacteria	$\leq 10^2$	per g or ml
Pseudomonas aeruginosa	n.d.	in 1 g or ml
Staphylococcus aureus	n.d.	in 1 g or ml

n.d. = not detectable

— A *coliform bacterial count* between $< 10^2$ and 10^4 CFU/g
— A *yeast and mold count* between 10^2 and 10^6 CFU/g

This microbial contamination is in the same range as that of vegetal foods. It is not so much caused by secondary contamination during processing, but is primarily due to the fact that plants have their own microbial flora. This was elegantly demonstrated by Schneider [95], who compared samples of the same three herbs in their fresh state and after work-up to dried material (Table 6). Due to this natural contamination, a majority of dried medicinal herb samples fails to meet the FIP requirements for microbial purity. This is particularly true for so-called mass drugs, such as peppermint, chamomile, melissa, and valerian [91,92,94]. Unfortunately, the technological possibilities to reduce the microbial content of dried herbs to levels below FIP limits are rather limited (Table 7). This has raised the question of whether it is sensible to submit crude herbal materials to vigorous germ-reducing treatment.

Effects of Processing
One important aspect of the FIP requirements for microbial purity is that these limits are intended for the quality control of finished medicinal products, whereas dried herbs are raw materials which still have to be worked up before they are ready for consumption. Extraction with an ethanolic solution may help to reduce the number of micro-organisms due to direct contact with the alcohol. Another noteworthy decontamination method is extraction with boiling water, which is the most common way of preparing medicinal teas [92,95].

The effects of the latter process were studied extensively by Leimbeck [91], who treated 184 dried herb samples by pouring boiling test liquid on the material (see Table 5 for microbiological details on the samples). This treatment produced a drastic reduction in nonsporing bacteria and molds, including *Escherichia coli*, *Klebsiella pneumoniae*, *Enterobacter cloacae*, and *Pseudomonas aeruginosa*, to < 10 CFU/g. Other investigators have obtained similar results [93,94,96,101]. In spite of these favorable data, it is not advisable to keep hotly extracted herbal teas

Table 5. Some representative large-scale studies on the microbial purity of crude herbal materials

Reference — Samples	Results
Lutomski and Kedzia 1980 [89]	
— 246 samples of 95 different crude herbal drugs	*Molds*: 10% < 10^2 CFU/g, 38% 10^2–10^3 CFU/g, 28% 10^3–10^4 CFU/g and 24% > 10^4 CFU/g
Schilcher 1982 [90]	
— 548 samples of seeds (Cucurbitae semen, Lini semen) — 221 samples of 38 other crude herbal materials (barks, flowers, leaves, fruits, herbs, roots, and rhizomes)	*Total aerobic count*: — seed samples: up to > 10^7 CFU/g (mean values in the range of 10^6 CFU/g) — other samples: variation from < 10^2 to > 10^7 CFU/g (> 80% of the mean values in the range of 10^4–10^6 CFU/g) *Escherichia coli*: — seed samples: positive in 37 samples (6.8%) — other samples: positive in 17 samples (7.7%) *Pathogenic bacteria*: occasional findings of potentially pathogenic organisms (such as *Proteus*, *Klebsiella*, enterococci and streptococci)
Leimbeck 1987 [91]	
— 184 samples of 56 different crude drugs	*Total bacterial count*: 85% > 10^4 CFU/g and 52% > 10^6 CFU/g *Yeasts and molds*: 36% > 10^4 CFU/g and 3% > 10^6 CFU/g *Coliform bacteria*: 58% > 10^4 CFU/g and 19% > 10^6 CFU/g *Staphylococcus aureus*: not detected *Escherichia coli*: detected in 12% of the samples *Salmonella* spp.: not detected *Pseudomonas aeruginosa*: detected in 11% of the samples
Frank 1989 [92]	
— 578 samples of crude herbal drugs	*Total viable count*: < 10^3 to > 10^8 CFU/g (most samples between 10^4 and 10^7 CFU/g) *Yeasts and molds*: up to 10^7 CFU/g (most samples between 10^3 and 10^5 CFU/g) *Coliform bacteria*: up to 10^8 CFU/g (most samples between 10^2 and 10^4 CFU/g) *Staphylococcus aureus*: detected in < 1.3% of the samples *Salmonella* spp.: detected in < 1.3% of 374 samples

Table 6. Microbial comparison of the same three herbs in their fresh state (f) and after drying (d) [95]

		Melissae folium	Rubi fruticosi folium	Salicis cortex
Total	f:	$5.10^5 - .10^6$	$3-8.10^4$	3.10^3
count	d:	$10^4 - 4.10^5$	3.10^3	$3.10^3 - 5.10^3$
Spore-forming	f:	$10^2 - 2.10^4$	10^3	6.10^2
organisms	d:	$3.10^3 - 2.10^4$	10^3	$1.10^3 - 5.10^3$
Coliform	f:	$10^2 - 4.10^5$	10^3	10^1
bacteria	d:	$10^2 - 2.10^4$	n.d.	n.d.
Yeasts and	f:	$n.d.-10^2$	n.d.	n.d.
molds	d:	$n.d.-10^2$	n.d.	$n.d.-10^3$

n.d. = not detected

Table 7. Established and potential methods to reduce the microbial content of dried herbs [92,94,96]

Method	Comments
Gaseous treatment with ethylene oxide	Has been widely used for the decontamination of crude dried herbs. However, there are plans to prohibit this treatment throughout the European Community because of the toxicological risks involved (see p. 31).
Heating	Is a very efficient germ-reducing process if properly validated. However, dry heat and autoclavation are not suitable for most herbal materials because volatile and thermolabile constituents are lost. Thermal processes also reduce the potency of mucilagenous drugs [97]. Pasteurization is often used to treat aqueous extracts, but this method is not appropriate for crude dried herbs. A new type of heat treatment is microwave heating [98,99], but its usefulness for dried plant materials has not been validated.
Gamma irradiation	Has been the subject of recent studies. Sinclulle et al. [100] showed that an irradiation dose of 10-15 kGy effectively decontaminated nine different crude drugs without an effect on the total level of characteristic constituents. Van Doorne et al. [96] reported that doses of 10 kGy or more can produce a good microbiological quality of senna leaves without the induction of any phytochemical change. Yet the prevailing German opinion is still reserved about the practical usefulness of this method. One argument is that more studies on the phytochemical effects of gamma irradiation are needed. Certain drug substances such as vitamins are known to be susceptible to chemical conversion by this method, so it is conceivable that certain botanical constituents might also be transformed. Another objection is that treatment of a herbal product with gamma irradiation would have to be declared on its package, and that this would discourage the users who expect a completely natural product [42,92].

for more than 24 h [102] because spore-forming species (*Bacillus, Clostridium perfringens*) are not effectively eliminated by boiling water [91,96,101]. A timely consumption is even more essential when a herbal tea has been prepared by cold maceration because this treatment has no decontaminating effect [92,94,96]. When Van Doorne et al. [96] extracted senna leaves with cold water and left the tea standing for 24 h, the microbial contamination increased from $< 10^2$ CFU/ml after 30 min to 10^3–10^5 CFU/ml after 24 h. In other words, when there are phytochemical considerations or other reasons to prefer cold extraction, the user should be carefully instructed to prepare each dose freshly instead of using the same macerate for a whole day. As a rule of thumb, cold macerates which are more than 4 h old should be regarded as unfit for consumption [92,94].

Pathogenicity of Micro-organisms

Another general reservation about the FIP requirements is that total counts of aerobic bacteria, yeasts, and molds are usually determined by ubiquitous, apathogenic micro-organisms. In other words, when the FIP limits for these parameters are exceeded, this does not imply that an actual health risk is involved [92]. This is also true for the total count of non-*Salmonella* enterobacteria, as this count may be largely due to apathogenic *Erwinia* species which habitually contaminate plants [101]. The only possible advantage of using these overall parameters is that an unusual pattern of contamination may be recognized more readily [92]. From the clinical point of view, however, it is much more relevant to know whether pathogenic microbes are present, such as *Staphylococcus aureus*, certain strains of *Escherichia coli*, *Salmonella* spp., *Shigella* spp., and *Pseudomonas aeruginosa* (see Table 8). *Listeria monocytogenes* should also be taken into account since infection with this gram-positive bacillus has been observed in a seriously ill 55-year-old man with multiple organ failure who had been taking several nonorthodox drug products besides his conventional medication (steroids, antacids, and cimetidine). He died from listeriosis that could definitely be traced to his use of alfalfa tablets [103].

Table 9 shows for some pathogens how many bacteria are needed to induce clinical illness. One should realize that these experimental data were obtained in relatively small series of healthy adults and cannot be extrapolated directly to assess the risk of real patients, since infectivity depends not only on the pathogenic bacterium but also on the age and underlying illness of the patient [109]. For instance, herbal remedies may be used by AIDS patients and cancer patients [110–112], and it is a well-known fact that HIV infection or intensive antitumor therapy may compromise the normal immune response. In other words, patients with AIDS or cancer are likely to be more susceptible to the microbial hazards of traditional medicines than relatively healthy users. That this is not some theoretical fear but an actual risk is evident from recent reports about disseminated *Salmonella arizona* infection in patients with AIDS and other debilitating diseases who had been consuming contaminated rattlesnake meat preparations [113,114].

Table 8. Some bacteria which should be taken into consideration in the microbiological evaluation of crude herbal drugs [91,92]

Micro-organism	Details
Staphylococcus aureus	Pathogenic, facultatively anaerobic, gram-positive bacterium. Produces a thermoresistant enterotoxin which is the most common cause of food poisoning. Such poisoning is usually the result of massive growth in foodstuffs. 10^5 bacteria per g food are said to be needed to produce an infection via the oral route.
Streptococcus spp.	Facultatively anaerobic, gram-positive bacteria. *S. faecalis* is usually apathogenic, but it can serve as indicator for fecal contamination. *S. pneumoniae* and *S. pyogenes* are pathogenic. Contamination may occur via excretion by symptomless carriers. Skin and mucosa are the most common routes of infection, especially when they are damaged.
Clostridium perfringens	Anaerobic, spore-forming, gram-positive bacterium which can serve as an indicator for fecal contamination. A pathogenic effect of oral intake is unlikely.
Escherichia coli	Facultatively anaerobic, gram-negative enterobacterium. Is usually apathogenic, but it can serve as indicator for fecal contamination. Some strains which can be differentiated serologically from apathogenic strains can produce enteritis, in particular in neonates and infants. See Table 9 for the infectivity of pathogenic strains in healthy adults.
Coliform bacteria	Facultatively anaerobic, gram-negative enterobacteria, such as *Klebsiella*, *Enterobacter*, and *Citrobacter*. These bacteria are usually apathogenic, but they can present a health threat when counts are very high.
Salmonella spp.	Facultatively anaerobic, gram-negative enterobacteria. Both *S. typhi* and *S. paratyphi* are pathogenic. See Table 9 for the infectivity of pathogenic species in healthy adults.
Shigella spp.	Facultatively anaerobic, gram-negative enterobacteria, such as *S. dysenteriae*, *S. ambigua* and *S. sonnei*. They are already pathogenic when small quantities are taken orally.
Pseudomonas aeruginosa	Pathogenic, facultatively anaerobic, gram-negative bacterium. Is primarily an infectant of wounds and mucosal areas and does not readily produce infection when taken orally (see Table 9).

One should also consider, however, that most sick people are allowed to consume foods that are potential sources of pathogens, usually in larger quantities than botanical medicines. It would therefore be rather unrealistic to apply microbiological regulations to herbal remedies that are much more strict than the standards limiting micro-organisms in common foodstuffs [92,109]. Furthermore, it should be repeated that vegetative cells, particularly those of gram-negative species, are very sensitive to heat and will thus be destroyed when

Table 9. Relationship between dose and infectivity of pathogenic bacteria in healthy subjects

Pathogen	Dose level	Results			Ref.
Escherichia coli[a]	7.0×10^6	mild symptoms developed in 7 of 11 subjects and none in 4 subjects; no definite diarrhea developed			[104]
	6.5×10^9	7 of 11 subjects became moderately or severely ill, and 4 subjects became slightly ill			
Pseudomonas aeruginosa	$< 10^4$ to $> 10^8$	Pseudomonas could not be detected in the stools at doses $< 10^4$ but could be recovered at doses $> 10^6$; no clinical illness occurred at doses up to 2×10^8 in 2 subjects			[105]
Salmonella spp.		Number of subjects	Positive stools	Clinical illness	
S. anatum	1.4×10^5	6	3	0	[106]
	5.9×10^5	6	4	2	
S. bareilly	1.3×10^5	6	5	1	[107]
	1.7×10^6	6	5	4	
S. derby	6.4×10^6	6	3	0	[107]
	1.5×10^7	6	4	3	
S. meleagrides	1.5×10^6	6	5	0	[106]
	1.0×10^7	6	5	2	
S. newport	1.5×10^5	6	3	1	[107]
	1.4×10^6	6	6	3	
S. pullorum	1.3×10^9	6	0	0	[108]
	7.6×10^9	6	6	6	

[a] Serotype 111, B_4 strains isolated from diarrheal infants

boiling water is used to prepare a medicinal tea from contaminated material [91,93,96].

Pharmacopoeial Requirements

There are thus several reasons why the FIP limits for microbial purity of nonsterile medicines are not suitable for the quality control of dried herbal materials. It is therefore gratifying that the German health authorities have recently created two categories of herbal drugs for which special pharmacopoeial limits have been established with respect to microbial contamination. These official requirements have been laid down in the 1989 Supplement to DAB 9, the latest edition of the *Deutsche Arzneibuch* (see Table 10).

Frank [92] has proposed upper limits for *Staphylococcus aureus* and *Pseudomonas aeruginosa*, namely $10^2/g$ in herbal tea mixtures and none in other internal preparations. In accordance with suggestions by other authors [91,101],

Table 10. Requirements for the microbial purity of herbal drugs established in the 1989 Supplement to DAB 9, the German pharmacopoeia [115]

Micro-organism	Limits per drug category	
	Category 4a[a]	Category 4b[b]
Aerobic bacteria	10^7/g	10^5/g
Yeasts and molds	10^4/g	10^3/g
Escherichia coli	10^2/g	10^1/g
Other enterobacteria	10^4/g	10^3/g
Salmonella	none	none

[a] *Drug category 4a*: Dried herbs and dried herbal mixtures for the preparation of medicinal teas, which undergo a germ reduction before use (e.g., by pouring boiling water on the material), as well as preparations for topical use that contain dried herbs

[b] *Drug category 4b*: Other preparations for internal use that contain dried herbs

however, the new German regulation does not provide separate limits for these pathogenic bacteria.

Transformation of Herbal Constituents

A special toxicological risk may arise when constituents of a medicinal plant are susceptible to chemical transformation by contaminating micro-organisms.

A well-established example is that the molding of dried sweet clover (*Melilotus officinalis*) can result in serious hemorrhagic activity. This medicinal herb contains coumarin, 3,4-dihydrocoumarin (= melilotine), o-coumaric acid, o-hydroxycoumaric acid, and the O-glycoside of o-coumaric acid (= melilotoside). Since withering leads to enzymatic glycoside hydrolysis, and the resulting o-coumaric acid is spontaneously transformed to coumarin, the dried herb strongly smells of coumarin [31]. Coumarin itself is devoid of anticoagulant effects in man [116] because an intact 4-hydroxycoumarin residue with a carbon constituent at the 3-position is an essential characteristic for the anticoagulant potential of coumarin derivatives [117]. Coumarin can be metabolized, however, by *Penicillium* molds, such as *P. nigricans* and *P. jensi*, and the transformation product dicoumarol is a 4-hydroxycoumarin derivative with potent anticoagulant effects [6]. Although poisoning by molded sweet clover has been observed almost exclusively in cattle [6], there is an unusual case report about abnormal clotting function and mild clinical bleeding in a young woman who had been drinking large amounts of a herbal tea prepared from sweet clover and other coumarin-containing ingredients [118]. Unfortunately, the possibility of coumarin transformation due to molding was not properly investigated, as the reporting physician was unaware of the exact phytochemistry and pharmacology of coumarin-yielding botanicals.

Microbial Toxins

Bacterial Endotoxins

As was pointed out earlier, a high bacterial count in botanical material usually remains without clinical consequences when the bacteria are apathogenic, and when the herb is used for the preparation of an oral dosage form (e.g., a medicinal tea). Heavy contamination of a crude herb with bacteria may lead to clinical effects, however, when the material is used for the production of a parenteral medicine because a high bacterial content of raw material entails the risk that a high concentration of bacterial endotoxins is present in the finished parenteral product. Most significant in this respect are the endotoxins originating from gram-negative bacteria. These endotoxins are outer cell-wall fragments which are chemically characterized as liposaccharides. Man is very sensitive to their pyrogenic activity. An intravenous dose of 3 ng/kg body weight to young healthy adults is sufficient to induce pyrogenic symptoms, such as a rise in temperature, chills, headache, joint pain, and restless legs [119]. The pyrogenic potency varies with the specific origin of the endotoxin. *Escherichia coli* endotoxin has consistently been shown to be the most potent one [120].

To prevent pyrogenic reactions, the European Pharmacopoeia requires that all parenterals with a volume over 15 ml be tested for the absence of pyrogens. This does not necessarily imply, however, that injection fluids with a smaller volume are incapable of producing a pyrogenic reaction [121].

Mexican 10-ml ampoules seized by US Customs Services and containing amygdalin (Laetrile) as their supposedly active ingredient were reported to contain high levels of endotoxins. Twenty of almost 6000 ampoules inspected visually showed apparent microbial growth. When ampoules containing visually clear solutions were submitted to the rabbit test for pyrogenicity, one of four seizure lots was positive at a therapeutic dose level of 100 mg/kg. Additional testing by means of the Limulus Amebocyte Lysate method confirmed the presence of a high level of endotoxin [122].

Becker et al. [121] assayed the bacterial and endotoxin content of four small-volume phytotherapeutic injection fluids on the German market after the use of such preparations had been associated with pyrogen-like side effects. None of the studied samples showed bacterial contamination, but each of the four brands tested had batches with substantial endotoxin levels (see Table 11). To investigate whether these endotoxins were primarily due to contamination of the botanical material or to secondary contamination during the manufacturing process, the researchers also tested the herbal ingredient of one of the injection fluids, namely the expressed sap of *Dionaea muscipula* (from which Carnivora injections are prepared). Twelve of 32 samples showed a bacterial count $> 10^4$/ml (8 samples with gram-negative bacteria and 4 samples with gram-positive bacteria). The mean endotoxin level of these 12 samples was higher (10^5 U/ml) than that of the 20 samples without heavy contamination (10^4 U/ml). Samples of sap expressed from plants cultured under sterile conditions yielded endotoxin levels < 1 U/ml.

Table 11. Endotoxin contamination and endotoxin-like activity of some German phytotherapeutic injection fluids [121]

Trade name	Botanical ingredient(s)	Results[a]
Pascotox forte- injektopas	*Echinacea angustifolia* (root)	Endotoxin level of 10^4 U/ml in 1 sample of a batch which had produced chills, fever, headache, and joint pain when given intravenously; levels between < 10 and 100 U/ml in 4 other samples
Esberitox N	*Thuja occidentalis* (herb) *Echinacea angustifolia* (root) *Echinacea purpura* (root) *Baptisia tinctoria* (root)	Endotoxin levels of 100 and 400 U/ml in samples of 2 batches which had produced pyrogen-like side effects when given intravenously; levels < 20 U/ml in 9 other samples
Carnivora[b]	*Dionaea muscipula*	Endotoxin levels up to 10^5 U/ml in 32 samples (mean value of 3000 U/ml)
Iscador M[c]	*Viscum album*	Endotoxin levels between 190 and 3800 U/ml in 6 samples

[a] Endotoxin levels are expressed in units/ml; 10^4 units correspond approximately to an endotoxin dose of 1.5 ng/kg body weight [121].
[b] Intramuscular use of this preparation has been associated with fever, shivers, and anaphylactic shock [123,124].
[c] Subcutaneous use of this preparation (the most common route of administration) has not been associated with serious pyrogenic effects [121]. Intravenous infusion of 0.21–0.38 mg/kg body weight has been reported to produce a fever reaction, headaches, very slight nausea, and chills, but an endotoxin level above the tolerance limit was not detected in the infusion [125].

These findings most certainly illustrate that parenteral phytotherapeutic preparations should be controlled for the absence of pyrogens even when their volume does not exceed 15 ml.

Mycotoxins

As has already been pointed out, heavy contamination of herbal material with yeasts and molds is itself not indicative of a health threat. There is always the possibility, however, that inappropriate drying procedures or storage of the material has resulted in the growth of mycotoxin-producing fungi [92]. Of particular concern is contamination with aflatoxin-producing strains, such as *Aspergillus* species. As this type of pollution is especially possible during storage in warm, humid conditions, it is most likely to occur in developing tropical countries where modern techniques of agriculture and storage are not generally available [126-128].

A large variety of mycotoxins has been identified. Among the important toxins occurring in feeds and foodstuffs are aflatoxins, sterigmatocystin, ochratoxin A, patulin, luteoskyrin, ergot alkaloids, citrinin, and zearalenone [6,89,129]. The aflatoxins are considered to be especially dangerous. A report about an outbreak of hepatitis in western India due to the consumption of maize contaminated heavily with *Aspergillus flavus* suggests that a daily intake of 2-6 mg aflatoxin (approximately 30-90 μg/kg bw) over a period of several weeks can be sufficient to produce fatal hepatitis [130]. Aflatoxins are mutagenic, and they produce hepatocarcinomas when given in very low doses to laboratory animals [131,132]. The most potent hepatocarcinogen in the aflatoxin group is aflatoxin B_1 [131], which has also been shown to have teratogenic and embryotoxic properties in numerous animals [133]. Another mycotoxin for which mutagenic and hepatotocarcinogenic activity has been reported is sterigmatocystin [134,135].

Pharmacopoeial limits for the presence of aflatoxins in medicines are not available, and the Joint FAO/WHO Expert Committee on Food Additives has not set an official threshold value for the occurrence of aflatoxins in foodstuffs. This committee states only that their presence in food should be reduced to the lowest practicable level [136]. A tentative upper limit may be derived from the requirement of the United States Food and Drug Administration (FDA) that the aflatoxin content of peanut butter should not exceed 20 ng/g [127]. When one assumes that no other contaminated foodstuffs are used, and that one sandwich with 30 g peanut butter may be consumed each day [127], this comes down to a maximum daily dose of 600 ng (10 ng/kg bw for an average 60-kg person). Such a threshold value is not too conservative, as it is in agreement with human data on the hepatocarcinogenicity of aflatoxins [131,132].

An age-adjusted excess of 10% in primary liver-cell cancer deaths was reported from the United States, where an area with an average intake of 13-197 ng/kg bw aflatoxin B_1 per day was compared to other areas with lower intakes of 0.2-0.3 ng/kg bw per day [137]. A recent overall analysis of data obtained from different studies in African and Asian regions revealed a highly significant correlation between the crude rate of hepatocellular carcinoma incidence and dietary aflatoxin B_1 intake when daily exposure levels varying from 3.5 to 183.7 ng/kg bw were compared (Table 12). Although the interpretation of such epidemiological data is seriously hampered, of course, by the existence of potentially confounding factors such as infection with hepatitis B virus [132,138], it would seem prudent to avoid daily exposure to aflatoxin levels of 10 ng/kg bw or more, in particular when most or all of the aflatoxin dose consists of aflatoxin B_1. This figure implies that dried medicinal herbs, which may be consumed in amounts of several grams per day, should be considered unfit for consumption when their aflatoxin contamination is in the range of 0.1 μg/g or more.

This roughly estimated threshold level of 0.1 μg/g is based on the assumption that the aflatoxin fraction passes completely from the crude material into the final dosage form. The actual degree of transition largely depends, however, on the

Table 12. Summarized results of studies measuring crude rates of hepatocellular carcinoma (HCC) and dietary aflatoxin B_1 intake [138]

Country	Area	Crude HCC rate (10^5/year)	Daily aflatoxin B_1 intake (ng/kg bw)
Kenya	High altitude	1.2	3.5
Thailand	Songkhla	2.0	5.0
Swaziland	Highveld	2.2	5.1
Kenya	Middle altitude	2.5	5.9
Swaziland	Middleveld	3.8	8.9
Kenya	Low altitude	4.0	10.0
Swaziland	Lebombo	4.3	15.4
Thailand	Ratburi	6.0	45.0
Transkei	Four districts	6.9	16.5
Mozambique	Manhica-Magude	5.9	20.3
Swaziland	Lowveld	9.2	43.1
Mozambique	Massinga	5.0	38.6
Mozambique	Inharrime	9.0	86.9
Mozambique	Inhambane	12.1	77.7
Mozambique	Morrumbene	15.5	87.7
Mozambique	Homoine-Maxixe	17.7	131.4
Mozambique	Zavala	14.0	183.7

specific method of preparation. Since aflatoxins are freely soluble in moderately polar organic solvents such as methanol[131], it seems likely that they may readily pass into ethanolic extracts. Extraction with water could be more difficult, since their solubility in this medium is only 10–20 μg/ml[131]. However, this relatively low solubility still allows more than 1 mg in a herbal tea cup of 150 ml. Moreover, little or no destruction of aflatoxins occurs under ordinary cooking conditions [131], so it can be expected that the aflatoxins are not destroyed when boiling water is poured on the herbal material. More research in this specific area is needed, in particular because Leimbeck [91] reported that aflatoxin B_1 could not be recovered from the aqueous phase after hot extraction of dried herbal material intentionally spiked with this toxin.

Several studies have shown that crude botanical drugs can be infested with *Aspergillus* strains producing aflatoxins (B_1, B_2, G_1, G_2) and/or sterigmatocystin [89,128,139–144]. The ability of isolated strains to produce aflatoxin B_1 varied from 0.15 μg/ml [139] to 1000 μg/ml in the culture filtrate [141]. Some research groups relied entirely on fungal counts and on mycotoxin-producing ability of isolates to assess the degree of mycotoxin contamination [89,140]. It seems doubtful, however, that these parameters always provide an accurate and reliable insight into actual mycotoxin levels [142,145]. One should bear in mind, for instance, that decontamination of material after mycotoxins have already been formed can reduce the fungal count without eliminating the toxins [92].

Some investigators have assayed their herbal drug samples directly for the presence of mycotoxins. As was to be expected, their results show considerable variation in the prevalence and intensity of mycotoxin contamination (Table 13).

Table 13. Aflatoxin levels in crude herbal drugs

Reference	Results
Hitokoto et al. 1978 [139]	No aflatoxin or sterigmatocystin detected in any of 49 herbal drug samples purchased from drugstores in Tokyo. When 69 of the isolates were assayed for aflatoxin production, a weakly positive result was obtained only once.
Hilal et al. 1986 [146] Hilal et al. 1987 [147]	This group of Egyptian investigators first reported the absence of aflatoxin B_1 in 27 locally purchased herbal tea samples and then discovered in a sequel study that 4 of 40 samples were contaminated with aflatoxin B_1. Unfortunately, the aflatoxin B_1 content of these samples was not quantitated.
Leimbeck 1987 [91]	No aflatoxins were recovered from 13 samples of 10 different crude herbal drugs, even though these samples were relatively heavily contaminated with *Aspergillus* in the range of 10^4–10^6 CFU/g.
Roy et al. 1988 [142]	These northern Indian researchers reported the isolation of toxigenic *Aspergillus flavus* strains from all 15 herbal drug samples that they studied. Chemical analysis revealed that 13 samples contained more than 0.1 μg/g aflatoxin B_1, despite the fact that the isolates elaborated aflatoxin B_1 in amounts of only 1–5 μg/ml of culture filtrate.
Kumari et al. 1989 [144]	In a sequel study, this research group recovered mean levels of 0.36 and 0.11 μg/g aflatoxin B_1 in contaminated seed samples of two Indian medicinal plants.

In one study performed in the northern part of India, 13 of 15 samples tested were found to contain more than 0.1 μg/g aflatoxin B_1, and 3 of these samples yielded even more than 1 μg/g [142]. These findings demonstrate the need to prevent aflatoxin contamination of medicinal plant material, especially in tropical and subtropical areas, by taking adequate processing measures such as rapid post-harvest drying and storage at low moisture levels [131]. This conclusion should be placed in the context, however, that the total daily aflatoxin burden in developing countries may be largely determined by dietary exposure, since foodstuffs may also be contaminated and are likely to be consumed in much larger quantities than botanical medicines.

Pesticides and Fumigation Agents

Pesticides

Potential Causes

Pesticides is the general denomination of compounds which are intended to be used for protection of plants against certain damaging influences, such as insects (insecticides), fungal diseases (fungicides), weeds (herbicides), and rodents (rodenticides). Although many countries have issued restricting regulations concerning the use of these substances, crude botanical drugs may still be contaminated by pesticide residues. Among the reasons for this type of contamination are [42,148–151]:

— Herbs can be imported from countries where restrictive rules are still absent or disregarded. This problem is complicated by the fact that the country from which a herb is imported is not necessarily the country of origin.
— Many herbs continue to be picked up from natural stands, where interventions to protect the general vegetation can lead to accidental contamination. For instance, a comparison of residual amounts of halogenated insecticides in Polish herbal raw materials over the period 1980–1984 revealed that average levels were substantially higher in 1982 than in the other four years. This seemed to be due to the plague of pests in Polish forests which required the use of considerable doses of insecticides. This probably caused excessive contamination of herbal materials collected from forests and adjoining areas [150].
— Large-scale cultivation of medicinal plants is not economically feasible without the use of pesticides. Moreover, the targets of pesticides may themselves be hazardous to health, so there may also be a toxicological reason to consider the application of a pesticide. For instance, it would be unwise to abandon an effective but carcinogenic fungicide without a careful comparison of its health risks to the potential risk of increased contamination by molds producing strongly carcinogenic aflatoxins [127]. It goes without saying, however, that one should always allow sufficient time between treatment and harvesting to avoid the intentional use of pesticides resulting in excessive contamination.
— Pesticides can persist for years in the environment and can thus lead to contamination of plants which have not been treated accidentaly or intentionally. It is obvious that it is very difficult to influence this type of contamination.

Different Classes of Contaminants

Analytical publications on pesticide residues in crude herbal materials indicate that the presence of chlorinated pesticides is quite common. Among the derivatives which have often been reported to occur are the following insecticides [148,150,152–160]:

— DDT (dichlorodiphenyltrichloroethane), its metabolites (such as DDE) and its methoxy congener DMDT
— γ-HCH (γ-hexachlorocyclohexane, lindane) and other HCH isomers (notably α-HCH and β-HCH)
— HCB (hexachlorobenzene)
— Cyclodiene derivatives, such as aldrin, dieldrin, heptachlor and its epoxide

Other potentially contaminating pesticides include organic phosphates, carbamate insecticides and herbicides, dithiocarbamate fungicides, and triazin herbicides [148,157,161,162]. In addition, polychlorinated biphenyls have been reported to occur in raw herbal material as the result of general environmental pollution [163].

For general information on the toxicity of these compounds, the reader is referred to textbooks on toxicology [e.g., 7,11,164]. Qualitative data about carcinogenic risk have recently been reviewed in the *Journal of the American Medical Association* [165] and are reproduced here in Table 14.

Levels of Contamination

With the exception of the pharmacopoeia in the former GDR [162], pharmacopoeias usually do not specify concrete limit values for pesticide residues in medicinal herbs. As a consequence, many investigators have compared their analytical data to limits that have been officially established for the food sector. A regulation which has been used most often for this purpose, particularly by researchers in the FRG, is the so-called *Höchstmengenverordnung* (HMVO) [90,152,153,156]. This food regulation provides, among other things, maximum allowable residue levels of pesticides in nonmedicinal tea and tea-like products (Table 15). When HMVO limits were applied to residual levels of pesticides in large test series, about 1 of every 4–6 crude medicinal herb samples did not meet these requirements (Table 16).

Toxicological Evaluation

Failure of a herb to comply with one or more HMVO limits does not necessarily mean that the herb in question poses a real health threat. For example, a herbal drug may contain 1 mg/kg lindane, which is twice the concentration allowed by the HMVO regulation. When the herb is usually consumed in doses up to 5 g per day, it can be calculated that a user with an average body weight of 60 kg is maximally exposed to 0.08 μg/kg per day. This is only 1% of 8 μg/kg per day, which is the acceptable daily intake (ADI) established for lindane by a joint effort of the FAO and the WHO [166]. It is therefore obvious that in this case the contamination by lindane does not entail a serious health risk, even though the HMVO limit for this pesticide is surpassed. To put it more generally, when an assessment of the actual toxicological risk of a contaminant is required, it is preferable to calculate how much of the compound is consumed per day by the user and to compare this calculated daily consumption to the ADI value of the FAO/WHO (Table 17). It should be noted that these ADI values indicate the total amount in the diet that can be safely taken each day. When this total dose would already be consumed in the form of a herbal drug, there would be no room left for exposure to dietary sources of the same pesticide.

An alternative approach is the use of ADI values to calculate maximum levels of contamination which are theoretically tolerable in crude herbs by means of the following general formula [161,162]:

$$\text{Theoretical maximally tolerable level (mg/kg)} = \frac{\text{ADI (mg/kg)} \times 60 \times \text{extraction factor}}{\text{average daily herb consumption (kg)} \times 100}$$

Table 14. Organic pollutants taken into account in the analytical and toxicological evaluation of environmental residues in herbal remedies [148,161,162]

Compound(s)	Carcinogenicity [165]
CHLORINATED INSECTICIDES	
Dichlorodiphenyl trichloroethane[a] (DDT)	DDT produces liver tumors in mice and promotes liver tumors in the rat, but evidence of carcinogenicity in humans is inadequate. Some studies have indicated that tissue levels of DDT in cancer patients were higher than those of patients dying of other causes.
Benzene hexachloride[b] (BHC, hexachloro-cyclohexane, HCH)	Although all three HCH isomers induce liver tumors in mice, and α-HCH promotes liver tumors in rats, more evidence of carcinogenicity in experimental animals is still needed. Evidence of carcinogenicity in humans is inadequate.
Hexachlorobenzene (HCB)	HCB produces thyroid neoplasms and liver tumors in rodents.
Cyclodiene derivatives (e.g., dieldrin, aldrin, endrin, chlordane, heptachlor)	These insecticides are hepatocarcinogenic in mice. Some compounds induce thyroid tumors, and most are suspected promoters. Rat studies are largely negative. Aldrin/dieldrin was carcinogenic in litters of mice and rats; dieldrin alone was carcinogenic in lungs and other sites in mice.
CHOLINESTERASE INHIBITORS	
Organic phosphate insecticides (e.g., malathion, parathion)	Results of long-term animal tests for carcinogenicity have been for the most part negative, perhaps because the organophosphates are highly toxic acutely and degrade rapidly.
Carbamates (e.g., carbaryl, aldicarb)	Carbaryl may be converted, while in the stomach, to its *N*-nitroso-derivative which is a potent carcinogen in the mouse.
OTHER PESTICIDES	
Dithiocarbamate fungicides (e.g., thiram, maneb, zineb)	The carcinogenic potential of thiram and its congeners is not well established. Ethylene thiourea, a main metabolite and degradation product of the bisdithiocarbamate derivatives maneb and zineb, induces thyroid and liver tumors in experimental animals.
Triazine herbicides (e.g., prometon, simazine)	
MISCELLANEOUS POLLUTANTS	
Polychlorinated biphenyls (PCBs)	Moderate repeated doses of PCBs have been associated with liver tumors in mice and bladder tumors in rats [164].

[a] DDT used to be one of the most widely applied insecticides, but its use is now prohibited or restricted in many countries. DDT and its metabolite dichlorodiphenyldichloroethane (DDE) accumulate in body fat [7,164].

[b] Technical BHC is a mixture of the α-, β-, γ- and δ-isomers of hexachlorocyclohexane. The γ-isomer is the most insecticidally active component and has become available as the insecticide lindane [164].

Table 15. Maximum residue levels of pesticides in nonmedicinal tea and tea-like products allowed by the German *Höchstmengenverordnung* (HMVO) regulations from 1978 [152] and 1982 [149]

Pesticide	Allowed maximum level
Total DDT (p,p'-DDT + o,p'-DDT + DDE)	1 mg/kg
Lindane (γ-hexachlorocyclohexane = γ-HCH)	0.5 mg/kg
Other HCH isomers (notably α-HCH and β-HCH)	0.2 mg/kg
Hexachlorobenzene	0.1 mg/kg
Aldrin + dieldrin	0.1 mg/kg
Heptachlor	0.1 mg/kg

Table 16. Residual levels of pesticides in some large test series of crude botanical drugs

Author(s) Samples	Results
Schilcher 1982 [90]	
2654 samples of > 120 different crude herbal drugs on the FRG market	26% of the samples did not comply with the HMVO food regulation[a]. Drugs tested at least 100 times showed the following rates of noncompliance: — Chamomillae flos (293 samples): 18% — Menthae piperitae folium (130 samples): 29% — Sennae folium (115 samples): 62% — Cucurbitae semen (132 samples): 69%[b] — Lini semen (221 samples): 28%
Ali 1983 [152] and 1987 [156]	
A total of 131 samples of 20 different crude herbal drugs on the FRG market	19% of all samples tested for 10 different chlorinated compounds did not comply with the HMVO food regulation[a]
Laboratorium Addipharma, quoted in Schilcher et al. 1987 [161]	
A total of 1125 samples of crude herbal drugs	16% of the samples did not comply with the HMVO food regulation[a]

[a] Compare Table 15.
[b] The high percentage of contamination of Cucurbitae semen samples was probably due to the extensive root system of the plant, which allows relatively much uptake of pesticides from the soil, and also to accumulation of the fat-soluble pesticides in the fat oil of the seed.

Table 17. Acceptable daily intake (ADI) values for pesticides, as established by FAO and WHO[166]

Pesticide	ADI value[a] (in mg/kg bw)		Comments[b]
Acephate	0.03	(1988)	
Aldicarb	0.005	(1982)	
Aldrin	0.0001	(1977)	For sum of aldrin and dieldrin
Aminocarb			Not cleared toxicologically
Amitraz	0.003	(1984)	
Amitrole	0.00003	(1977)	Uses of amitrole should be restricted to those where residues in food would not be expected to occur
Anilazine	0.1	(1989)	
Azinphos-ethyl			Not cleared toxicologically
Azinphos-methyl	0.0025	(1968)	
Azocyclotin	0.003	(1981)	
Benalaxyl	0.05	(1987)	
Bendiocarb	0.004	(1984)	
Benomyl	0.02	(1983)	
Binapacryl			ADI withdrawn (1982)
Bioresmethrin			Not cleared toxicologically
Bitertanol	0.01	(1988)	
Bromophos	0.04	(1977)	
Bromophos-ethyl	0.003	(1975)	
Bromopropylate	0.008	(1973)	
Butocarboxim			Not cleared toxicologically
sec-Butylamine			TADI withdrawn (1984)
Camphechlor			Not cleared toxicologically
Captafol			TADI withdrawn (1985)
Captan	0.1	(1984)	
Carbaryl	0.01	(1973)	
Carbendazim	0.01	(1983)	
Carbofuran	0.01	(1982)	
Carbon disulfide			Not cleared toxicologically
Carbon tetrachloride			Not cleared toxicologically
Carbophenothion	0.0005	(1979)	
Carbosulfan	0.01	(1986)	
Cartap	0.1	(1978)	
Chinomethionat	0.006	(1987)	
Chlordane	0.0005	(1986)	
Chlordimeform			TADI withdrawn (1987)
Chlorfenvinphos	0.002	(1971)	
Chlormequat	0.05	(1972)	
Chlorobenzilate	0.02	(1980)	
Chlorothalonil	0.003		TADI (1987–1990)
Chlorpyrifos	0.01	(1982)	
Chlorpyrifos-methyl	0.01	(1975)	
Clofentezine	0.02	(1986)	
Coumaphos			TADI withdrawn (1980)
Crufomate	0.1	(1968)	
Cyanofenphos			TADI withdrawn (1983)
Cyfluthrin	0.02	(1987)	
Cyhalothrin	0.02	(1984)	
Cyhexatin	0.008	(1981)	
Cypermethrin	0.05	(1981)	

Table 17. (*Continued*)

Pesticide	ADI value[a] (in mg/kg bw)		Comments[b]
2,4-D	0.3	(1975)	
Daminozide	0.5	(1989)	For damozide containing less than 30 mg 1,1-dimethylhydra-zine/kg
DDT	0.02	(1984)	
Deltamethrin	0.01	(1982)	
Demeton			ADI withdrawn (1982)
Demeton-S-methyl	0.0003	(1989)	For sum of demeton-S-methyl, demeton-S-methylsulfon, and oxydemeton-methyl
Demeton-S-methylsulfon	0.0003	(1989)	For sum of demeton-S-methyl, demeton-S-methylsulfon, and oxydemeton-methyl
Dialifos			ADI withdrawn (1982)
Diazinon	0.002	(1970)	
1.2-Dibromoethane			Not cleared toxicologically
Dichlofluanid	0.3	(1983)	
1.2-Dichloroethane			Not cleared toxicologically
Dichlorvos	0.004	(1977)	
Dicloran	0.03	(1977)	
Dicofol	0.025	(1968)	
Dieldrin	0.0001	(1977)	For sum of aldrin and dieldrin
Diflubenzuron	0.02	(1985)	
Dimethipin	0.02	(1988)	
Dimethoate	0.01	(1987)	
Dinocap	0.001	(1989)	
Dioxathion	0.0015	(1968)	
Diphenyl	0.125		
Diphenylamine	0.02	(1984)	
Diquat	0.008	(1977)	For diquat cation
Disulfoton	0.002	(1975)	
Dodine	0.01	(1976)	
Edifenphos	0.003	(1981)	
Endosulfan	0.006	(1989)	
Endrin	0.0002	(1970)	
Ethephon			Not cleared toxicologically
Ethiofencarb	0.1	(1982)	
Ethion	0.006		TADI (extended to 1990)
Ethoprophos	0.0003	(1987)	
Ethoxyquin	0.06	(1969)	
Ethylenethiourea	0.002		TADI (extended to 1993)
Etrimfos	0.003	(1982)	
Fenamiphos	0.0005	(1987)	
Fenbutatin oxide	0.03	(1977)	
Fenchlorphos	0.01	(1968)	
Fenitrothion	0.005	(1988)	
Fensulfothion	0.0003	(1982)	
Fenthion	0.001	(1980)	
Fentin	0.0005	(1970)	
Fenvalerate	0.02	(1986)	
Ferbam	0.02	(1980)	For sum of ferbam and ziram

Table 17. (*Continued*)

Pesticide	ADI value[a] (in mg/kg bw)		Comments[b]
Flucythrinate	0.02	(1985)	
Flusilazole	0.001	(1989)	
Folpet	0.01		TADI (1986–1990)
Formothion	0.02	(1973)	
Glyphosate	0.3	(1986)	
Guazatine	0.03	(1978)	
Heptachlor	0.0005	(1970)	
Hexachlorobenzene			Previous conditional ADI withdrawn (1978)
Hydrogen cyanide	0.05	(1965)	
Hydrogen phosphide			ADI not necessary: good usage practices should ensure that residues are not present at time of consumption
Imazalil	0.01	(1986)	
Inorganic bromide	1	(1988)	
Iprodione	0.3	(1977)	
Isofenphos	0.001	(1986)	
Lindane	0.008	(1989)	
Malathion	0.02	(1966)	
Maleic hydrazide	5	(1984)	Based on Na or K salt, 99.9% pure and containing not more than 1 mg hydrazine/kg
Mancozeb	0.05	(1980)	For sum of mancozeb, maneb, and zineb; not more than 0.002 mg/kg bw present as ethylenethiourea
Maneb	0.05	(1980)	For sum of mancozeb, maneb, and zineb; not more than 0.002 mg/kg bw present as ethylenethiourea
Mecarbam	0.002	(1986)	
Metalaxyl	0.03	(1982)	
Methacrifos	0.003		TADI (1988–1990)
Methamidophos	0.0006	(1985)	
Methidathion	0.005	(1975)	
Methiocarb	0.001	(1987)	
Methomyl	0.03	(1989)	
Methoprene	0.1	(1987)	
Methyl bromide			Not cleared toxicologically
Mevinphos	0.0015	(1972)	
Monocrotophos	0.0006	(1975)	
Nitrofen			Not cleared toxicologically
Omethoate	0.0003	(1985)	
Ortho-phenylphenol	0.02		TADI (extended to 1990)
Oxamyl	0.03	(1984)	
Oxydemeton-methyl	0.0003	(1989)	For sum of demeton-S-methyl, demeton-S-methylsulfon, and oxydemeton-methyl
Paclobutrazol	0.1	(1988)	
Paraquat	0.004	(1986)	For paraquat cation; equivalent to 0.006 mg paraquat dichloride/kg bw

Table 17. (*Continued*)

Pesticide	ADI value[a] (in mg/kg bw)		Comments[b]
Parathion	0.005	(1967)	
Parathion-methyl	0.02	(1984)	
Permethrin	0.05	(1987)	For the nominal 40% *cis*-, 60% *trans*- and 25% *cis*-, 75% *trans*- materials only
Phenothrin	0.07	(1988)	For "d-phenothrin"
Phenthoate	0.003	(1984)	
Phorate	0.0002	(1985)	
Phosalone	0.006	(1972)	
Phosmet	0.02	(1979)	
Phosphamidon	0.0005	(1986)	
Phoxim	0.001	(1984)	
Piperonyl butoxide	0.03	(1972)	
Pirimicarb	0.02	(1982)	
Pirimiphos-methyl	0.01	(1976)	
Prochloraz	0.01	(1983)	
Procymidone	0.1	(1989)	
Propamocarb	0.1	(1986)	
Propargite	0.15	(1982)	
Propiconazole	0.04	(1987)	
Propineb			TADI withdrawn (1985)
Propoxur	0.02	(1989)	
Propylenethiourea			Not cleared toxicologically
Pyrazophos			Not cleared toxicologically
Pyrethrins	0.04	(1972)	
Quintozene	0.007	(1977)	
2,4,5,-T	0.03	(1981)	Based on 2,4,5-T containing not more than 0.01 mg TCDD/kg
Tecnazene	0.01	(1983)	
Terbufos	0.0002	(1989)	
Thiabendazole	0.3	(1977)	
Thiodicarb	0.03	(1986)	
Thiometon	0.003	(1979)	
Thiophanate-methyl	0.08	(1977)	
Thiram			TADI withdrawn (1985)
Tolylfluanid	0.1	(1988)	
Triadimefon	0.03	(1985)	
Triadimenol	0.05	(1989)	
Triazophos	0.0002		TADI (extended to 1990)
Trichlorfon	0.01	(1978)	
Triforine	0.02	(1978)	
Vamidothion	0.008	(1988)	
Vinclozolin	0.07	(1988)	
Zineb	0.05	(1980)	For sum of mancozeb, maneb, and zineb; not more than 0.002 mg/kg bw present as ethylenethiourea
Ziram	0.02	(1980)	For sum of ferbam and ziram

[a] The year of estimation or confirmation of the ADI value by the Joint Meeting on Pesticide Residues of the FAO and WHO (JMPR) is shown in parenthesis.

[b] TADI = Temporary acceptable daily intake. The year of withdrawal, current period or most recent extension by the Joint Meeting on Pesticide Residues of the FAO and WHO (JMPR) is shown in parenthesis.

The factor 60 in the numerator stands for the body weight of the average user in kilograms, while the factor 100 in the denominator is a general safety factor to compensate for unforeseen risks, such as a higher susceptibility of sick persons or special age groups [162]. An extraction factor has also been added because finished herbal preparations may contain a lower amount of pesticide than the crude herbs from which they have been prepared.

Effects of Processing

Ali [152] analyzed the levels of 10 chlorinated compounds in 80 samples of 11 different crude herbal drugs on the German market. Subsequently he prepared teas from 75 of these samples by extracting 2 g with 150 ml boiling water and assayed the resulting teas for the presence of the chlorinated pesticides [149]. Only 1.6% of the assays showed that more than 50% of pesticide had passed into the tea. In these sporadic cases the crude drug was not heavily contaminated. The highest recovery was 82% of α-HCH in a tea prepared from a Betulae folium sample contaminated with 0.03 mg/kg. In the majority of cases passage into the tea was relatively low: 90% of the assays revealed a passage of only 0%–25% (see Table 18 for average values on individual pesticides). In view of the poor solubility of chlorinated pesticides in water, these results are far from surprising. Ali [156] corroborated his findings in a sequel study on teas prepared from 45 samples of 13 different crude herbal drugs. The majority of measurements (85%) showed a passage of 0%–25%, and a recovery of more than 50% was observed only sporadically (1.1% of the assays).

The level of contamination is not only reduced by extraction with boiling water but also by ethanolic extraction [90,162]. Dry herbal dosage forms may also contain lower levels of pesticides than their crude ingredients. When Pluta [150,158] tested 266 Polish samples of raw herbal materials and 199 samples of herbal mixtures for the preparation of infusions and decoctions, 50 samples (10.8%) yielded 1.5–10 mg/kg of p,p' DDT plus its metabolites p,p'-DDE and p,p'-DDD, and 12 samples (2.6%) contained 10–15 mg/kg. In contrast, not a single sample of 78 herbal granulates for direct consumption contained more than 0.5 mg/kg of p,p'-DDT plus metabolites. Probably the main reasons for this difference were the composition of the granulates (30% of which consisted of pure pilular mass) and the technological processing [158].

Fumigation Agents

Residues in medicinal herbs do not always originate from contamination with pesticides and environmental pollutants but may also result from treatment with fumigation agents, such as ethylene oxide, methyl bromide, and phosphine [148].

Ethylene oxide has undoubtedly been the most important representative of this group. It has been widely used for the decontamination and disinfestation (i.e., the extermination of insects) of crude dried herbs [96,167]. In 1982, Schilcher [90] reported residual concentrations up to 22 mg/kg in 68 samples of dried herbs

Table 18. Relative passage of chlorinated pesticides from crude herbal drugs into medicinal teas prepared by extraction with boiling water [149]

Crude drug (number of samples)	Relative passage (mean values in %)									
	op-DDT	pp-DDT	DDE	γ-HCH	α-HCH	β-HCH	HCB	Aldrin	Dieldrin	Heptachlor
HERBS										
Equiseti herba (12)	7	8	6	22	9	5	10	5	6	4
LEAVES										
Sennae folium (8)	6	9	11	4	3	4	10	7	5	6
Betulae folium (9)	11	12	19	36	33	–	28	32	28	23
Menthae pip. folium (7)	6	16	10	19	17	9	10	10	5	5
FLOWERS										
Hibisci flos (4)	5	25	14	21	15	18	11	5	11	12
Chamomillae flos (11)	16	17	20	30	11	9	9	34	17	23
FRUITS										
Carvi fructus (4)	5	12	5	5	31	2	7	5	5	5
Foeniculi fructus (6)	5	15	25	20	12	9	5	14	9	10
Anisi fructus (6)	10	24	8	34	9	24	13	5	5	5
Sennae fructus (6)	9	10	6	9	17	13	10	5	9	5

that had been treated with ethylene oxide at the wholesale stage. Schilcher himself treated more than 45 samples of five different herbal drugs with ethylene oxide 750 g/m^3 for 6 h and recovered mean residual levels between 3 and 75 mg/kg 9 days later [90].

Ethylene oxide is by no means without toxicological risks. It has alkylating properties and reacts with water to form ethylene glycol and with chloride ion to form ethylene chlorhydrin, both of which are toxic reaction products [164,168]. Residues in medical devices sterilized with ethylene oxide have been associated with serious acute effects in patients, such as sensitization and anaphylactoid reactions during hemodialysis [169]. Occupational exposure to ethylene oxide has been associated with an increased frequency of spontaneous abortion in hospital personnel [170]. Even more serious are the concerns about the mutagenic and carcinogenic potential of the compound. It has mutagenic properties in various test systems, and monkey studies have shown that it induces chromosomal aberrations and sister chromatid exchanges. It is carcinogenic in rats and mice, and there is epidemiological evidence to suggest that ethylene oxide may be carcinogenic in man as well [168,171]. For instance, an increased incidence of leukemia and gastric cancer has been observed among workers in Sweden occupationally exposed to the gas [172]. In addition to these problems, treatment with ethylene oxide may affect the phytochemical composition of crude herbs [173–175], thereby forming new compounds with pharmacological and toxicological properties that are insufficiently known [92]. Because of the toxicological risks involved, health authorities in the Federal Republic of Germany issued special recommendations in 1986 to restrict the gaseous treatment of herbal drugs with ethylene oxide (see Table 19). The European Community announced that this treatment would be completely banned from January 1, 1990 [92], but this measure was later postponed for 1 year [177].

A promising alternative method for the disinfestation of medicinal plants which is currently under investigation is the so-called pressure/expansion (PEX) procedure, which consists of pressure treatment with carbon dioxide [178,179].

Radioactivity

Introduction

Medicinal plants may be exposed to radionuclides, such as Sr-90. If need be, herbal remedies should therefore be tested for residual levels of radioactivity [39,90,162].

Table 19. Recommendations of the FRG health authorities (1986) concerning the gaseous treatment of herbal drugs with ethylene oxide [176][a]

— Treatment of herbal mixtures and fresh plants is prohibited, as is the treatment of dried herbs that will be submitted to further processing (extraction).
— Treatment is prohibited, when the total count is lower than 5×10^4 CFU/g, or when the yeast and mold count is lower than 5×10^2 CFU/g.
— Herbs that are intended for tea preparation by the user (extraction with boiling water) or for application on the intact skin may be treated only when the total count exceeds 5×10^5 CFU/g.
— The concentration of ethylene oxide in the treatment room should be no more than 250 g/m^3. This limit may be raised to 500 g/m^3 for individual species and batches on the condition that the absence of toxic reaction products is properly demonstrated.
— No residual ethylene oxide should be detectable after the desorption period (with a detection sensitivity of at least 1 mg/kg), and a limit value of 150 mg/kg should be observed for halogenated ethylene hydrins. Irrespective of this limit, the tolerable daily amount of halogenated ethylene hydrins should be established at 1 mg per day.
— Repeated treatment is prohibited.

---

[a] According to Schilcher [148], the careful use of ethylene oxide also requires that the residual humidity of the herbal drug is < 10%, and that the drug is aired repeatedly after treatment. The low humidity is needed because ethylene chlorhydrin can be found in larger amounts when the dried herb contains more than 10% of water and has a high mineral content as well [90].

Some years ago, no research data on this subject were available. This situation was changed drastically, however, by the tragic nuclear reactor accident at Chernobyl on April 26, 1986. This disaster raised such concerns about fallout exposure of medicinal herbs that several research groups in Austria and the FRG started to investigate the contamination with radioactivity of crude herbs and their extracted preparations [180–186]. In a study performed immediately after the Chernobyl accident, the following isotopes were measured: Cs-134, Cs-137, Ru-103, and I-131. The investigators pointed out, however, that the observed levels of I-131 (up to 3626 Bq/kg) were without practical relevance, as this contaminant will have lost all its radioactivity by the time that the herbal drug reaches the patient [180]. Subsequent studies have therefore been restricted to the more persistent major isotopes Cs-134 and Cs-137 and to the minor radionuclide Ru-103.

Levels of Contamination

The researchers needed threshold values to put their results into perspective. The only official limits available at that time were the maximum allowable Cs-134/Cs-137 concentrations of 370 Bq/kg for milk and 600 Bq/kg for other fresh foodstuffs that had been established by the EC. An expert committee in the FRG questioned whether it was appropriate to transfer such values for fresh foods to dried herbal ingredients for medicinal teas which were likely to be taken in lower doses and for shorter periods of time, but the committee failed to come up with an alternative limit [187].

For want of something better and to avoid that herbs surpassing the legal limit for foodstuffs would be sold in pharmacies, the Zentrallaboratorium Deutscher Apotheker (Central Laboratory of German Pharmacists) decided to retain the EC limit of 600 Bq/kg. It calculated that herbs satisfying this upper value were unlikely to represent a real health risk: even when the crude drug contains 600 Bq/kg, and all this radioactivity is extracted, the contamination of 1 l tea prepared from 15 g is still less than 10 Bq/l, much lower than the EC limit of 370 Bq/l for milk. The daily use of 1 l of the tea would result in an exposure of about 6 mrem per year, whereas natural radiation provides an annual dose of 200–500 mrem [183,188].

A considerable proportion of herbal samples gathered in Austria and Bavaria shortly after the Chernobyl disaster showed radioactivity levels over 600 Bq/kg, and in the first year after the nuclear accident several crude herbal drugs destined for the FRG market were found to exceed this limit (see Table 20).

The studies on Austrian medicinal plants showed that contamination varied with herb, habitat, and time of harvesting [180,181]. An impressive drop in the levels of radioactivity was seen when samples of different crops of the same plant collected at the same habitat were compared with each other (see Table 21). On average, drugs consisting of leaves were more prone to contamination than those

Table 20. Levels of radioactivity in crude herbal drugs after the nuclear reactor accident at Chernobyl

Research group — Reference	Type of herbal drugs studied — Results
Kartnig c.s. — Kartnig et al. 1986 [180]	*Crude herbal drugs harvested in Austria*[a] — 61.5% of 39 samples of 15 drugs harvested between 2.5.86 and 9.7.86 had a level > 600 Bq/kg; the highest value was 40 000 Bq/kg (Melissae folium) — none of 10 samples of 3 drugs harvested between 4.6.86 and 30.6.86 (so-called 2nd crop) had a level > 600 Bq/kg (cf. Table 21)
— Kartnig and Zödl 1987 [184]	— none of 7 samples of 4 drugs harvested in 1987 had a level > 600 Bq/kg (cf. Table 21)
Kopp and Kubelka — Kopp and Kubelka 1986 [181]	*Crude herbal drugs collected in Austria*[b] — 75.0% of 28 samples of 22 drugs collected between 2.6.86 and 22.6.86 had a level > 600 Bq/kg; the highest value was 10 105 Bq/kg (Sambuci flos)
Pratzel and Reinelt — Pratzel and Reinelt 1986 [182]	*Crude herbal drugs collected in Bavaria*[a] — 51.4% of 35 drugs (a total of 298 samples with 1–27 samples/drug) collected in 7.86/8.86 had a *mean* level > 600 Bq/kg; the highest value was 15 394 Bq/kg (thyme)
Zentrallabor Deutscher Apotheker — Blume et al. 1987 [183]	*Crude herbal drugs available on or destined for the FRG market*[c] — None of 49 drugs available on the FRG market between 7.86 and 12.86 had a level > 600 Bq/kg — Three of 9 drugs from other countries presumably destined for the FRG market had a level > 600 Bq/kg; the highest value was 3100 Bq/kg (Bulgarian Nasturtii herba)
— Anonymous 1987 [185]	— None of 59 drugs available on the FRG market between 1.87 and 5.87 had a level > 600 Bq/kg — Seven drugs of unspecified origin destined for the FRG market had a level > 600 Bq/kg; the highest value was 6410 Bq/kg (Veronicae herba)

[a] Cs contamination and Ru-103 levels were determined separately by these research groups [180,182]. The results presented here refer to total Cs contamination (Cs-134/Cs-137 levels) without the inclusion of Ru-103 contamination.
[b] The results presented here refer to unspecified levels of radioactivity [181].
[c] The detection method used by the Zentrallabor Deutscher Apotheker determined Ru-103 and Ru-106 in addition to the major radionuclides Cs-134 and Cs-137 [183]. The results presented here therefore refer to total Cs levels with the inclusion of Ru contamination.

Table 21. Variation of Cs-134/Cs-137 radioactivity with crop in Melissae folium cultivated in the Austrian Steiermark area [180,184]

Habitat	Crop[a]	Cs-134/Cs-137 con-tamination (Bq/kg)
Petersdorf I	first crop 1986 (10.5.86/13.6.86)	16 687
	second crop 1986 (4.6.86/18.7.86)	188.7
	first crop 1987	15.5
Hochenegg	first crop 1986 (10.5.86/12.6.86)	40 000
	second crop 1986[b] (30.6.86/11.7.86)	99.9
	first crop 1987	21.1

[a] Times of harvesting and analysis indicated in parentheses
[b] Melissae herba instead of Melissae folium

consisting of flowers. This finding was not unexpected, since generally the plants were not yet in full bloom at the time of the fallout [180].

Effects of Processing

Usually, traditional teas prepared from contaminated medicinal herb samples do not contain all the radioactivity that was present in the crude material (see Table 22). The few available data on tinctures suggest that the passage of radioactivity is also incomplete when an alcoholic extraction fluid is used [180]. Particularly low levels of radioactivity (with a maximal passage rate of only 5.4%) have been reported for essential oils obtained from contaminated herbs by means of steam distillation [186].

Toxic Metals

Introduction

There are two major reasons why it has become necessary to monitor levels of toxic metals in herbal drugs:

— Contamination of the general environment with toxic metals has increased [189]. The sources of this environmental pollution are quite varied, ranging from industrial and traffic emissions to the use of purification mud and agricultural expedients, such as cadmium-containing dung, organic mercury fungicides, and the insecticide lead arsenate [161,164,190].

Table 22. Passage of radioactivity in crude herbal drugs into medicinal teas

Reference	Results
Kopp and Kubelka 1986 [181]	Extraction rates up to 50% were observed following the preparation of teas from 26 herbal samples. The samples belonged to 20 different plant species and were contaminated with 289 to 10 105 Bq/kg of unspecified radioactivity. Only 2 finished teas showed a contamination level over 10 Bq/l; the highest value (approximately 30 Bq/l) was found in the tea prepared from the most heavily contaminated herb sample (Sambuci flos).
Pratzel and Reinelt 1986 [182]	Teas of 16 different contaminated drugs were prepared by covering each herb with water and boiling the mixture for a short while. The passage of Cs isotopes was ≤ 50% in 7 cases (with a lowest value of 6% for Equiseti herba), 51%–90% in 6 cases, and > 90% in the remaining 3 cases (up to 100% for Hyperici herba).
Ali and Ihrig 1987 [186]	Cs passages varied between 5% and 68%, when 24 samples of 16 different drugs (contaminated with 361 to 6410 Bq/kg) were extracted with boiling water. Eight teas contained ≤ 25%, 9 teas 26%–50%, and 7 teas > 50%. Six tea samples had a level over 10 Bq/l, with a maximum of 23 Bq/l (Veronicae herba).

— Exotic herbal remedies, particularly those of Asian origin, have been repeatedly reported to contain toxic levels of heavy metals and/or arsenic.

As these two types of contamination are quite different, both in their nature and in their health risks, they will be treated separately. Some general toxicological information about the major metals involved is provided in Table 23.

Environmental Pollution

Levels of Environmental Contamination

Investigators in the FRG have performed several studies on residual levels of toxic metals in medicinal herbs [90,156,161,189,196]. As concrete threshold limits could not be found in the European Pharmacopoeia or the German pharmacopoeia, the researchers took limit values of the so-called *Zentrale Erfassungs- und Bewertungsstelle für Umweltchemikalien* (ZEBS) as a point of reference. The national ZEBS regulation offers maximum allowable values for herb-like food products, such as grains and vegetables (Table 24). It should be noted that the limits usually refer to the fresh weight of foodstuffs destined for consumption, whereas medicinal herbs are generally tested in their dried form [148].

Crude medicinal herb samples were found to exceed the threshold values of the ZEBS regulation quite often (Table 25). Failure to meet these limits does not imply, however, that a real health risk is involved. Comparison of test results with

Table 23. Some metallic contaminants that have been taken into account in the quality assurance and/or toxicological evaluation of herbal remedies [90, 189, 191, 192]

Metal	Chronic toxicity problems [11, 164]
Lead [193]	Although chronic plumbism can express itself in various ways, three major clinical syndromes can be recognized: — Alimentary type: anorexia, metallic taste, constipation, and severe abdominal cramps — Neuromuscular type: peripheral neuritis — Cerebral type: encephalopathy Other signs of chronic lead poisoning include renal dysfunction, anemia, mild jaundice, facial pallor, a gingival lead line, and basophilic stippling of red blood cells. Blood lead levels as low as 2 μmol/l have been associated with subtle psychological changes and also with decreased sperm count and abnormal sperm morphology. Lead is clearly teratogenic in laboratory animals. In man, the reproductive system appears to be very sensitive to chronic lead exposure. Cognitive developmental deficits have been observed in infants born with cord blood lead levels $\geq$ 0.5 μmol/l.
Cadmium [194]	Renal injuries are common among chronically exposed workers. Other recognized sequelae of chronic respiratory exposure are liver damage, anemia, severe emphysema, and yellow-stained teeth. Chronic cadmium poisoning may also lead to signs of a disturbed calcium metabolism (osteomalacia, decreased bone density, hypercalcinuria, renal stones). Exposure to cadmium has been associated with increased incidence of respiratory and prostatic cancers, but evidence is still limited, especially for prostatic cancer.
Mercury [148]	The poisonous actions are usually associated with the mercuric ion, but alkyl mercurials, such as methyl mercury, have toxic effects due to the parent compound and can be more toxic than inorganic mercurials. In chronic exposure to mercury compounds the kidney is a major target organ. Another predominant sign of chronic mercurialism is neurotoxicity. Peripheral neuropathies have been described, but the principal target of damage is the CNS (e.g., tremors, impaired motor control, sensory disturbances, psychic and behavioral changes). Other symptoms include metallic taste, stomatitis, salivation, diarrhea, and discoloration of the anterior lens surface. All forms of mercury are teratogenic in animal tests. Cases of human fetal poisonings have mostly been traced to mercury vapor and organic mercurials, especially methyl mercury.
Arsenic [195]	Among the manifestations of chronic poisoning are anorexia, gastrointestinal disturbances, fever, persistent headache, pallor, weakness, alopecia, coryza-like symptoms, and skin afflictions. Renal damage, hepatomegaly and severe blood dyscrasias have been described, as have nervous symptoms (peripheral neuritis, encephalopathy) in advanced poisoning. Arsenic crosses the placental barrier, and acute maternal arsenic poisoning has been incriminated in neonatal death. Inorganic arsenic compounds are established carcinogens in man. Occupational and medicinal exposures to arsenical products have been associated with lung cancer (due to chronic inhalation), skin cancer and visceral cancers.
Thallium	Repeated ingestion of small quantities may produce effects similar to the subacute symptoms of acute poisoning, such as gastrointestinal disturbances, salivation, gingival discoloration, peripheral polyneuritis, signs of encephalopathy, skin reactions, hepatorenal injury, and alopecia.

Table 24. Maximum allowed levels of heavy metals in foodstuffs, according to the FRG *Zentrale Erfassungs-und Bewertungsstelle für Umweltchemikalien* (ZEBS) regulation [161]

Metal	Year of ZEBS	Maximum allowed level per type of foodstuff (mg/kg)				
		Grain	Rye/rice	Fruit/root vegetables	Leafy vegetables	Sprout vegetables
Lead						
	1979	0.5	–	0.5	1.2	1.2
	1986	–	0.4	0.25	0.8	0.5
Cadmium						
	1979	0.1	–	0.1	0.1	0.1
	1986	–	0.1	0.1	0.1	0.1
Mercury						
	1979	0.03	–	–	–	–
	1986	–	0.03	0.05	0.05	0.05

Table 25. Residual levels of toxic metals in some large test series of crude botanical drugs

Author(s) Samples	Results[a]
Schilcher 1982 [90]	
120 linseed samples and 222 samples of other crude herbal drugs on the FRG market	*Lead:* — linseed samples: 11% between 0.6 and 1.2 mg/kg and 42% > 1.2 mg/kg — other samples: 22% between 0.6 and 1.2 mg/kg and 49% > 1.2 mg/kg *Cadmium:* — linseed samples: 58% > 0.10 mg/kg — other samples: 35% > 0.10 mg/kg *Mercury:* — linseed samples: 7% > 0.03 mg/kg — other samples: 14% > 0.03 mg/kg
Ali 1983 [189] and 1987 [156]	
A total of 131 samples of 20 different crude herbal drugs on the FRG market	*Lead:* 21% of the samples between 0.6 and 1.2 mg/kg and 22% > 1.2 mg/kg; the highest value was 6.1 mg/kg in a sample of Urticae herba. *Cadmium:* 40% of the samples contained > 0.10 mg/kg; the highest value was 0.85 mg/kg in a sample of Hyperici herba. *Thallium:* All 80 samples tested for this metal contained less than 0.01 mg/kg.

[a] The results are expressed in terms of the limit values for grains and vegetables of the FRG ZEBS regulation from 1979 (see Table 24).

the ZEBS values should merely be considered as a tool of quality assurance for the timely detection of potentially undesirable contamination [148, 161].

In the experience of Schilcher and associates [161,196], herbal drugs occurring wild show more anomalous values than cultivated herbs, in particular with respect to lead levels. The reason is, of course, that drugs grown wild are more difficult to control for all the potential ways of environmental pollution. As was to be expected, the research group also demonstrated that the levels of lead and cadmium in the same crude herb may vary considerably with plant part and habitat (Table 26).

Toxicological Evaluation

Just as the FAO/WHO ADI values for pesticides are a good starting point for the risk assessment of pesticide levels in botanical drugs, it is preferable to base the risk evaluation of metal residues in herbs on the so-called provisional weekly tolerable intake (PTWI) values for toxic metals that have been established by the same two organizations (Table 27). Mutatis mutandis, the formula given in the section on pesticides for the calculation of theoretical maximally tolerable contamination levels from ADI values, can also be used to derive similar levels for metal residues [161,162]:

Table 26. Variation in lead and cadmium levels with plant part and habitat in *Achillea millefolium* and *Hypericum perforatum* grown wild [196]

METAL	Level of contamination (in mg/kg)					
Medicinal plant	Habitat	Total herb	Flower	Leaf	Stem	Root
LEAD						
Achillea millefolium	Median strip	8.41	4.66	23.73	1.34	4.59
	Road-side	2.37	2.33	8.90	1.25	4.16
Hypericum perforatum	Median strip	11.97	5.77	17.82	2.32	4.57
	Road-side	1.77	1.85	5.96	1.05	5.06
CADMIUM						
Achillea millefolium	Median strip	0.34	0.13	0.78	0.33	0.44
	Road-side	1.48	0.89	2.17	1.33	2.57
Hypericum perforatum	Median strip	0.37	0.38	0.54	0.32	0.85
	Road-side	5.62	6.97	7.43	3.74	3.30

Table 27. Provisional tolerable weekly intake (PTWI) values
for toxic metals, as established by FAO and WHO

Metal	PTWI value (μg/kg/week)	Reference
Lead	50[a]	197
Cadmium	7	198
Mercury	5[b]	197
Arsenic (inorganic)	15[c]	198

[a] For children, the PTWI value has been set at 25 μg/kg per week [199].
[b] But no more than 3.3 μg/kg per week in the form of methyl mercury [198].
[c] This PTWI does not refer to organoarsenicals, as the organoarsenic compounds naturally occurring in marine products are considerably less toxic than inorganic arsenicals [198].

$$\text{Theoretical maximally tolerable level (mg/kg)} = \frac{\text{PTWI (mg/kg)} \times 60 \times \text{extraction factor}}{\text{average weekly herb consumption (kg)} \times 100}$$

When PTWIs are used for the toxicological evaluation of metal residues in herbal drugs, the following points deserve special consideration:

— The safety margin between a PTWI and the weekly exposure that produces deleterious effects can be relatively small. For instance, the critical organ in relation to the toxic effects of chronic ingestion of small amounts of cadmium is the kidney. Intakes as low as 140 255 μg/day have been associated with low molecular weight proteinuria (without specific histological changes) in the elderly. Yet the PTWI for cadmium has been set at 7 μg/kg/week, i.e., 60 μg/day for a person with an average body weight of 60 kg [198].
— Experts are still debating whether PTWI values can be used in general or whether they should be applied only to healthy adults, with the exclusion of risk groups such as chronically ill patients, pregnant women, and breast-feeding mothers [161]. With respect to lead, a special pediatric PTWI of 25 μg/kg per week has been established, which is only half the PTWI value for adults (see Table 27).
— As PTWI values refer to total dietary intakes, it is impossible to determine the acceptability of a certain contamination level in a botanical drug without considering the normal dietary exposure to the metal in question. As is illustrated by Table 28, where results of recent studies from seven different countries are shown, the normal daily diet may provide a substantial portion of the tolerable daily amount that can be derived from the PTWI. It should also be realized that there may be large regional differences in the level of dietary

Table 28. Comparison of tolerable daily amounts (TDA) of toxic metals with actual dietary intakes measured in seven different countries [200]

Studied country	Mean dietary intake (μg/day)			
	Lead (TDA = 429 μg)[a]	Cadmium (TDA = 60 μg)[a]	Mercury (TDA = 43 μg)[a]	Arsenic[b] (TDA = 129 μg)[a]
The Netherlands	32 (7%)	21 (35%)	0.7 (2%)	38 (29%)
Belgium	179 (42%)	18 (30%)	13.5 (31%)	45 (35%)
United Kingdom	115 (27%)	20 (33%)	ND	129 (100%)
Sweden	27 (6%)	10 (17%)	ND	ND
Finland	66 (15%)	13 (22%)	ND	ND
United States	82 (19%)	33 (55%)	5 (12%)	65 (50%)
Canada	54 (13%)	14 (23%)	ND	17 (13%)

[a] Tolerable daily amounts (TDA) derived from the FAO/WHO provisional tolerable weekly intake values (Table 27) for an average body weight of 60 kg
[b] The data on arsenic should be interpreted with caution, because there is a substantial toxicological difference between inorganic arsenic and organoarsenicals in seafoods [198]. In the United Kingdom, for instance, only a small part of the daily arsenic intake seems to consist of inorganic arsenic [201].

exposure to a toxic metal. For instance, the dietary load of cadmium in the FRG averaged 42% of the PTWI value in 1982, but loads up to 80% of the PTWI were found regionally [148].

On the other hand, however, it should be considered that the PTWI limits are adhered to on a longer term basis, and that short-term exposure to levels exceeding the PTWI is not necessarily a cause for concern, provided the individual's intake averaged over longer periods of time does not exceed the level set [198].

Thallium
Most studies on residual levels of toxic metals in medicinal herbs have focused on lead, cadmium, and mercury [148,156,161]. In one study, where samples of crude botanical drugs were analyzed for thallium concentrations, all 80 samples tested contained less than 0.01 mg/kg [189].

An FAO/WHO PTWI value for thallium is not available. The current dietary intake of this toxic element in the United Kingdom, which is estimated to be 5 μg/day, is not regarded as a cause for concern [202]. A clue about unsafe levels of subchronic thallium exposure can be found in a recent report on endemic thallotoxicosis in a Chinese province, which was in all probability caused by the consumption of cabbage grown on polluted soil. Poisoning occurred after the protracted use of large amounts of cabbage (e.g., 0.5 kg daily for 1 month or more) providing 41.7 mg/kg thallium. In contrast, the use of cabbage contaminated with 5.6 mg/kg was not associated with toxic symptoms [203].

Effects of Processing

The effects of extraction with boiling water were studied extensively by Ali [149,156], who analyzed the lead and cadmium levels in 120 samples of 19 crude drugs and in finished teas prepared from these samples. Passage into the tea was above 50% in only 12% of the lead assays and 8% of the cadmium tests. The majority of tea samples (67% and 71% for lead and cadmium, respectively) showed a relatively low extraction of 25% or less (see Table 29 for average extraction percentages per crude drug). Individual extraction values ranged from 0.1% to 87% for lead, and the passage rates of cadmium varied from 1% to 68%. These large variations may well be connected to different ways of contamination. When a herbal drug is contaminated at its surface with inorganic salts, it is likely that a relatively large proportion will dissolve in the hot water. Passage into a tea is relatively low, however, when metal traces are organically bound in the plant cell [149,156].

Incomplete extraction with boiling water was also observed by Schilcher et al. [161]. This research group found that the washing of plants while they are still

Table 29. Relative passage of heavy metals from crude herbal drugs into medicinal teas prepared by extraction with boiling water [149,156]

Crude drug (number of samples)	Relative passage (mean values in %)	
	Lead	Cadmium
HERBS		
Equiseti herba (13)	22	23
Hyperici herba (5)	12	19
Millefolii herba (5)	15	24
Thymi herba (6)	9	28
Urticae herba (7)	9	25
LEAVES		
Sennae folium (8)	33	50
Betulae folium (9)	16	15
Menthae piperitae folium (8)	20	28
Melissae folium (1)	15	19
LEAVES + FLOWERS		
Crataegi folia cum floribus (1)	9	8
FLOWERS		
Hibisci flos (4)	37	49
Chamomillae flos (16)	36	18
Malvae flos (4)	13	13
Crataegi flos (4)	9	6
Tiliae flos (1)	11	19
FRUITS		
Carvi fructus (4)	73	25
Foeniculi fructus (6)	40	16
Anisi fructus (10)	29	19
Sennae fructus (8)	4	9

Table 30. Effect of washing on the lead and cadmium levels of some fresh medicinal herbs [161]

Medicinal herb	Level of contamination (in mg/kg)		
	Metal	Unwashed	Washed
Taraxaci	Lead	0.283	0.197 (70%)
herba	Cadmium	0.057	0.039 (68%)
Urtical	Lead	0.248	0.198 (80%)
herba	Cadmium	0.016	0.0113 (71%)
Plantaginis	Lead	0.201	0.164 (82%)
herba	Cadmium	0.080	0.067 (84%)

fresh, may remove about 15%–30% of a heavy metal contaminant (see Table 30). In other experiments the group showed that the passage of lead and cadmium into the extraction fluid decreased as the polarity of the extraction fluid decreased [196]. Thus there can be little doubt that ethanolic extraction of crude drug herbs likewise results in incomplete passage of heavy metals.

Cadmium in Linseed
A few botanical drugs are not used in processed form but as raw materials so that the user cannot benefit from the fact that extracts contain less in heavy metals than their crude ingredients. A most notable example is linseed. This drug is relatively often contaminated with cadmium levels > 0.1 mg/kg (see Table 25), and it may be taken in considerable amounts up to 40–50 g/day [148,149].

Ali [156,189] tested 11 linseed samples and found cadmium concentrations up to 0.6 mg/kg. When 40–50 g linseed is consumed each day, this level results in a daily exposure to 30 μg cadmium, i.e., 50% of the tolerable daily amount of 60 μg/day for persons with an average body weight of 60 kg (see Table 28). This percentage is certainly a cause for concern since a normal diet already provides 17%–55% of the tolerable cadmium dose (Table 28) and may regionally yield even up to 80% of this amount [148]. On the basis of similar calculations, the health authorities in the FRG have recently set the maximally tolerable level of cadmium in linseed at 0.3 mg/kg [204].

Arsenic in Kelp
The presence of arsenic in kelp products came to attention when abnormally high urinary levels of arsenic were observed in two female patients. This finding was traced to the use of health food tablets prepared from kelp, and chemical determinations confirmed that significant amounts of arsenic can occur in such preparations [205]. The investigators did not sufficiently recognize, however, that arsenic can be present in marine organisms in the form of organoarsenicals that are less toxic than inorganic arsenic [206]. For instance, organoarsenic compounds naturally occurring in fish are excreted very rapidly by man, and there have been no reports of ill effects among populations, whose consumption of large

quantities of fish results in organoarsenical intakes of about 0.05 mg/kg per day. In view of such data, the FAO and WHO have established a PTWI only for inorganic arsenic without assigning such a value to organic arsenicals [198].

The toxicological difference between inorganic arsenic and organoarsenicals has been properly acknowledged in a recent British study on 16 different kelp tablets and capsules. Fifteen products were on sale in the United Kingdom as food supplements and health foods while the remaining product was a kelp capsule available in Australia. All products were analyzed for total and "reducible" arsenic levels (the latter level reflected the total of inorganic arsenic and some unstable organoarsenic species and was thus regarded as an indicator of maximum inorganic arsenic content). The products from Britain yielded total arsenic levels between 2 and 45 μg/g, and their reducible arsenic concentrations were only 0.01–0.45 μg/g. Potential daily intakes of reducible arsenic (based on maximum manufacturers' dose recommendations) ranged from 0.05 to 9 μg. In sharp contrast, the Australian capsule contained 120 and 50 μg/g of total and reducible arsenic, respectively, and the maximum dose recommended by the manufacturer would provide 700 μg of reducible arsenic [201]. This unusually high value is more than five times the tolerable daily amount (TDA) of 129 μg that can be calculated from the FAO/WHO PTWI value for inorganic arsenic (see Table 28).

Toxic Metals in Exotic Remedies[1]

Publications about unacceptable levels of toxic metals in exotic herbal remedies have regularly appeared in the medical and pharmaceutical literature. One report described an outbreak of arsenic poisoning in Singapore, and at least four reports attribute lead poisoning to the use of an oriental herbal medicines (see Table 31 for clinical and chemical details).

Potential sources of contamination include lead-releasing brewing pots [213], grinding weights [210], and other metal utensils. In India, the recommended procedure to give botanical medicines known as Bal Jivan Chamcho to children is to turn them into a paste, which is spread on a spatula-shaped spoon and allowed to dry. The dried material is then soaked in milk or water for several minutes, after which the liquid is to be taken by the child. When the spoon has a high lead content, toxic amounts of lead leach into the herbal preparation [192]. It is also possible, however, that the toxic metal is not an accidental contaminant. According to Yeung [214], several Chinese herbal formulas contain arsenic and mercury salts as intentional ingredients (see Table 32). There have also been reports about lead poisoning by Chinese folk medicines adulterated with lead oxide and by Chinese face powders containing lead carbonate [213].

The deliberate incorporation of metal salts or oxides into the composition of traditional medicines and cosmetics is observed in various parts of the world. Notorious examples, many of which have actually been associated with lead or arsenic poisonings, are reviewed in Table 33.

[1] See also the note added in proof on p. 261

Table 31. Reports about unacceptable levels of arsenic and heavy metals in Far Eastern herbal remedies

Author(s)	Clincal and chemical details
Tay and Seah 1975 [191]	In Singapore, arsenic poisoning was observed in 74 patients who had been using Chinese herbal medicines providing a high inorganic arsenic intake. Among the various symptoms noted were sensorimotor polyneuropathy, psychosis, acute toxic hepatits, anemia, transient albuminuria, skin cancers, and internal malignancies. Three patients died from spreading arsenic-induced carcinomas and one from ventricular arrhythmia. Of those remaining alive, 12% were moderately disabled. Forty-seven patients (64%) had taken an antiasthmatic herbal pill called Sin Lak, which contained 12 mg/g arsenic sulfide. This pill provided an arsenic intake of about 10.3 mg/day when used as recommended. Another 28 brands of Chinese herbal preparations with high concentrations (ranging from 45 μg/g to 107 mg/) of arsenic sulfide or trioxide were identified. These preparations resulted in daily exposures to 0.5–3.3 mg arsenic.
Chan et al. 1977 [207]	A 4-month-old boy presented at a Hong Kong hospital with a history of fever, cough, anorexia, vomiting, and a grand mal seizure. On physical examination he was comatose with repeated tonic-clonic convulsions. His whole blood lead level was 137 μg/100g and the 24-h urinary lead excretion was 52 μg. Since birth the boy had been treated with several Chinese herbal medicines (16 unit dose packages of Po Ying Tan, 5 packages of Chun Chu Mu, and one package each of Po Lung Yuen and Siu Fun San). All these medicines were found to contain lead. The highest content was found in samples of the Po Ying Tan preparation: a mean of 7.5 mg/dose with a range of 4.004–9.44 mg (implying a total lead intake via this drug of 64–151 mg). Samples of six other Po Ying Tan brands showed lead levels from 0.012 to 0.07 mg/dose.
Lightfoote et al. 1977 [208]	A 59-year-old woman in the United States developed anemia, diffuse pain, insomnia, irritability, and paranoia as well as difficulty using her hands. Her 24-h urinary lead excretion was 1044 μg. Four months before, she had been instructed by a herbalist-acupuncturist to take 30 Chinese herbal pills per day. Since the pills showed a lead content of 0.5 mg per bill, this advice amounted to a lead intake of 15 mg/day.
Chung et al. 1980 [209]	This South Korean case report describes lead poisoning (abdominal pain, anemia, and a urinary lead level of 739.4 μg/l) due to a herbal medicine containing a high concentration of lead.
Yu and Yeung 1987 [210]	A semiconscious 2-month-old boy was admitted with repeated convulsions to a Hong Kong hospital. Subsequent investigations showed a blood lead level of 195 μg/dl and a 24-h urinary lead excretion of 20.7 mg. Since the 4th day of his life he had been treated with a herbal powder mixture with a total and leachable lead content of 23.3% and 15.6%, respectively. At least 0.2 g of this powder had been painted onto his buccal mucosa twice a week, resulting in a lead intake of 62.4 mg/week. A survey by the Hong Kong Medical and Health Department showed that 2 of 44 patent herbal medications contained > 30 μg/pill of lead and would provide > 3 mg/week when taken in recommended doses (i.e. more than the provisional weekly tolerable intake for lead established by FAO/WHO).
Anonymous 1989 [211]	Chuifong tokuwan pills (Nan Ling Pharmaceutical Company; Hong Kong) illegally sold in Texas contained not only synthetic Western drugs (diazepam, indomethacin, hydrochlorothiazide, mefenamic acid, dexametha-

Table 31. (*Continued*)

Author(s)	Clinical and chemical details
	sone) but also lead and cadmium. When 93 persons who had ingested these pills were tested for exposure to these heavy metals, none showed elevated levels of lead, but 22 (24%) had abnormally high urinary cadmium levels over 2.5 µg/l ml, and 39 (42%) showed elevated urine values for retinol-binding protein, a low molecular weight protein indicative of renal tubular dysfunction.
De Smet and Elferink 1990 [212]	Two Chinese herbal preparations available on the Dutch market (Tien Wang Pu Hsin Wan pills and Bi Yan Pian tablets) were found to contain 0.03 mg legd per piece and would exceed the FAO/WHO PTWI for lead of 3 mg/week when used in recommended doses.

Table 32. Occurrence of arsenic and mercury salts in Chinese herbal formulas compiled by Yeung [214]

Formula	Salt(s)	Providing[a]
An-Kung-Niu-Huang-Wan (Bezoar Resurrection pills)	Arsenic disulfide Red mercuric sulfide	48 mg/g As 45 mg/g Hg
Chen-Ling-Tan (Pills for Shocking the Spirits)	Red mercuric sulfide	37 mg/g Hg
Chi-Chu-Wan (Sedative Pills with Magnetite and Cinnabar)	Red mercuric sulfide	97 mg/g Hg
Chi-Li-San (Anti-bruises Powder)	Red mercuric sulfide	60 mg/g Hg
Chih-Pao-Dan (The Most Precious Pellets)	Arsenic disulfide Red mercuric sulfide	16 mg/g As 20 mg/g Hg
Chou-Che-Wan (The Boat and Carriage Pills)	Mercurous chloride	8 mg/g Hg
Chu-Sha-An-Shen-Wan (Cinnabar Sedative Pills)	Red mercuric sulfide	12 mg/g Hg
Liu-Shen-Wan (Pills of Six Miraculous Drugs)	Arsenic disulfide	N.C.
Niu-Huang-Chieh-Tu-Pian (Antiphlogistic Pills with Bos Calculus)	Arsenic disulfide	N.C.
Shu-ching-huo-hsieh-tang (Decoction for Removing Blood Stasis in the Channels	Red mercuric sulfide	10 mg/g Hg
Tien-Wang-Pu-Hsin-Tan (The King's Mind-Easing Tonic Pills)	Red mercuric sulfide	13 mg/g Hg
Tzu-Hsueh-Tan (Purple Snowy Powder)	Red mercuric sulfide	12 mg/g Hg

[a] Expressed as milligrams of As or Hg per gram of total active ingredients.
N.C. = Not calculable.

Table 33. Non-Western folk medicines that are known or suspected to contain poisonous metal compounds as intentional ingredients

Medicine	Details
Azarcón [215–219]	This Mexican folk remedy consists of lead tetraoxide (over 90% lead by weight). It is used among Hispanic populations in the United States for relief of abdominal distress in children. It has been associated with several cases of lead poisoning. In at least one case it was the suspected cause of fatal encephalopathy.
Greta [217,219]	This remedy resembles azarcón both in its folk uses and health risks. It consists of lead oxide (over 90% lead by weight).
Pay-loo-ah [220–223]	Pay-loo-ah preparations are used by Laotian Hmong and Mien refugees living in the United States. They can have arsenic levels of 70%–80% and lead levels up to 90%. Their consumption has been associated with arsenic poisonings and lead poisonings.
Surma [192,224–226]	Surma powders originating from India and Pakistan are brought into the United Kingdom, where they are used by Asian families. They can contain over 80% of lead as lead sulfide. They are applied as a cosmetic to the conjunctival surface of infants and children, who may transfer the powder to the mouth by wiping the eyes and then sucking the fingers. This can result in abnormally high blood lead concentrations and has been associated with fatal encephalopathy.
Al kohl [227]	In Kuwait, lead poisonings have resulted from the use of this traditional preparation in children. It is applied as an eye cosmetic (in a manner similar to surma) or as a pack on the raw umbilical stump. The principal component is lead sulfide, and lead levels up to 91.8% have been recovered.
Tiro [228]	This preparation has lead sulfide as its major ingredient and may contain up to 81.1% of lead. It is used in Nigeria as an eye medicine and cosmetic similar to surma and al kohl in other parts of the world.
Kushta [192,229]	Just as surma powders, kushta medicines originate from India and Pakistan. They are often used as aphrodisiacs. Their composition is mainly oxidized metals (e.g., lead, mercury, arsenic, zinc) ground together with various herbs. Lead contents up to 72.8% have been reported. Since kushta medicines are directly ingested, they are potentially far more hazardous than surma powders.
Bhasam [230]	Bhasams are medicines prepared by repeated oxidation of ores, which are commonly used in India by ayurvedic practitioners. Arsenic contents up to 67 µg/g have been reported.
Sikor [231]	This mineral clay substance is relatively rich in lead and arsenic and may also contain cadmium, mercury, and other metals. It is traditionally taken by many Asians living in the United Kingdom as a remedy for indigestion and as a tonic during pregnancy.

Synthetic and Animal Drug Substances

Synthetic Drug Substances[1]

Certain botanical remedies are not purely of herbal origin but also contain one or more potent synthetic drug substances, which may substantially add to their risk profile. When such products are officially registered as prescription drugs, and when their synthetic components are disclosed on the product label, health care providers can be on guard against the adverse reaction profile of the nonherbal component(s). However, there is a continuous stream of literature reports from the 1970s up to the present day that potent synthetic drug substances are sometimes incorporated in Asian herbal medicines without being declared (see Table 34). Notorious examples are Chuifong Toukuwan pills from Hong Kong, Singapore or Taiwan [211,232–236,241,244] and Amborum Special F syrup (also labeled as ASFO Natural Herbs Tea) from Sri Lanka or the United States [239,243].

The adulterants belong to various pharmacological classes (see Table 35). Their serious health implications have been highlighted by cushingoid effects or withdrawal symptoms because of a hidden corticosteroid [234,236,240,247] and by life-threatening and even fatal agranulocytosis due to the incorporation of phenylbutazone and aminophenazone [232,233].

Although most incriminated herbal remedies appear to be of Asian origin, there is also evidence that Western products are occasionally adulterated unscrupulously with potent nonherbal agents [248]. A recent report from the United States warned against diethylpropion, chlordiazepoxide, and diazepam in diet capsules purchased by mail order from France, which were labeled to consist only of herbal materials, mineral salts, beta carotene, and lactose [249].

Animal Drug Substances

The undeclared occurrence of thyroid hormones in a botanical remedy was recently discovered when several United States residents developed thyrotoxicosis following the use of a purportedly herbal slimming capsule adulterated with thyroid, diethylpropion, and hydrochlorothiazide. The product had been imported into the United States from Peru [250].

Over the years, thyroid hormones have been repeatedly incorporated in nonorthodox drug programs for weight reduction [251–254]. Although it is well recognized that these hormones can help to reduce weight, primarily by increasing metabolic rate, they have no place in the therapy of obese euthyroid patients. When dietary intake of protein and calcium is inadequate, they may induce worrisome catabolic losses of these muscular and skeletal components, and the weight loss is not sustained after termination of therapy. Furthermore, the large doses needed for weight reduction may suppress endogenous thyroid

---

[1] See also the note added in proof on p. 261.

Table 34. Adulteration of Asian herbal medicines with synthetic drug substances: chemical and clinical reports

Reference	Preparation(s)	Chemical and clinical details[a]
Ries and Sahud 1975 [232]	— Chuifong Toukuwan Nan Lien — Long Life Brand Ginseng Hui Sheng Tsaitsaowan — Sanlungpai Ginseng Hui Sheng Tsaitsaowan — Fonsuning Tongwan — Lilongpai Fonsuning — Hippo Brand secret Formula Chui Fung Eng (Nan Lien Pharm. Co., Taiwan and Hong Kong)	All 6 brands contained amino-phenazone and phenylbutazone. Three of the brands (with 23–43 mg and 17–34 mg, respectively) produced life-threatening agranulocytosis in 4 patients, when taken in doses of 8–12 pills/day. One patient died.
Brooks and Lowenthal 1977 [233]	— Chuifong Toukuwan (Hong Kong)	One patient developed agranul-ocytosis after starting treat-ment with 12 pills per day. Analysis of different batches showed varying amounts of amino-phenazone, phenylbutazone, and phenacetin.[b]
Uitdehaag et al. 1979 [234]	— Chuifong-Toukuwan (Hong Kong)	One patient developed Cushing's syndrome from 12 pills/day. The pills contained dexamethasone (0.112 mg), indomethacin (7.5 mg), hydrochlorothiazide, and diazepam (see next entry).
Anonymous 1979 [235]	— Chuifong Toukuwan (Nan Lien Pharm. Co., Hong Kong)	Dexamethasone 0.112 mg Indomethacin 7.3–8.3 mg Hydrochlorothiazide 4.1 mg Diazepam 0.45 mg (Dose: 12 pills/day)
	— Chuifong Toukuwan (Nan Lien Pharm. Co., Singapore)	Prednisolone 0.4 mg Hydrochlorothiazide 4.0 mg Chlordiazepoxide 0.5 mg Chlorpheniramine 1.3 mg[c] Thiaminedisulphide 5.0 mg (Dose: 12 pills/day)
	— Chuifong Toukuwan (Shou Sing Pharm. Co. Taiwan)	Aminophenazone 8 mg Phenylbutazone 0.6–6.0 mg Thiamine (Dose: 12 pills/day)
	— Chihshiton (Yi Chung Tai Med. Manuf. Co., Taiwan)	Paracetamol 8.1 mg Ethaverine 0.26 mg[d] Chlorzoxazone 2.0 mg Diazepam 0.55 mg Caffeine 1.9 mg Thiamine (Dose: 18 pills/day)

Table 34. (*Continued*)

Reference	Preparation(s)	Chemical and clinical details[a]
Forster et al. 1979 [236]	— Chuei-Fong-Tou-Geu-Wan	One patient developed a low plasma cortisol concentration and a cushingoid look.
Morice 1986 [237]	— Dumcap capsules (Duzcap Pharmacy, Pakistan)	Prednisolone 4 mg Betamethasone (Dose: 3 capsules/day)
Morice 1987 [238]	— Deecap capsules (Shaham Homeo Pharmacy, Pakistan)	Prednisolone
Steinigen 1987 [239]	— Amborum special-F syrup[e] (Sri Lal, United States)	Dexamethasone 0.02–0.2 mg/ml[f]
Bury et al. 1987 [240]	— Unmarked green capsules (Chinese herbalist, Kuala Lumpur) — #3 Colds and Flu — #6 Arthritis (Medical practitioner, Sri Lanka)	Phenylbutazone One patient gained weight and became moonfaced Powder #3 contained prednisolone (0.5 mg/g) and paracetamol (63 mg/g). Powder #6 contained similar amounts of both drugs as well as phenylbutazone (42 mg/g).
De Smet and Elferink 1987 [241]	— Chuifong Toukuwan (Nan Lien)	Indomethacin Hydrochlorothiazide Diazepam
Anonymous 1988 [242]	— Thong Yen Obat China (Lim Yik Kong)	Prednisolone
Anonymous 1988 [243]	— ASFO Natural Herbs Tea[g] (Sri Lal, Sri Lanka)	Betamethasone 0.1–0.5 mg/ml
Anonymous 1989 [211]	— Chuifong Tokuwan[h] (Nan Lien Pharm. Co., Hong Kong)	Dexamethasone Indomethacin Mefenamic acid Hydrochlorothiazide Diazepam[i]
Tay and Johnston 1989 [244]	— Nan Lien Chui Fong Toukuwan — Dr. Tong Shap Yee's asthma pills — Leung Pui Kee Cough (Hong Kong)	Diazepam 0.6 mg Theophylline 12 mg Bromhexine 0.7 mg
De Smet et al. 1990 [245]	— Cow's Head Brand Tung Shueh (Ta Ang Pharm. Co., Taiwan)	One patient developed a low plasma cortisol concentration. Each pill contained 0.09 mg dexamethasone (dose: 12 pills/day).

Table 34. (*Continued*)

Reference	Preparation(s)	Chemical and clinical details[a]
Yuen and Lau-Cam 1985 [246]	— Unspecified Chinese herbal preparations	Phenazone, propyphenazone, and methyltestosterone have also been identified as adulterants of Chinese herbal products.

[a] Unless stated otherwise, quantities refer to one pill or capsule.
[b] In addition to these synthetic compounds, the pills also contained mercuric sulfide.
[c] Calculated as the maleate.
[d] Calculated as the hydrochloride.
[e] Also labeled as Formula Nr. 9, Hautwaschmittel Cureall-6, Kayankal forte, Asforte, Herbal Tea Syrup, or Natural Herbs Tea syrup.
[f] Prednisolone and prednisone had been isolated from earlier samples.
[g] ASFO stands for Amborum Special Forte. This latter product had already been shown to be adulterated with corticosteroids, e.g., with dexamethasone 0.02–0.2 mg/ml [239].
[h] Repackaged and relabeled as The Miracle Herb – Mother Nature's Finest.
[i] In addition to synthetic drugs, the pills also contained lead and cadmium (see Table 31).

function and have potentially dangerous effects on the heart, such as tachyarrhythmias and cardiomegaly [255,256]

Consumer Information

Introduction

The preceding sections have amply reviewed the health risks that are associated with the adulteration and/or contamination of herbal remedies by toxic botanicals, micro-organisms and their toxins, radioactive isotopes, pesticides, fumigation agents, toxic metals, and nonherbal drug substances. There is more to the quality control of herbal remedies, however, than the classical approach to check the identity, quantity, and purity of herbal raw materials and their finished preparations. In modern medicine it is considered a must to provide each medicinal product with adequate consumer information. Such information is sometimes described as the software that is needed to make the hardware (i.e., the product itself) perform in the way it should. It has become generally recognized, for instance, that inappropriate drug taking and adverse drug reactions may be reduced if patients are properly informed [257–259]. In other words, assurance of the safety of a herbal drug requires not only that the quality of the herbal remedy itself is monitored, but also that the quality of the consumer information on that herbal remedy is assessed.

Table 35. Adulteration of Asian herbal medicines with synthetic drug substances: pharmacological classification

Pharmacological class	Substance	References
Analgesic and anti-inflammatory agents	Aminophenazone (= Aminopyrine)	[232,233,235]
	Indomethacin	[211,234,235,241]
	Mefenamic acid	[211]
	Paracetamol (= Acetaminophen)	[235,240]
	Phenacetin	[233]
	Phenazone (= Antipyrine)	[246]
	Phenylbutazone	[232,233,235,240]
	Propyphenazone (= Isopropyl-antipyrine)	[246]
Antihistamines	Chlorpheniramine	[235]
Corticosteroids	Betamethasone	[211,237,243]
	Dexamethasone	[234,235,239,245]
	Prednisolone	[235,237–240,242]
	Prednisone	[239]
Diuretics	Hydrochlorothiazide	[211,234,235,241]
Mucolytic cough agents	Bromhexine	[244]
Muscle relaxants	Chlorzoxazone	[235]
Sex hormones	Methyltestosterone	[246]
Smooth muscle relaxants	Ethaverine	[235]
Tranquillizers	Chlordiazepoxide	[235]
	Diazepam	[211,234,235,241,244]
Vitamins	Thiamine (= Vitamin B_1)	[235]
Xanthines	Caffeine	[235]
	Theophylline	[244]

Special Considerations

There are two special aspects of botanical remedies that make the availability of objective and reliable consumer information all the more essential for this particular category of medicines. The first one is that in most if not all countries the majority of herbal preparations has a nonprescription status (e.g., [26,34,44,,260–262]). It is obvious that stringent demands are to be made on the product information of a herbal remedy when it can be purchased by members of the public on their own initiative and without the intervention of an orthodox health care provider. The second important aspect of botanical remedies is that the health authorities in certain countries do not permit any labeling claim of therapeutic utility of a traditional herbal medicine unless there is conclusive evidence that the product is both efficacious and safe. This does not prevent herbal drug sellers, however, from marketing herbal medicines under the guise of food supplements or nutritional products. To prevent seizure of these goods, no claim of effectiveness in any medical condition appears in or on the package of such products [34,44]. This lack of therapeutic detail is compensated by making available to the buyer a variety of promotional pamphlets and booklets that are sold side-by-side with the products but do not qualify legally as part of the labeling, as they do not directly accompany the products. Unfortunately, such sources are all too often written for the mere purpose of selling products. They tend to advocate all the allegedly favorable features of botanical drugs, even if this entails the reiteration of outdated information, while the potential dangers are minimized, intentionally or out of ignorance [263]. Needless to say, it is vital to counterbalance this assortment of uncritical writings by providing the user with scientifically accurate product information.

The following example may serve to illustrate how relevant it is to have appropriate consumer information on botanical remedies. Kelp preparations are widely advocated as harmless antiobesity agents. The underlying belief is that the iodine in the kelp stimulates the production of iodine-containing thyroid hormones which are known to affect metabolic processes. There is no evidence, however, that overweight consumers without iodine deficiency actually benefit from this supposed mechanism [44,264,265]. Weight loss has been observed in some kelp users, but in these particular cases the weight reduction was a sign that thyrotoxicosis had developed (see Table 36). This iatrogenic condition is associated with well-known cardiac risks and should therefore be avoided [255]. In other words, instead of ignoring this risk or reinforcing antiobesity claims, the labeling of a kelp product should advise the user to consult a physician or to discontinue the medication in the not-so-likely event that weight loss develops together with other symptoms of hyperthyroidism (see Table 36).

Basic Requirements

The general rule that written drug information for consumers should always be presented at a level which is comprehensible to them is of special importance in the cgse of botanical remedies, as most of these medicines are nonprescription products. This means that the information provided must be devoid, as much as possible, of scientific and medical terminology [259].

With respect to the contents of herbal product information, a useful outline can be derived from two recent booklets of the European Proprietary Medicines Manufacturer's Association (EPMMA). In these booklets, the following details about identity, origin, storage, purposes, directions for use, dosage, warnings, and precautions are listed as essential elements of product information on nonprescription medicines [270,271]:

— Name of the product
— Name and quantity of the active ingredient(s) in the product
— Net weight, fluid measure, or number of contents of the package

Table 36. Case reports of hyperthyroidism in users of kelp products

Reference	Details
Liewendahl and Gordin 1974 [266]	— A 38-year-old female with a family history of toxic goiter developed nervousness, insomnia, fatigue, increased sweating, tremor of the hands, and goiter after the regular ingestion of 4 seaweed tablets a day (estimated daily intake of 1–2 mg iodine) for a period of over 2 years.
Skare and Frey 1980 [267]	— A 52-year-old male with a family history of goiter had a pulse rate of 100/min, weight loss, fine finger tremor, and lid lag without goiter after the daily consumption of one spoonful of dried kelp powder (approximately 10 mg iodine according to the producer) for about 1 year. — A 36-year-old male with a family history of hypothyroidism showed weight loss, fine finger tremor, and lid lag without goiter after the sporadic use of dried kelp (partly as an admixture to bread dough) for some years.
Shilo and Hirsch 1986 [268]	— A 72-year-old female without a family history of thyroid disease presented with weight loss, excess sweating, fatigue, several soft stools a day, and goiter. During the previous year she had been taking 4–6 kelp tablets (each tablet containing 0.7 mg iodine) per day.
De Smet et al. 1990 [269]	— A 50-year-old female without a family history of thyroid disease presented with a tense feeling, palpitations, insomnia, heat intolerance, weight loss, nervousness, and heavy perspiration without goiter after the daily use of 6 kelp tablets (200 mg of kelp each) for 2 months.

— Name and address of the person responsible for putting the product on the market
— Marketing authorization number and batch number
— Information about proper storage (including storing medicines safely away from children) and expiry date
— Purposes for which the product is intended to be used
— Directions for use explaining how the product is to be taken or applied
— How much to use (including separate instructions, if appropriate, for adults and children, and a general reminder to take no more than the recommended dosage on the label)
— Instructions on how to use the product correctly and safely (including advice about those occasions when the use of the medicine may be inappropriate, e.g., during pregnancy, and a reminder to see a doctor if symptoms continue for longer than usual)

These EPPMA requirements are relevant not only for synthetic medicines for self-medication but also for botanical remedies. This becomes particularly evident when they are compared to some of the orthodox concerns about herbal therapies that have been identified (on basis of case histories and the like) in recent volumes of the *Side Effects of Drugs Annuals* (see Table 37).

Table 37. Some of the arguments that underlie current orthodox concern about the safety of botanical medicines [27,32,36,37]

Argument	Examples
The identity of the herbal ingredients should not be kept secret.	— Sellers of herbal remedies may refuse to reveal the exact composition of their tea mixtures [26]. Such a reluctant attitude deprives customers with a history of sensitivity reactions of the possibility to recognize a sensitizing ingredient in time.
	— Inadequate labeling also interferes with the proper evaluation and recording of adverse effects. For instance, a recent report about allergic contact dermatitis due to the topical use of a Chinese herbal drug named Yunnan Paiyao complained that the identity of the allergen(s) remained obscure since the nature of the ingredients was not specified by the supplier of the product [272].
More attention should be paid to instability problems and to storage conditions.	— An analysis of Norwegian kelp tablets revealed that tablets taken from the bottom of a fresh packet contained 1250 μg iodine a piece whereas tablets taken from the surface layer only contained 115 μg. The tablets yielded no iodine at all after they had been stored in the laboratory for 1.5 years [273]. Unfortunately, the paper did not specify under which storage conditions the latter result was obtained.
	— Herbs valued for their essential oil should not be kept in containers made from polyethylene, polypropylene, or polyvinyl chloride since essential oils are rapidly absorbed by these materials [42].
	— A 10-year-old girl was poisoned by her elder sister who had prepared a herbal cough tea from *Datura* leaves which she had found in the kitchen cupboard while the parents were away [274].
Undeclared ingredients can lead to unforeseen reactions.	— Adulteration or contamination of oriental products with toxic metals and synthetic drug substances is reviewed elsewhere in this chapter (see Tables 31 and 34). The presence of a marketing authorization number might help attentive consumers to distinguish between officially approved products and untested imported preparations.
Consumers must receive clear directions for use.	— Users of herbal bulk-forming laxatives should be clearly instructed to take their products with sufficient water immediately with the preparation [275,276] and without exceeding the recommended dose [277] to avoid the risk of serious esophageal obstruction.
	— The microbiological need to consume cold macerates within a few hours after their preparation is discussed in the section on micro-organisms.
Ineffective herbal healing can produce serious sequelae when it replaces essential orthodox therapy.	— In self-limiting diseases, the recommendation of a herbal remedy with unproven efficacy may remain without serious consequences. However, when it comes to disorders that need adequate drug treatment to prevent life-threatening complications (e.g., epilepsy), it may be quite dangerous to claim that an

Table 37. (*Continued*)

Argument	Examples
	unproven botanical cure is effective. This is particularly hazardous when the herbal agent is regarded as a substitute for orthodox drug therapy. A recent questionnaire study among Dutch general practitioners revealed that several patients had stopped their orthodox medication on the advice of an alternative healer. In one particular case, a 40-year-old woman with a suspected mammary carcinoma was given alternative treatment without informing her family doctor. When the patient finally came to her family doctor after 1 year of alternative therapy, her carcinoma turned out to be inoperable [278].
More information is needed on pediatric dosage requirements.	— A recent analysis of inquiries received by the Welsh Drug Information Centre (which has specialized in information on alternative medicines) has made clear that there is a substantial need for information on the pediatric dosing of herbal remedies [279].
Overconsumption by uninformed users can substantially increase the health risks of herbal drugs.	— The ingestion of large doses of pennyroyal oil for the induction of abortion has been associated with serious hepatotoxicity [280] and fatal poisoning [281]. — A fairly recent Australian case report describes coma and persistent neuropathy after an overdose of herbal laxative tablets containing podophyllin [282].
While herbal healers and consumers may readily recognize gross symptoms of acute toxicity, such as skin reactions, they are likely to oversee more subtle effects, such as hepatotoxicity, teratogenicity, and carcinogenicity.	— Herbal preparations containing low levels or trace amounts of pyrrolizidine alkaloids can produce veno-occlusive liver disease when taken for a prolonged period [13,54,283,284]. Their regular consumption during pregnancy can also affect the liver of the unborn child [36,285,286]. — The aristolochic acids occurring in *Aristolochia* species [287] have mutagenic properties [288], and they are strongly carcinogenic in rodents [289,290]. A distressing detail is that their carcinogenicity was discovered some years ago by accident in a study that was not intended or designed to demonstrate such activity [291]. Since aristocholic acids may pass into mother's milk [292], they may also endanger the breast-fed infant.
The possibility of drug interactions between herbal remedies and orthodox medicines should more often be taken into account.	— The oriental herbal drug karela (*Momordica charantia*) has hypoglycemic properties [293,294] and can thus potentiate conventional antidiabetic therapy [295]. — Guar gum (a bulk-forming fiber advocated as an antidiabetic medicine and slimming aid) was shown to decrease both the peak concentration of phenoxymethylpenicillin and its area under the serum curve by about 25% when taken together with the antibiotic [296]. Another bulk-forming fibrous slimming aid, glucomannan, was reported to reduce the plasma levels of glibenclamide [297].

Examples

A noteworthy compilation of consumer-friendly drug information texts is the second volume of the annually appearing *USP Dispensing Information* [298]. Although most texts are devoted to synthetic drugs and would be considered by some as being too long for unabridged use as a package insert, they are an inspiring source on how to write herbal product information in lay language. One of the few texts in this book which deals with a botanical drug is shown here in Table 38.

Readers familiar with the German language should consult the monographs of the so-called Kommission E, which is the Federal Committee for Phytotherapy in Germany [299]. This committee has been established for the particular purpose of submitting herbal remedies to a benefit/risk evaluation. The result of each evaluation is reported in a monograph which serves as a scientific touchstone when a marketing license is sought for a new botanical medicine, or when the license of an already existing product must be renewed. When the committee reaches a positive decision, the monograph provides concise information about denomination, constituents, uses, contraindications, side effects, drug interactions, dosage, directions for use, and actions (see Table 39 for an example). In the case of a negative judgement, the monograph explains why the risks are considered to outweigh the potential benefits of the herb.

Another useful source on herbal product information is the German collection of so-called *Standardzulassungen* [300], for which another federal committee is responsible. These *Standardzulassungen* specify under what standardized con-

Table 38. Consumer-oriented drug information on oral ipecac in the second volume of the *USP Dispensing Information*[a]

Ipecac (IP-e-kak) is used in the emergency treatment of certain kinds of poisoning. Only the syrup form of ipecac should be used. It is used to cause vomiting of the poison.

A bottle of ipecac labeled as being Ipecac Fluidextract or Ipecac Tincture should not be used. These dosage forms are too strong and may cause serious side effects or death. Only ipecac syrup contains the proper strength of ipecac for treating poisonings.

Ordinarily, this medicine should not be used if strychnine, corrosives such as alkalies (lye) and strong acids, or petroleum distillates such as kerosene, gasoline, coal oil, fuel oil, paint thinner, or cleaning fluid have been swallowed since it may cause seizures, additional injury to the throat, or pneumonia.

Ipecac should not be used to cause vomiting as a means of losing weight. If used regularly for this purpose, serious heart problems or even death may occur.

This medicine in amounts of more than 1 ounce is available only with your doctor's prescription. It is available in ½- and 1-ounce bottles without a prescription. However, before using ipecac syrup, call your doctor, a poison control center, or an emergency room for advice.

Remember:
- *Keep all medicines out of the reach of children.*
- In order for this medicine to work, it must be used as directed. *If you are using this medicine without a prescription, it is very important to follow the directions on the label.*
- *If you have any questions* about the following information or if you want more information about this medicine or your medical problem, *ask your doctor, nurse, or pharmacist.*

Table 38. (*Continued*)

Before Using This Medicine

Before using this medicine to cause vomiting in poisoning, call your doctor, a poison control center, or an emergency room for advice. It is a good idea to have these telephone numbers readily available. Be sure to tell them:

— if you are *pregnant.* Studies with ipecac have not been done in either humans or animals.

— if you have heart disease. There is an increased risk of heart problems such as unusually fast heartbeat if the ipecac is not vomited.

— if this medicine is to be given to a *child.* Infants and very young children are at a greater risk of choking with their own vomit (or getting vomit in their lungs). Therefore, it is especially important to call a doctor, a poison control center, or an emergency room for instructions before giving ipecac.

— if this medicine is to be taken by a person *65 years of age or older.* This medicine has been tested and has not been shown to cause different side effects or problems in older people than it does in younger adults.

Proper Use of This Medicine

It is very important that you take this medicine only as directed. Do not take more of it and do not take it more often than recommended on the label, unless otherwise directed. When too much ipecac is used, it can cause damage to the heart and other muscles, and may even cause death.

Do not give this medicine to unconscious or very drowsy persons, since the vomited material may enter the lungs and cause pneumonia.

To help this medicine cause vomiting of the poison, adults should drink 1 full glass (8 ounces) of water, and children should drink ½ to 1 full glass (4 to 8 ounces) of water immediately after taking this medicine. Water may be given first in the case of a small or scared child.

Do not take this medicine with milk, milk products, or with carbonated beverages. Milk or milk products may prevent this medicine from working properly, and carbonated beverages may cause swelling of the stomach.

If vomiting does not occur within 20 minutes after you have taken the first dose of this medicine, take a second dose. If vomiting does not occur after you have taken the second dose, you must immediately see your doctor or go to an emergency room.

If you have been told to take both this medicine activated charcoal to treat the poisoning, *do not take the activated charcoal until after you have taken this medicine to cause vomiting.*

To store this medicine:

● *Keep out of the reach of children* since overdose is very dangerous in children.

● Store away from heat and direct light.

● Keep the syrup from freezing.

● Do not keep outdated medicine or medicine no longer needed. Be sure that any discarded medicine is out of the reach of children.

● Do not keep a bottle of ipecac that has been opened. Ipecac may evaporate over a period of time. It is best to replace it with a new one.

Side Effects of This Medicine

Along with its needed effects, a medicine may cause some unwanted effects. Although side effects usually do not occur with recommended doses of ipecac, if they do occur they may need medical attention.

Check with your doctor as soon as possible if any of the following side effects occur:

Symptoms of overdose (may also occur if ipecac is taken regularly)

Diarrhea

Nausea or vomiting (continuing more than 30 minutes)

Stomach cramps or pain

Troubled breathing

Unusual tiredness or weakness

Unusually fast or irregular heartbeat

Weakness, aching, and stiffness of muscles, especially those of the neck, arms, and legs

Other side effects not listed above may also occur in some patients. If you notice any other effects, check with your doctor.

ᵃCopyright, The USP Convention, Inc. Permission granted for copying from the USP DI Volume II, 10th edition [298]

Table 39. Extract of the monograph on gentian root issued by the so-called Kommission E, the Federal Committee for Phytotherapy in Germany [299]

Uses
 Digestive complaints, such as lack of appetite, feeling of fullness, flatulence.

Contraindications
 Gastric and duodenal ulcers.

Side effects
 Headaches may occasionally occur in predisposed individuals.

Interactions with other agents
 None known.

Dosage
 Unless prescribed otherwise: average single dose: 1 g drug; average daily dose: 3 g drug.
 Preparations corresponding to their bitter value.

Mode of administration
 Small-cut drug and dry extracts for infusions, bitter tasting dosage forms for oral use.

Actions
 The essential active substances are the bitter principles in the drug. They lead to a reflectory stimulation of salivary and gastric secretion through stimulation of the taste receptors.
 Gentian root is therefore considered not only an amarum (purum), but also a roborans and tonic.
 There is evidence from animal experiments that the amount of bronchial secretion may be increased.

ditions certain finished products (herbal as well as nonherbal) are admissible to the German drug market without the submission of a full registration dossier to the health authorities. One of the conditions is that the product be provided with the package insert text that is given by the *Standardzulassung*. An example of a text on a herbal drug is given in Table 40.

Many Kommission E monographs and package inserts of the *Standardzulassungen* have been reproduced in the recently updated textbook *Teedrogen* [42].

General Cautionary Leaflet

The Royal Dutch Association for the Advancement of Pharmacy recently decided to develop a general leaflet on the safe use of botanical remedies because of the following arguments [1]:

— The Dutch health authorities do not adequately monitor the quality of the product information on herbal medicines.
— When a herbal product is known to have serious toxicity in its normal dose range, the product should be banned from the market, regardless of the quality of its product information. In other words, efforts to improve consumer information on individual herbal products tend to increase the safety of the most innocuous part of the herbal drug market.

Table 40. Package insert text for Chinchona bark in the German *Standardzulassungen* [300]

Uses
   For gastric complaints, e.g., due to deficient production of digestive juices; as appetite stimulant.

Contraindications
   Pregnancy, hypersensitivity to quinine, gastric or intestinal ulcers.

Side effects
   Ingestion of quinine containing medicines may occasionally lead to hypersensitivity reactions, such as skin allergies or fever. An increased bleeding tendency may be observed in rare cases due to a reduced number of thrombocytes (thrombocytopenia). In these cases a physician should be consulted without delay. Warning: overdosage or prolonged application of quinine containing medicines may lead to nausea, vomiting, and diarrhea, and also to auditory and visual disturbances.

Dosage and mode of administration
   About ½ a teaspoonful (0.5–1 g) of Chinchona bark is covered with boiling water (about 150 ml) and poured through a tea strainer 10 min later.
   Unless prescribed otherwise, a cup of freshly prepared infusion is taken more than once per day 0.5 h before the meal.

Direction
   Protect from light and moisture during storage.

The leaflet provides a series of cautionary notes which are largely based on the orthodox concerns about herbal therapies that have been listed in Table 37. It is not meant to hearten those readers who already have a critical attitude toward herbal remedies but to educate uninformed and credulous users of botanical medicines about the potential health risks of such products. To reach this particular audience, the leaflet deliberately speaks about phytotherapy in a sympathetic tone (see Table 41).

Table 41. Text of a Dutch cautionary leaflet on the safe use of botanical remedies [1]

The Safe Use of Herbal Remedies
Back to Nature
A lot of our medicines today are chemically prepared, unlike in the past when this was quite different. In the old days, all drugs originated from nature. Pills, powders, potions, and ointments were prepared from medicinal plants; a variety of loose-leaf herbs were used to prepare teas. All of these botanical drugs are known as "herbal remedies." With the advent and advancement of chemically prepared drugs, the use of herbal remedies decreased substantially, but nowadays botanical drugs have become "fashionable" once again. Many people today favor natural products.

Difference with homeopathic medicines
Herbal remedies are often confused with homeopathic medicines, yet there are major differences in use and preparation. Herbal remedies can be used in precisely the same way as chemically prepared drugs. Their action is always opposed to the disease or complaint, e.g., a laxative herb is used against constipation. In homeopathy, however, a laxative herb is used to treat diarrhea ("like cures like"). To give the herb a homeopathic action, it must be diluted first in a special way ("potentization"). This dilution results in a homeopathic medicine with properties different from those of the herb itself. A herbal remedy is not diluted in a homeopathic way and therefore retains the action (and any adverse effects) of the original herb.

There are two different kinds of herbal remedies: (a) strongly acting herbal remedies. These have strong reactions in quite small amounts. They are to be dispensed only and exclusively on prescription. (b) Mildly acting herbal remedies. These are available without prescription from pharmacies and health food stores. Follow the safety tips given in this leaflet, and such mildly acting remedies may be used for self-medication without difficulty.

Safety Tips
Buy herbal remedies from reliable and trusted sources. Never bring herbal remedies from far-away countries. Never order them by mail from abroad because you will have no guarantee whatever that you are buying a safe product. The purity of herbal remedies is not carefully controlled everywhere in the world. Moreover, you should buy herbal remedies only from outlets where you may go back if necessary.

Purchase a herbal remedy only if the package clearly states which herb(s) it contains. Do not trust herbal remedies in which the composition is kept secret. Check before you buy anything that the package states which herbal ingredients have been used to prepare the product. When it is a "ready-to-use" medicine, you should also be able to see who prepared the agent (the manufacturer).

Always ask for the exact directions for use. You are entitled to proper and correct directions for use, informing you of how often you may take the remedy, and how much you should take per dose. In the case of a herbal tea, you should also be informed about the proper method of preparation, e.g., how much herb and (boiling) water you should use and how long the tea should be left to "draw". Buy your products only where this information is given.

Do not collect herbs in the wild, unless you are well able to distinguish poisonous and innocuous herbs from one another. Just as with wild mushrooms and toadstools, poisonous and nonpoisonous herbs can look very much alike. A mistake might be fatal!

Store herbal remedies with care. Herbal remedies should be stored carefully, in exactly the same way as other drugs, i.e., in a cool, dry environment, which is safe from children's hands. A "ready-to-use" product can best be stored in the package in which you have bought it. For the storage of a loose-leaf tea, a tightly closed tin is suitable. A plastic container is not suitable for the storage of herbs, particularly when they are strong-smelling herbs, because plastic may absorb the volatile oil of these herbs.

Do not use herbal remedies which you have kept for years. Every herbal remedy purchased should give an indication (on its packaging) of how long it may be kept. Many loose-leaf herbs begin to loose their activity when you keep them for more than one year. "Ready-to-use" herbal remedies are not infinitely storable either. Your pharmacist can give you advice if you are unsure whether a herbal remedy is still active after a long storage period.

Do not use herbal remedies for serious illnesses. Mildly acting herbal remedies are not meant for serious diseases, such as diabetes, hypertension, or epilepsy. If you suffer from such a serious condition, you should consult your physician and

Table 41. (*Continued*)

not try to "play doctor" yourself, because there is a high element of risk. You should also not depend on mildly acting herbs in the case of cancer.

Stop using a herbal remedy if you start experiencing side effects. Some people have the idea that drugs from a chemical factory can be damaging whereas natural products can not. They also think that herbal medicines cannot have adverse effects, but this is not the case. Herbal remedies can also have side effects, such as skin eruptions or stomach ache. If such a complaint occurs, you should stop using the herbal remedy to enable the side effects to clear.

Do not exceed the dose range stated in the directions for use. All too often, one is inclined to think that if a small amount of natural product is doing good, a larger dose would be even better. However, a herbal remedy will not be better for you if you take it upon yourself to exceed the stated dose. Quite the contrary: there are herbs which have serious consequences if you consume too large quantities. Therefore, always take herbal remedies according to the directions for use (as with any medicine). If the remedy is not helping your ailment, it is far better to stop the treatment than to raise the dosage yourself.

Do not use herbal remedies for prolonged periods. Mildly acting herbal remedies are innocuous if used in the recommended dosage for short periods. Unfortunately, we do not yet know whether all remedies are safe to consume over a continuous period of months or years. Therefore, it is always better to err on the side of caution and refrain from taking a herbal remedy for an extended period unless you have previously sought the advice of your physician or pharmacist.

If you are pregnant or breast feeding and want to use a herbal remedy, do this only after consulting your physician or pharmacist. Certain herbal remedies should definitely not be used during pregnancy. There is also a large group of herbal remedies which cannot be entirely guaranteed to be without effect on your unborn child. Always, therefore, consult your physician or pharmacist if you are pregnant and wish to use a particular herbal remedy. Also, if you are breast feeding, it is best to ask for expert advice first.

Your physician or pharmacist must always be informed if you are using a herbal remedy simultaneously with other medicines. It is vital that this information is available, as it is a known fact that certain herbal remedies can affect (either by increasing or decreasing) the action of other medicines.

Points to Remember, in Brief

- Buy herbal remedies from reliable and trusted sources.
- Purchase a herbal remedy only if the package clearly states which herb(s) it contains.
- Always ask for the exact directions for use.
- Do not collect herbs in the wild unless you are well able to distinguish poisonous and innocuous herbs from one another.
- Store herbal remedies with care.
- Do not use herbal remedies which you have kept for years.
- Do not use herbal remedies for serious illnesses.
- Stop using a herbal remedy if you start experiencing side effects.
- Do not exceed the dose range stated in the directions for use.
- Do not use herbal remedies for prolonged periods.
- If you are pregnant or breast feeding and want to use a herbal remedy, do this only after consulting your physician or pharmacist.
- Your physician or pharmacist must always be informed if you are using a herbal remedy simultaneously with other medicines.

References

1. De Smet PAGM (1989) Dutch patient information on the safe use of herbal remedies. Int Pharm J 3:98–101
2. Lewin L (1962) Gifte und Vergiftungen. Lehrbuch der Toxikologie. Fünfte unveränderte Ausgabe. Ulm/Donau: Karl F. Haug Verlag
3. Kingsbury JM (1964) Poisonous plants of the United States and Canada. Englewood Cliffs: Prentice-Hall
4. Gessner O, Orzechowski G (1974) Gift- und Arzneipflanzen von Mitteleuropa, 3rd edn. Heidelberg: Carl Winter Universitätsverlag
5. Der Marderosian A, Liberti LE (1988) Natural product medicine. A scientific guide to foods, drugs, cosmetics. Philadelphia: George F. Stickley Company
6. Cheeke PR, Shull LR (1985) Natural toxicants in feeds and poisonous plants. Westport: AVI Publishing Company
7. Wirth W, Gloxhuber C (1985) Toxikologie für Ärzte, Naturwissenschaftler und Apotheker. 4th edn. Stuttgart: Georg Thieme Verlag
8. Lampe KF, McCann MA (1985) AMA Handbook of Poisonous and Injurious Plants. Chicago: American Medical Association
9. Moeschlin S (1986) Klinik und Therapie der Vergiftungen. 7th edn. Stuttgart: Georg Thieme Verlag
10. Frohne D, Pfänder HJ (1987) Giftpflanzen. 3rd edn. Stuttgart: Wissenschaftliche Verlagsgesellschaft
11. Dreisbach RH, Robertson WO (1987) Handbook of Poisoning. 12th edn. Norwalk: Appleton & Lange
12. Teuscher E, Lindequist U (1988) Biogene Gifte. Biologie – Chemie – Pharmakologie. Berlin: Akademie-Verlag
13. Weston CFM, Cooper BT, Davies JD, Levine DF (1987) Veno-occlusive disease of the liver secondary to ingestion of comfrey. Br Med J 295:183
14. Lewis WH (1978) Reporting adverse reactions to herbal ingestants. JAMA 240:109–110
15. Anonymous (1979) Toxic reactions to plant products sold in health food stores. Med Lett Drugs Ther 21:29
16. Spoerke DG (1980) Herbal medication: use and misuse. Hosp Form 15:941–951
17. Röder E (1982) Nebenwirkungen von Heilpflanzen. Dtsch Apot Ztg 122:2081–2092
18. Larkin T (1983) Herbs are often more toxic than magical. FDA Consumer 17 (October):5–10
19. Penn RG (1983) Adverse reactions to herbal medicines. Adv Drug React Bull no 102:376–379
20. Eichler I (1984) Probleme und potentielle Gefahren der Phytotherapie. Österreich Ärzteztg 39:869–875
21. Fossati C, Fanzio G (1985) Effetti tossici da piante medicinali. Clin Ter 112:249–259
22. Penn RG (1986) Adverse reactions to herbal and other unorthodox medicines. In: D'Arcy PF, Griffin JP (eds) Iatrogenic diseases. 3rd edn. Oxford: Oxford University Press, pp 898–918
23. Anderson LA, Phillipson JD (1986) Herbal medicine, education and the pharmacist. Pharm J 236:303–311
24. Boyd EL, Tjolsen E (1986) Herbal teas and remedies: are they safe? J Pharm Technol 2:153–159
25. Anonymous (1986) Herbal medicines – safe and effective? Drug Ther Bull 24:97–100
26. De Smet PAGM (1987) Kruidenmiddelen en volksgezondheid. Pharm Weekbl 122:1069–1071
27. De Smet PAGM, Vulto AG (1987) Drugs used in non-orthodox medicine. In: Dukes MNG (ed) Side Effects of Drugs – Annual 11. Amsterdam: Elsevier, pp 422–431
28. Anonymous (1987) Hoffnung auf Kräutermittel? Anspruch und Wirklichkeit im Abgleich. Arznei-telegram no 3:26–29
29. Corrigan D (1987) Phytotherapy. Int Pharm J 1:96–101
30. Ridker PM (1987) Toxic effects of herbal teas. Arch Environ Health 42:133–136
31. Vulto AG, De Smet PAGM (1988) Drugs used in non-orthodox medicine. In: Dukes MNG (ed) Meyler's side effects of drugs. 11th edn. Amsterdam: Elsevier, pp 999–1032
32. De Smet PAGM, Vulto AG (1988) Drugs used in non-orthodox medicine. In: Dukes MNG, Beeley L (eds) Side effects of drugs – Annual 12. Amsterdam: Elsevier, pp 402–415
33. Thesen R (1988) Phytotherapeutika – nicht immer harmlos. Pharm Ztg 133:38–43

34. Chandler RF (1988) Herbal medicines. In: Krogh C, Clarke C, Ebbs HL, Shaughnessy C, Welbanks L (eds) Self-medication. A reference for health professionals. Ottawa: Canadian Pharmaceutical Association, pp 517–532
35. Moulds RFW, McNeil JJ (1988) Herbal preparations – to regulate or not to regulate? Med J Aust 149:572–574
36. De Smet PAGM (1989) Drugs used in non-orthodox medicine. In: Dukes MNG, Beeley L (eds) Side effects of drugs – Annual 13. Amsterdam: Elsevier, pp 442–473
37. De Smet PAGM (1990) Drugs used in non-orthodox medicine. In: Dukes MNG, Beeley L (eds) Side effects of drugs – Annual 14. Amsterdam: Elsevier pp 429–451
38. De Smet PAGM (1991) Is there any danger in using traditional remedies? J Ethnopharmacol, 32:43–50
39. Anonymous (1989) Quality of herbal remedies. In: The rules governing medicinal products in the European Community, vol III. Guidelines on the quality, safety and efficacy of medicinal products for human use. Luxembourg: Office for Official Publications of the European Communities, pp 31–37
40. Anonymous (1976) Mikrobiologische Reinheit von Arzneimitteln, die nicht steril sein müssen. Prüfmethoden. Pharm Acta Helv 51:41–49
41. Schilcher H (1985) Rückstandsanalytik bei Drogen und Drogenzubereitungen. Fresenius Z Analyt Chem 321:342–351
42. Wichtl M (ed) Teedrogen (1988) Ein Handbuch für die Praxis auf wissenschaftlicher Grundlage, 2nd edn. Stuttgart: Wissenschaftliche Verlagsgesellschaft
43. Ulmann RM (1985) Wie wiedt er in de kruidenhof? Pharm Weekbl 120:482–483
44. Tyler VE (1987) The new honest herbal. A sensible guide to herbs and related remedies. 2nd edn. Philadelphia: George F. Stickley Company
45. Bauer R, Khan IA, Wagner H (1987) Echinacea. Nachweis einer Verfälschung von Echinacea purpurea (L.) Moench mit Parthenium integrifolium L. Dtsch Apoth Ztg 127:1325–1330
46. Siegel RK (1977) Kola, ginseng and mislabeled herbs. JAMA 237:25
47. Hoppe HA (1975) Drogenkunde, vol 1. Angiospermen, 8th edn. Berlin: Walter de Gruyter
48. Anonymous (1977) Poisoning associated with herbal teas – Arizona, Washington. MMWR 26:257–258
49. Stillman AE, Huxtable R, Consroe P, Kohnen P, Smith S (1977) Hepatic veno-occlusive disease due to pyrrolizidine (Senecio) poisoning in Arizona. Gastroenterology 73:349–352
50. Fox DW, Hart MC, Bergeson PS, Jarrett PB, Stillman AE, Huxtable RJ (1978) Pyrrolizidine (Senecio) intoxication mimicking Reye syndrome. J Pediatr 93:980–982
51. Huxtable RJ (1980) Herbal teas and toxins: novel aspects of pyrrolizidine poisoning in the United States. Perspect Biol Med 24:1–14
52. Schier W, Schultze W (1987) Aktuelle Verfälschungen bei Arzneidrogen. Dtsch Apoth Ztg 127:2717–2721
53. Zänglein A, Schultze W, Kubeczka K-H (1989) Steranis und Shikimi. Zur Unterscheidung der Früchte von Illicium verum Hook.f. und Illicium anisatum L. I. Morphologisch-anatomische Unterscheidungsmerkmale. Dtsch Apoth Ztg 129:2819–2829
54. McGee JO'D, Patrick RS, Wood CB, Blumgart LH (1976) A case of veno-occulusive disease of the liver in Britain associated with herbal tea consumption. J Clin Pathol 29:788–794
55. Hegnauer R (1964) Chemotaxonomie der Pflanzen, vol 3. Dicotyledoneae: Acanthaceae – Cyrillaceae. Basel: Birkhäuser Verlag
56. Anonymous (1988) Pyrrolizidine Alkaloids. Environmental Health Criteria 80. Geneva: World Health Organization
57. Bryson PD, Watanabe AS, Rumack BH, Murphy RC (1978) Burdock root tea poisoning. Case report involving a commercial preparation. JAMA 239:2157
58. Bryson PD (1978) Burdock root tea poisoning. JAMA 240:1586
59. Anonymous (1984) Belladonna-haltige Klettenwurzeltees in Frankreich. Dtsch Apoth Ztg 124:390
60. Rhoads PM, Tong TG, Banner Jr W, Anderson R (1984–85) Anticholinergic poisonings associated with commercial burdock root tea. Clin Toxicol 22:581–584
61. Scholz H, Kascha S, Zingerle H, Atropin-Vergiftung durch "Gesundheitstee". Fortschr Med 98:1525–1526
62. Anonymous (1983) Poisoned comfrey tea warning. Pharm J 230:173

64   Peter A.G.M. De Smet

63. Galizia EJ (1983) Clinical curio: hallucinations in elderly tea drinkers. Br Med J 287:979
64. Routledge PA, Spriggs TLB (1989) Atropine as possible contaminant of comfrey tea. Lancet 1:963–964
65. Awang DVC, Kindack DG (1989) Atropine as possible contaminant of comfrey tea. Lancet 2:44
66. Wagner H, Bladt S, Zgainski EM (1983) Drogenanalyse. Berlin: Springer Verlag
67. Kubeczka K-H, Bohn I, Radix Pimpinellae und ihre aktuellen Verfälschungen. Dtsch Apoth Ztg 125:399–402
68. Berghöfer R, Hölzl J (1986) Johanniskraut (Hypericum perforatum L.). Prüfung auf Verfälschung. Dtsch Apoth Ztg 126:2569–2573
69. Veit M, Czygan F-C, Frank B, Hofmann D, Worlicek B (1989) Schachtelhalmkraut. Reinheits- und Identitätsuntersuchungen mit Hilfe der HPLC. Dtsch Apoth Ztg 129:1591–1598
70. Schier W, Sachsa B, Schultze W (1989) Aktuelle Verfälschungen von Arzneidrogen. Sennes- blätter und Hohlzahnkraut. Dtsch Apoth Ztg 129:1193–1197
71. Schier W, Sachsa B, Schultze W (1989) Aktuelle Verfälschungen von Arzneidrogen. Baldrian- wurzel, Enzianwurzel und Nieswurzelstock. Dtsch Apoth Ztg 129:1540–1542
72. Schier W, Sachsa B, Schultze W (1990) Aktuelle Verfälschungen von Arzneidrogen. Bären- traubblätter und Sauerampferkraut. Dtsch Apoth Ztg 130:463–465
73. Liberti LE, Der Marderosian A (1978) Evaluation of commercial ginseng products. J Pharm Sci 67:1487–1489
74. Reynolds JEF, Parfitt K, Parsons AV, Sweetman SC (eds) (1989) Martindale The Extra Phar- macopoeia. 29th edn. London: The Pharmaceutical Press
75. Senff H, Kuhlwein A, Kalveram KJ, Hausen BM (1989) Asthma bronchiale durch Inhalation mit Echter Kamille (Chamomilla recutita [L.] Rauschert). Allergologie 12:51–53
76. Hausen BM, Busker E, Carle R (1984) Über das Sensibilierungsvermögen von Compositenarten. VII. Experimentelle Untersuchungen mit Auszügen und Inhaltsstoffen von Chamomilla recutita (L.) Rauschert und Anthemis cotula L. Planta Med 50:229–234
77. Abel G (1987) Chromosomenschädigende Wirkung von β-Asaron in menschlichen Lym- phocyten. Planta Med, pp 251–253
78. Göggelman W, Schimmer O (1983) Mutagenicity testing of β-asarone and commercial calamus drugs with Salmonella typhimurium. Mutat Res 121:191–194
79. Habermann RT (1971) Carcinogenicity of beta asarone in rats in a two-year feeding study. Report to the Food and Drug Administration dated June 16, 1971
80. Stahl E, Keller K (1981) Zur Klassifizierung handelsüblicher Kalmusdrogen. Planta Med 43:128–140
81. Keller K, Odenthal KP, Leng-Peschlow E (1985) Spasmolytische Wirkung des Isoasaronfreien Kalmus. Planta Med, pp 6–9
82. Mauz Ch, Candrian U, Lüthy J, Schlatter Ch, Sery V, Kuhn G, Kade F (1985) Methode zur Entfernung von Pyrrolizidin-Alkaloiden aus Arzneipflanzenextrakten. Pharm Acta Helv 60:256–259
83. Van de Dungen FM, Vermeulen NPE, Fischer FC, 't Hart LA, Gijbels MJM (1987) Removal of pyrrolizidine alkaloids from Symphytum tinctures — their toxicity towards isolated hepatocytes. Pharm Weekbl Sci Ed 9:222
84. Keller K (1990) Bundes Gesundheits Amt, Berlin. Personal communication
85. Bain RJI (1985) Accidental digitalis poisoning due to drinking herbal tea. Br Med J 290:1624
86. Caravaca Magariños F, Cubero Gomez JJ, Arrobas Vaca M, Pizarro Montero JL, Pimentel Leo JJ, Fernandez Alonzo J, Sanchez Casado E (1985) Afectacion renal y hepática en la intoxicacion por Atractylis gummifera. Nefrologia 5:205–210
87. Kallings LO, Ringertz O, Silverstolpe L, Ernerfeldt F (1966) Microbiological contamination of medical preparations. Acta Pharm Suec 3:219–228
88. Anonymous (1972) Mikrobiologische Reinheit von Arzneimitteln, die nicht steril sein müssen. Zbl Pharm 111:675–687
89. Lutomski J, Kedzia B (1980) Mycoflora of crude drugs. Estimation of mould contaminations and their toxicity. Planta Med 40:212–217
90. Schilcher H (1982) Rückstände und Verunreinigungen bei Drogen und Drogenzubereitungen. 19. Mitteilung: Zur Wertbestimmung und Qualitätsprüfung von Drogen. Planta Med 44:65–77
91. Leimbeck R (1987) Teedrogen — Wie steht es mit der mikrobiologischen Qualität? Dtsch Apoth Ztg 127:1221–1226

92. Frank B (1989) Mikroorganismen in Drogen. Der mikrobiologische Status von Drogen und Drogenzubereitungen und seine Beurteilung. Dtsch Apoth Ztg 129:617–623

93. Y de M, Van Rillaer E, De Mayer-Cleempoel S (1981) Mikrobiologisch onderzoek van thee en kruidenthee's. Arch Belg Méd Soc 39:488–497

94. Härtling C (1987) Beitrag zur Frage des mikrobiellen Zustandes pflanzlicher Drogen – Fakten und Folgerungen. Pharm Ztg 132:643–644

95. Schneider E (1987) Keimbesiedlung von frischen Arzneipflanzen und von Drogen. Veränderugen der Keimzahlen von Drogen während der Gewinnung und Verarbeitung. Dtsch Apoth Ztg 127:1683–1686

96. Van Doorne H, Bosch EH, Zwaving JH, Elema ET (1988) Gamma irradiation of Sennae Folium. Microbiological and phytochemical studies. Pharm Weekbl Sci Ed 10:217–220

97. Graf E, Scheer R (1980) Keimzahlverminderung in Drogen und Hilfstoffen. Pharm Ind 42:732–744

98. Gröning R, Janske U (1985) Keimzahlreduzierung durch Mikrowellen. Pharm Ztg 130:2621–2625

99. Gröning R, Janske U (1987) Keimzahlreduzierung durch Mikrowellen – mikrowellenspezifische Effekte. Pharmazie 42:167–168

100. Sincholle D, Cotta M, Guedon D, Coll R (1987) Plantes médicinales et décontamination. Pharm Acta Helv 62:14–18

101. Lenoble M, Fourniat J, Bourlioux P, Paris M, Maghami P, German A (1980) Contrôle de la qualité microbiologique d'échantillons de *Mentha piperita* de diverses origines géographiques. Ann Pharm Franc 38:333–342

102. Boer YB (1990) Laboratory of Dutch Pharmacists, The Hague. Personal communication

103. Farber JM, Carter AO, Varughese PV, Ashton FE, Ewan EP (1990) Listeriosis traced to the consumption of alfalfa tablets and soft cheese. New Engl J Med 322:338

104. Ferguson WW, June RC (1952) Experiments of feeding adult volunteers with *Escherichia coli* 111, B₄, a coliform organism associated with infant diarrhea. Am J Hyg 55:155–169

105. Buck AC, Cooke EM (1969) The fate of ingested *Pseudomonas aeruginosa* in normal persons. J Med Microbiol 2:521–525

106. McCullough NB, Eisele CW (1951) Experimental human salmonellosis. I. Pathogenicity of strains of *Salmonella meleagridis* and *Salmonella anatum* obtained from spray-dried whole egg. J Infect Dis 88:278–289

107. McCullough NB, Eisele CW (1951) Experimental human salmonellosis. III. Pathogenicity of strains of *Salmonella newport*, *Salmonella derby*, and *Salmonella bareilly* obtained from spray-dried whole egg. J Infect Dis 89:209–213

108. McCullough NB, Eisele CW (1951) Experimental human salmonellosis. IV. Pathogenicity of strains of *Salmonella pullorum* obtained from spray-dried whole egg. J Infect Dis 88:259–265

109. Schneller GH (1977) Microbial testing of oral dosage forms. Presentation at the FIP Congress, The Hague, 7 September 1977

110. Anonymous (1988) Fraudulent AIDS product. JAMA 259:178

111. Danielson KJ, Stewart DE, Lippert GP (1988) Unconventional cancer remedies. Can Med Assoc J 138:1005–1011

112. Umstead GS (1988) Unapproved drug therapies. Geriatrics, arthritis and cancer. J Pharm Technol 4:97–106

113. Riley KB, Antoniskis D, Maris R, Leedom JM (1988) Rattlesnake capsule-associated *Salmonella arizona* infections. Arch Intern Med 148:1207–1210

114. Bhatt BD, Zuckerman MJ, Foland JA, Polly SM, Marwah RK (1989) Disseminated *Salmonella arizona* infection associated with rattlesnake meat ingestion. Am J Gastroenterol 84:433–435

115. Krüger D (1989) Was ist neu aus mikrobiologischer Sicht? Dtsch Apoth Ztg 129(Suppl 16):21–24

116. Ritschel WA, Brady ME, Tan HSI, Hoffmann KA, Yiu IM, Grummich KW (1977) Pharmacokinetics of coumarin and its 7-hydroxymetabolites upon intravenous and peroral administration of coumarin in man. Eur J Clin Pharmacol 12:457–461

117. O'Reilley (1980) Anticoagulant, antithrombotic, and thrombolytic drugs. In: Goodman LS, Gilman A (eds) The pharmacological basis of therapeutics, 6th ed. New York: MacMillan, pp 1347–1366

118. Hogan III RP (1983) Hemorrhagic diathesis caused by drinking an herbal tea. JAMA 249:2679–2680
119. Fritsch H, Krecke HJ, Becker B, Urbaschek B, Nowotny A (1968) Zur Erzeugung einer Endotoxintoleranz durch detoxifiziertes Endotoxin (Endotoxoid) beim Menschen. Verh Dtsch Ges Inn Med 74:1151–1154
120. Baggerman C (1986) Endotoxins in large volume parenterals. A focus on physicochemical parameters related to their detection and removal. PhD thesis. Leiden: State University
121. Becker KP, Ditter B, Nimsky C, Urbaschek R, Urbaschek B (1988) Untersuchungen zum Endotoxingehalt von Phytopharmaka. Korrelation zu klinisch beobachteten Nebenwirkungen. Dtsch Med Wschr 113:83–87
122. Davignon JP, Trissel LA, Kleinman LM (1978) Pharmaceutical assessment of amygdalin (Laetrile) products. Cancer Treat Rep 62:99–104
123. Stadler HW, Dietzel U, Sauer R (1985) Erfahrungen mit einem "Onkophytotherapeutikum". Dtsch Med Wochenschr 110:1184–1185
124. Dietzel U, Sauer R, Reichardt U (1985) Erfahrungen mit Carnivora. Fortschr Med 103:760–761
125. Hajto T (1986) Immunomodulatory effects of Iscador: a *Viscum album* preparation. Oncology 43(Suppl 1):51–65
126. Anonymous (1975) More on the aflatoxin-hepatoma story. Br Med J 2:647–648
127. Ames BN, Magaw R, Gold LS (1987) Ranking possible carcinogenic hazards. Science 236:271–280
128. Roy AK, Chourasia HK (1989) Effect of temperature on aflatoxin production in *Mucuna pruriens* seeds. Appl Environ Microbiol 55:531–532
129. Watson DH (1985) Toxic fungal metabolites in food. CRC Crit Rev Food Sci Nutr 22:177–198
130. Krishnamachari KAVR, Bhat RV, Nagarajan V, Tilak TBG (1975) Hepatitis due to aflatoxicosis. Lancet 1:1061–1063
131. Anonymous (1976) Aflatoxins. IARC Monographs 10:51–72
132. Anonymous (1987) Aflatoxins. IARC Monographs. Suppl 7:83–87
133. Geissler F, Faustman EM (1988) Developmental toxicity of aflatoxin B_1 in the rodent embryo in vitro: contribution of exogenous biotransformation systems to toxicity. Teratology 37:101–111
134. Anonymous (1976) Sterigmatocystin. IARC Monographs 10:245–251
135. Maekawa A, Kajiwara T, Odashima S, Kurata H (1979) Hepatic changes in male ACI/N rats on low dietary levels of sterigmatocystin. Gann 70:777–781
136. Anonymous (1987) Evaluation of certain food additives and contaminants. 31st Report of the Joint FAO/WHO Expert Committee on Food Additives. Technical Report Series 759. Geneva: World Health Organization
137. Stoloff L (1983) Aflatoxin as a cause of primary liver-cell cancer in the United States: a probability study. Nutr Cancer 5:165–186
138. Van Rensburg SJ, Cook-Mozaffari P, Van Schalkwyk DJ, Van der Watt JJ, Vincent TJ, Purchase IF (1985) Hepatocellular carcinoma and dietary aflatoxin in Mozambique and Transkei. Br J Cancer 51:713–726
139. Hitokoto H, Morozumi S, Wauke T, Sakai S, Kurata H (1978) Fungal contamination and mycotoxin detection of powdered herbal drugs. Appl Environ Microbiol 36:252–256
140. Yamazaki M, Horie Y, Itokawa H (1980) On the toxigenic fungi contaminating drugs. I. Mycoflora of commercially available crude drugs and productivity of mycotoxins in some species. Yakugaku Zasshi 100:61–68
141. Ichinoe M, Kartastisna A, Hirai K, Teshima R, Ikebuchi H (1988) Aflatoxin production of *Aspergillus flavus* isolated from Indonesian crude herbal drugs. Eisei Shikenjo Hokoku (106)25–29
142. Roy AK, Sinha KK, Chourasia HK (1988) Aflatoxin contamination of some common drug plants. Appl Environ Microbiol 54:842–843
143. Roy AK, Prasad MM, Kumari N, Chourasia HK (1988) Studies on association of mycoflora with drug-plants and aflatoxin producing potentiality of *Aspergillus flavus*. Ind Phytopathol 41:261–262
144. Kumari V, Chourasia HK, Roy AK (1989) Aflatoxin contamination in seeds of medicinal value. Curr Sci 58:512–513

145. Blaser P, Schmidt-Lorenz W (1981) *Aspergillus flavus* Kontamination von Nüssen, Mandeln und Mais mit bekannten Aflatoxin-Gehalten. Lebensmitt Wissensch Technol 14:252–259
146. Hilal SH, Sayed AM, Mahmoud II, El-Kirsh T (1986) Study of mutagenic/carcinogenic activity of certain medicinal teas in Egypt as determined by the *Salmonella* test. Egypt J Pharm Sci 27:235–245
147. Hilal SH, Soliman FM, Mahmoud II, El-Kersh TA (1987) Quantitative study of the mutagenic activity of folkloric Egyptian herbs. II. Lecture presented at the 47th International Congress of Pharmaceutical Sciences of the Fédération Internationale Pharmaceutique, Amsterdam: 31 August – 4 September 1987
148. Schilcher H (1985) Rückstandbelastung von Drogen und Drogenzubereitungen. Dtsch Apoth Ztg 125:47–52
149. Ali SL (1985) Bestimmung der Pestizidrückstände und toxischen Metallspuren in Teeaufgüssen aus Arzneidrogen. Pharm Ztg 130:1927–1932
150. Pluta J (1988) Studies on contamination of vegetable drugs with halogen derivative pesticides. I. Changes of concentrations of halogen derivatives in herbal raw materials within the period of 1980–1984. Pharmazie 43:121–123
151. Ditzel P (1989) Arzneidrogen – wie stark sind sie mit Pestiziden und Schwermetallen belastet? Dtsch Apoth Ztg 129:2394–2396
152. Ali SL (1983) Bestimmung der pestiziden Rückstände und anderer bedenklicher Verunreinigungen – wie toxische Metallspuren – in Arzneipflanzen. I. Mitt: Pestizid-Rückstände in Arzneidrogen. Pharm Ind 45:1154–1156
153. Kwon SK, Dicke W, Thier H-P (1986) Pestizidrückstände in drei Drogen aus Südkorea. Planta Medica pp 155–156
154. Benecke R, Thieme H, Brotka J (1986) Untersuchung pflanzlicher Drogen auf Rückstände von Organochlorverbindungen. Pharmazie 41:133–137
155. Benecke R, Brotka J, Wijsbeek J, Franke JP, Bruins AP, De Zeeuw RA (1986) Untersuchung pflanzlicher Drogen auf Rückstände von Organochlorverbindungen. 2. Mitteilung. Identifizierung der Rückständen von DDT und seinen Analogen durch Vergleich von Gaschromatographie an gepackter und Kapillarsäule sowie GC/MS-Kopplung. Pharmazie 41:499–501
156. Ali SL (1987) Bestimmung der Pestizidrückstände und toxischen Schwermetallspuren in Arzneidrogen und deren Teeaufgüssen. Pharm Ztg 132:633–638
157. Benecke R, Ennet D, Frauenberger H (1987) Rückstände von Pflanzenschutzmitteln in Drogen von wildwachsenden Arzneipflanzen. Pharmazie 42:869–871
158. Pluta J (1988) Studies on contamination of vegetable drugs with halogen derivative pesticides. II. Concentrations of halogen derivative pesticides in vegetable blends and herbal granulated products produced in Poland in 1980–1984. Pharmazie 43:348–351
159. Pluta J (1989) Studies on concentration of halogen derivatives in herbal products from various regions of Poland. Pharmazie 44:222–224
160. Benecke R, Ortwein J, Ennet D, Frauenberger H (1989) Rückstände von Lindan und DDT in Drogen von wildwachsenden Arzneipflanzen aus forstwirtschaftlich genutzen Waldgebieten. 2. Mitteilung. Pharmazie 44:562–564
161. Schilcher H, Peters H, Wank H (1987) Pestizide und Schwermetalle in Arzneipflanzen und Arzneipflanzen-Zubereitungen. Pharm Ind 49:203–211
162. Ennet D (1989) Fremdstoffe in pflanzlichen Arzneimitteln. Pharmazie 44:383–386
163. Benecke R, Brotka J, Wijsbeek J, Franke JP, Bruins AP, De Zeeuw RA (1988) Untersuchung pflanzlicher Drogen auf Rückstände von Organochlorverbindungen. 3. Mitteilung. Identifizierung von Rückständen polychlorierter Biphenyle durch Vergleich von Gaschromatographie an gepackter und Kapillarsäule sowie GC/MS-Kopplung. Pharmazie 43:123–125
164. Gosselin RE, Smith RP, Hodge HC, Braddock JE (1984) Clinical Toxicology of Commercial Products. 5th edn Baltimore: Williams & Wilkins
165. Council on Scientific Affairs (1988) Cancer risk of pesticides in agricultural workers. JAMA 260:959–966
166. Anonymous (1990) Guide to codex maximum limits for pesticide residues. Rijswijk: Dutch Secretariat for Codex Alimentarius Commission (April 1990)

167. Schilcher H (1970) Begasung von getrockneten Arzneipflanzen mit T-Gas/Äthylenoxid. Planta Med 18:101–113
168. Anonymous (1986) Ethylene oxide – a human carcinogen? Lancet 2:201–202
169. Nicholls A (1986) Ethylene oxide and anaphylaxis during haemodialysis. Br Med J 292:1221–1222
170. Hemminki K, Mutanen P, Saloniemi I, Niemi M-L, Vainio H (1982) Spontaneous abortions in hospital staff engaged in sterilising instruments with chemical agents. Br Med J 285:1461–1463
171. Anonymous (1987) Ethylene oxide. IARC Monographs. Suppl 7:205–207
172. Hogstedt C, Aringer L, Gustavsson A (1986) Epidemiological support for ethylene oxide as a cancer-causing agent. JAMA 255:1575–1578
173. Samuelsson G, Yman B-M, Diding N (1968) Ethylene oxide treatment of crude drugs. II. Influence on drugs containing glycosides. Acta Pharm Suec 5:183–198
174. Samuelsson G, Yman B-M, Diding N (1968) Ethylene oxide treatment of crude drugs. III. Influence on drugs containing alkaloids. Acta Pharm Suec 5:199–204
175. Samuelsson G, Yman B-M, Diding N (1968) Ethylene oxide treatment of crude drugs. IV. Influence on drugs containing volatile oils, mucilages and starch. Acta Pharm Suec 5:205–214
176. Anonymous (1986) Empfehlungen zur Verwendung von Ethylenoxid. Dtsch Apoth Ztg 126:659–660
177. Ihrig M (1989) Qualitätsmangel bei pflanzlichen Arzneimitteln vom ZL überprüft. Pharm Ztg 134:3074–3082
178. Stahl E, Rau G, Adolphi H (1985) Entwesung von Drogen durch Kohlendioxid-Druckbehandlung (PEX-Verfahren). Pharm Ind 47:528–530
179. Pohlen W, Rau G, Finkenzeller E (1989) Erste praktische Erfahrungen mit einem Verfahren zur Druckentwesung mit Kohlendioxid. Pharm Ind 51:917–918
180. Kartnig T, Hiermann A, Zödl M, Still F (1986) Untersuchungen über die Strahlenbelastung von Drogen aus steirischen Arzneipflanzenkulturen. Österreich Apoth Ztg 40:697–700
181. Kopp B, Kubelka W (1986) Arzneipflanzen – radioaktiv? Österreich Apoth Ztg 40:646–647
182. Pratzel H, Reinelt D (1986) Radioaktive Belastung von Arzneipflanzen – differenzierte Ergebnisse der Untersuchung in Bayern. Dtsch Apoth Ztg 126:1957–1958
183. Blume H, Ali SL, Ihrig M (1987) Die radioaktive Belastung von Teedrogen und anderen natürlichen Produkten aus Apotheken. Pharm Ztg 132:85–87
184. Kartnig T, Zödl M (1987) Untersuchungen über die Strahlenbelastung von Drogen aus steirischen Arzneipflanzenkulturen. 2. Mitteilung – 1 Jahr nach Tschernobyl. Österreich Apoth Ztg 41:742–743
185. Anonymous (1987) Die radioaktive Belastung von Teedrogen und anderen natürlichen Produkten aus Apotheken. Pharm Ztg 132:1690–1691
186. Ali SL, Ihrig M (1987) Die radioaktive Belastung von wässrigen Zubereitungen und ätherischen Ölen aus kontaminierten Drogen. Pharm Ztg 132:2537
187. Anonymous (1986) Strahlenbelastete Arzneimittel – Ein gesundheitliches Risiko? Pharm Ztg 131:3007–3010
188. Anonymous (1987) Radioaktive Belastung von Arzneitees unbedenklich. Apotheker Zeitung 3(5):5
189. Ali SL (1983) Bestimmung der pestiziden Rückstände und anderer bedenklicher Veruntreinigungen – wie toxische Metallspuren – in Arzneipflanzen. 2. Mitteilung. Bestimmung von toxischen Metallspuren in Arzneidrogen. Pharm Ind 45:1294–1295
190. Schilcher H (1983) Contamination of natural products with pesticides and heavy metals. In: Breimer DD, Speiser P (eds) Topics in pharmaceutical sciences 1983. Amsterdam: Elsevier Science Publishers, pp 417–423
191. Tay C-H, Seah C-S (1975) Arsenic poisoning from anti-asthmatic herbal preparations. Med J Aust 2:424–428
192. Aslam M, Davis SS, Healy MA (1979) Heavy metals in some Asian medicines and cosmetics. Publ Health (London) 93:274–284
193. Rempel D (1989) The lead-exposed worker. JAMA 262:532–534
194. Anonymous (1987) Cadmium and cadmium compounds. IARC Monographs. Suppl 7:139–142
195. Anonymous (1987) Arsenic and arsenic compounds. IARC Monographs. Suppl 7:100–106

196. Peters H, Schilcher H (1986) Schwermetallbelastung von Arzneidrogen und deren Zuberei-tungen. Planta Med, pp 521–522
197. Anonymous (1978) Evaluation of certain food additives and contaminants. 22nd Report of the Joint FAO/WHO Expert Committee on Food Additives. Technical Report Series 631. Geneva: World Health Organization
198. Anonymous (1989) Evaluation of certain food additives and contaminants. 33rd Report of the Joint FAO/WHO Expert Committee on Food Additives. Technical Report Series 776. Geneva: World Health Organization
199. Anonymous (1987) Evaluation of certain food additives and contaminants. 30th Report of the Joint FAO/WHO Expert Committee on Food Additives. Technical Report Series 751. Geneva: World Health Organization
200. Van Dokkum W, De Vos RH, Muys T, Wesstra JA (1989) Minerals and trace elements in total diets in The Netherlands. Br J Nutr 61:7–15
201. Norman JA, Pickford CJ, Sanders TW, Waller M (1987) Human intake of arsenic and iodine from seaweed-based food supplements and health foods available in the UK. Food Addit Contam 5:103–109
202. Sherlock JC, Smart GA (1986) Thallium in foods and the diet. Food Add Contamin 3:363–370
203. Dai-xing Z, Ding-nan L (1985) Chronic thallium poisoning in a rural area of Guizhou province, China. J Environment Health 48:14–18
204. Anonymous (1988) Zuviel Cadmium in Leinsamen. Dtsch Apoth Ztg 128:145–146
205. Walkiw O, Douglas DE (1975) Health food supplements prepared from kelp — a source of elevated urinary arsenic. Clin Toxicol 8:325–331
206. Phillips DJ, Depledge MH (1985) Metabolic pathways involving arsenic in marine organisms a unifying hypothesis. Mar Environ Res 17:1–12
207. Chan H, Yeh Y-Y, Billmeier GJ, Evans WE (1977) Lead poisoning from ingestion of Chinese herbal medicine. Clin Toxicol 10:273–281
208. Lightfoote J, Blair J, Cohen JR (1977) Lead intoxication in an adult caused by Chinese herbal medication. JAMA 238:1539
209. Chung JG, Yoon YB, Kim CY (1980) A case of lead-poisoning by herb medicine. J Korean Med Assoc 23:517–522
210. Yu ECL, Yeung CY (1987) Lead encephalopathy due to herbal medicine. Chin Med J 100:915
211. Anonymous (1989) Cadmium and lead exposure associated with pharmaceuticals imported from Asia — Texas. MMWR 38:612–614
212. De Smet PAGM, Elferink F (1990) Te veel lood in Chinese kruidenpillen. Pharm Weekbl 125:169
213. Chia BL, Leng CK, Hsii FP, Yap MHL, Lee YK (1973) Lead poisoning from contaminated opium. Br Med J 1:354
214. Yeung H-C (1985) Handbook of Chinese Herbs and Formulas, vol II. Los Angeles
215. Anonymous (1981) Use of lead tetroxide as a folk remedy for gastrointestinal illness. MMWR 30:546–547
216. Anonymous (1982) Lead poisoning from lead tetroxide used as a folk remedy — Colorado. MMWR 30:647–648
217. Anonymous (1983) Lead poisoning from Mexican folk remedies — California. JAMA 250:3149
218. Bose A, Vashistha K, O'Loughlin BJ (1983) Azarcón por empacho — another cause of lead toxicity. Pediatrics 72:106–108
219. Baer RD, Ackerman A (1988) Toxic Mexican folk remedies for the treatment of empacho: the case of azarcon, greta, and albayalde. J Ethnopharmacol 24:31–39
220. Anonymous (1983) Folk remedy-associated lead poisoning in Hmong children. JAMA 250:3149–3150
221. Anonymous (1984) Nonfatal arsenic poisoning in three Hmong patients — Minnesota. MMWR 33:347–349
222. Levitt C, Godes J, Eberhardt M, Ing R, Simpson JM (1984) Sources of lead poisoning. JAMA 252:3127–3128
223. D'Alauro F, Lin-Fu JS, Ecker TJ (1984) Toxic metal contamination of folk remedy. JAMA 252:3127

224. Warley MA, Blackledge P, O'Gorman P (1968) Lead poisoning from eye cosmetic. Br Med J 1:117
225. Ali AR, Smales ORC, Aslam M (1978) Surma and lead poisoning. Br Med J 2:915–916
226. Aslam M, Healy MA, Davis SS, Ali AR (1980) Surma and blood lead in children. Lancet 1:658–659
227. Fernando NP, Healy MA, Aslam M, Davis SS, Hussein A (1981) Lead poisoning and traditional practices: the consequences for world health. A study in Kuwait. Publ Health (London) 95:250–260
228. Healy MA, Aslam M, Bamgboye OA (1984) Traditional medicine and lead-containing preparations in Nigeria. Publ Health (London) 98:26–32
229. Haq I, Asghar M (1989) Lead content of somonal preparations — "Kushtas". J Ethnopharmacol 26:287–291
230. Datta DV, Mitra SK, Chhuttani PN, Chakravarti RN (1979) Chronic oral arsenic intoxication as a possible aetiological factor in idiopathic portal hypertension (non-cirrhotic portal fibrosis) in India. Gut 20:378–384
231. Middleton JD (1989) Sikor: an unquantified health hazard. Br Med J 298:407–408
232. Ries CA, Sahud MA (1975) Agranulocytosis caused by Chinese herbal medicines. Dangers of medications containing aminopyrine and phenylbutazone. JAMA 231:352–355
233. Brooks PM, Lowenthal RM (1977) Chinese herbal arthritis cure and agranulocytosis. Med J Aust 2:860–861
234. Uitdehaag CMJ, Hekster YA, van de Putte LBA, Waas RJM, Bertels B, Huysse H, Slijkhuis C, Smits HM (1979) Chinese pillen, Cushingsyndroom en geneesmiddelenonderzoek. Ned T Geneesk 123:1009–1011
235. Anoniem (1979) Nader onderzoek van de zg. Chinese pil. Ned T Geneeskd 123:1347
236. Forster PJG, Calverley M, Hubball S, McConkey B (1979) Chuei-Fong-Tou-Geu-Wan in rheumatoid arthritis. Br Med J 2:308
237. Morice A (1986) Adulterated "homoeopathic" cure for asthma. Lancet 1:862–863
238. Morice A (1987) Adulteration of homoeopathic remedies. Lancet 1:635
239. Steinigen M (1987) Erneute Warnung vor Amborum special-F. Dtsch Ap Ztg 127:21
240. Bury RW, Fullinfaw RO, Barraclough D, Muirden KD, Moulds RFW (1987) Problems with herbal medicines. Med J Aust 146:324–325
241. De Smet PAGM, Elferink F (1988) Chinese pillen nog steeds verontreinigd. Ned T Geneesk 132:407–408
242. Anonymous (1988) Asthma-Wundermittel "Thong Yen Obat China/Lim Yok Kong". Pharm Ztg 133(21):7
243. Anonymous (1988) "ASFO" — natural herbs tea. Pharm Ztg 133(40):6–7
244. Tay SAB, Johnston MA (1989) Quality of imported herbal products. Med J Aust 151:52
245. De Smet PAGM, Elferink F, Kerremans ALM, Meyboom RHB (1990) Dexamethason in oosterse Cow's Head Brand Tung Shueh pillen. Pharm Weekbl 125:414–415
246. Yuen S, Lau-Cam CA (1985) Thin-layer chromatographic screening procedure for undeclared synthetic drugs in chinese herbal preparations. J Chromatogr 329:107–112
247. Offerhaus L (1978) Waarschuwing voor Cushing-syndroom en onttrekkingsverschijnselen bij Hongkong-pilgebruikers. Ned T Geneeskd 122:1633
248. Vulto AG, Buurma H (1984) Drugs used in non-orthodox medicine. In: Dukes MNG (eds) Side effects of drugs. Amsterdam: Elsevier, pp 886–907
249. Ambre JJ, Rahmanian M (1988) Prescription drugs in a mail order diet aid. J Am Med Assoc 260:925
250. Braunstein GD, Koblin R, Sugawara M, Pekary AE, Hershman JM (1986) Unintentional thyrotoxicosis factitia due to a diet pill. West J Med 145:388–391
251. Jelliffe RW, Hill D, Tatter D, Lewis Jr E (1969) Death from weight-control pills. A case report with objective postmortem confirmation. JAMA 208:1843–1847
252. Anonymous (1984) Neues "Wundermittel" für Übergewichtige? Pharm Ztg 129:2104–2105
253. Langford HG, Nicholas WC (1987) Dangerous and expensive ways to lose weight. J Miss State Med Assoc 28:99–100
254. Anonymous (1989) Gefährliche und irrationale Zusammensetzungen bei Magistralrezepturen gegen Übergewicht. Schweiz Apoth Ztg 127:353

255. Rivlin RS (1975) Therapy of obesity with hormones. N Engl J Med 292:26-29
256. American Medical Association Department of Drugs, Division of Drugs and Technology (1986) AMA Drug Evaluations. 6th edn. Chicago: American Medical Association
257. Volans GN (1987) Monitoring the safety of over the counter drugs. Br Med J 295:797-798
258. Regner MJ, Hermann F, Ried LD (1987) Effectiveness of a printed leaflet for enabling patients to use digoxin side-effect information. Drug Intell Clin Pharm 21:200-204
259. Hielema A, Lelie-Van der Zande A, De Smet P (1989) The professional pharmaceutical association as a source of patient-oriented drug information. In: Bogaert M, Vander Stichele R, Kaufman J-R, Lefebvre R (eds) Patient package insert as a source of drug information. Amsterdam: Excerpta Medica, pp 131-137
260. Ammon HPT (1988) Möglichkeiten und Grenzen: Selbstmedikation mit Phytopharmaka. Pharm Ztg 133(40):36
261. Blasius H, Jahn H (1988) Aufbereitung und Nachzulassung in verschiedenen EG-Ländern. Auf dem Weg zum gemeinsamen Arzneimittelmarkt in Europa. Dtsch Apoth Ztg 128:1153-1158
262. Levin LS, Beske F, Fry J (1988) Self-medication in Europe. Report on a study of the role of non-prescription medicines. Copenhagen: World Health Organization, Regional Office for Europe
263. Tyler VE (1987) Herbal medicine in America. Planta Med, pp 1-4
264. Hayes Jr AH, Schweiker RS (1982) Weight control drug products for over-the-counter human use; establishment of a monograph. Fed Reg 47:8466-8484
265. Björvell H, Roessner S (1987) Long-term effects of commonly available weight reducing programmes in Sweden. Int J Obes 11:67-71
266. Liewendahl K, Gordin A (1974) Iodine-induced toxic diffuse goitre. Acta Med Scand 196:237-239
267. Skare S, Frey HMM (1980) Iodine induced thyrotoxicosis in apparently normal thyroid glands. Acta Endocrinol (Copenh) 94:332-336
268. Shilo S, Hirsch HJ (1986) Iodine-induced hyperthyroidism in a patient with a normal thyroid gland. Postgrad Med J 62:661-662
269. De Smet PAGM, Stricker BHC, Wilderink F, Wiersinga WM (1990) Hyperthyreoidie tijdens het gebruik van kelptabletten. Ned T Geneeskd 134:1058-1059
270. Anonymous (1988) The role of consumer information. AESGP – Association Européenne des Spécialités Pharmaceutiques Grand Public. Luton: White Crescent Press
271. Anonymous (undated) Passport to Europe. Proposals for completion of the internal market for non-prescription medicines. AESGP – Association Européenne des Spécialités Pharmaceutiques Grand Public. Luton: White Crescent Press
272. Lee TY, Lam TH (1987) Allergic contact dermatitis to Yunnan Paiyao. Contact Derm 17:59 60
273. Liewendahl K, Turula M (1972) Iodide-induced goitre and hypothyroidism in a patient with chronic lymphocytic thyroiditis. Acta Endocrinol 71:289-296
274. Mebs D, Schmidt K, Raudonat HW, Schenk F (1988) Vergiftung durch "Hustentee". Dtsch Med Wschr 113:1457
275. Sandeman DR, Clements MR, Perrins EJ (1980) Oesophageal obstruction due to hygroscopic gum laxative. Lancet 1:364-365
276. Noble JA, Grannis FW Jr (1984) Acute esophageal obstruction by a psyllium-based bulk laxative. Chest 86:800
277. Sauerbruch T, Kuntzen O, Unger W (1980) Agiolax bolus in the esophagus. Report of two cases. Endoscopy 12:83-5
278. Hoekstra DFJ (1988) Onzorgvuldig handelen door alternatieve genesers en de wet. Medisch Contact 43:711-714
279. Baldwin CA, Anderson LA, Phillipson JD, Spencer MG (1987) Drug information – herbal concern. Pharm J 239(no. 6452): R13-R14
280. Sullivan Jr JB, Rumack BH, Thomas Jr H, Peterson RG, Bryson P (1979) Pennyroyal oil poisoning and hepatotoxicity. JAMA 242:2873-2874
281. Vallance WB (1955) Pennyroyal poisoning. A fatal case. Lancet 4:850-851
282. Dobb GJ, Edis RH (1984) Coma and neuropathy after ingestion of herbal laxative containing podophyllin. Med J Aust 140:495-496
283. Ridker PM, Ohkuma S, McDermott WV, Trey C, Huxtable RJ (1985) Hepatic venocclusive

disease associated with the consumption of pyrrolizidine-containing dietary supplements. Gastroenterology 88:1050–1054

284. Bach N, Thung SN, Schaffner F (1989) Comfrey herb tea-induced hepatic veno-occlusive disease. Am J Med 87:97–99
285. Roulet M, Laurini R, Rivier L, Calame A (1988) Hepatic veno-occlusive disease in newborn infant of a woman drinking herbal tea. J Pediatr 112:433–436
286. Spang R (1989) Toxicity of tea containing pyrrolizidine alkaloids. J Pediatrics 115:1025
287. Mix DB, Guinaudeau H, Shamma M (1982) The aristolochic acids and aristolactams. J Nat Prod 45:657–666
288. Mengs Y, Klein M (1988) Genotoxic effects of aristolochic acid in the mouse micronucleus test. Planta Med 54:502–503
289. Mengs U, Lang W, Poch J-A (1982) The carcinogenic action of aristolochic acid in rats. Arch Toxicol 51:107–119
290. Mengs U (1988) Tumour induction in mice following exposure to aristolochic acid. Arch Toxicol 61:504–505
291. Anonymous (1981) Zum Zulassungswiderruf Aristolochiasäure-haltiger Fertigarzneimittel. Pharm Ztg 126:1373–1374
292. Schulz M, Weist F, Gemählich M (1971) Dünnschichtchromatographischer Nachweis der Aristolochia-Säure in verschiedenen Körperflüssigkeiten. Arzneim Forsch 21:934–936
293. Leatherdale BA, Panesar RK, Singh G, Atkins TW, Bailey CJ, Bignell AH (1981) Improvement in glucose tolerance due to Momordica charantia (karela). Br Med J 282:1823–1824
294. Welihinda J, Karunanayake EH, Sheriff MHR, Jayasinghe KSA (1986) Effect of Momordica charantia on the glucose tolerance in maturity onset diabetes. J Ethnopharmacol 17:277–282
295. Aslam M, Stockley IH (1979) Interaction between curry ingredient (karela) and drug (chlorpropamide) Lancet 1:607
296. Huupponen R, Seppälä P, Iisalo E (1984) Effect of guar gum, a fibre preparation, on digoxin and penicillin absorption in man. Eur J Clin Pharmacol 26:279–281
297. Shima K, Tanaka A, Ikegami H, Tabata M, Sawazaki N, Kumahara Y (1983) Effect of dietary fiber, glucomannan, on absorption of sulfonylurea in man. Horm Metabol Res 15:1–3
298. Anonymous (1990) USP Dispensing information, vol II. Advice for the patient. Drug information in lay language. 10th edn. Rockville: The United States Pharmacopeial Convention
299. Anonymous (1990) Bekanntmachung über die Zulassung und Registrierung von Arzneimitteln. Bundesanzeiger (herausgegeben von Bundesminister der Justiz). 3.1.1984 (no 1); 5.12.1984 (no 228); 15.5.1985 (no 90); 21.8.1985 (no 154); 30.11.1985 (no 223); 13.3.1986 (no 50); 18.9.1986 (no 173); 24.9.1986 (no 177a); 23.4.1987 (no 76); 15.10.1987 (no 193a); 5.5.1988 (no 85); 6.7.1988 (no 122); 2.3.1989 (no 43); 27.4.1989 (no 80); 1.2.1990 (no 22a); 12.3.1990 (no 50)
300. Braun R (ed) (1989) Standardzulassungen für Fertigarzneimittel. Text und Kommentar. Stuttgart: Deutscher Apotheker Verlag

Allium sativum

C.-P. Siegers

Botany

Allium sativum L. belongs to the Alliaceae (Lilianae). The vernacular name is garlic.

The family Alliaceae also includes common onions (*Allium cepa* L. var. *cepa*), shallots (*Allium cepa* L. var. *ascalonicum*), leek (*Allium ampeloprasum* L. var. *porrum*), and chives (*Allium schoenoprasum* L.) [1].

Chemistry

The bulb of *Allium sativum* contains alliin and degradation products such as allicin, polysulfides, ajoenes, mercaptanes, thioglycosides, thiosulfinates, and adenosin. The sulfur-containing degradation products of alliin have been detected mainly in garlic oil [2–4]. In a recently published investigation [5] selenium has been found in appreciable amounts in garlic and garlic preparations which can serve as a sufficient supply of this biologically active trace element.

Pharmacology and Uses

Extracts from garlic bulbs or garlic oil have been reported to exert bactericidal [6–9], antiviral [10], and fungicidal activities [11–16], to decrease serum lipid and cholesterol contents [17–19], to prolong bleeding and clotting time [20,21], to inhibit collagen-induced platelet-aggregation [22–25], and to increase fibrinolytic activities [21,26,27].

Preparations of garlic extracts or garlic oil are used as an adjuvant in the treatment of mild forms of hyperlipidemia [28].

Adverse Reaction Profile

General Animal Data

Acute toxicity of allicin is characterized by LD_{50} values of 120 mg/kg s.c. and 60 mg/kg i.v. in mice [29]. For garlic extracts LD_{50} values between 0.5 ml/kg and > 30 ml/kg p.o., i.p., and s.c. have been reported in rats and mice [30,31]. In chronic toxicity studies with garlic oil or garlic extracts in rats, growth retardation and stomach injury [32,33] as well as anemia in rats, cats, and dogs have been observed [34–36].

Allergic Reactions

Exposure to garlic has been reported repeatedly (e.g., [37–42]) to evoke allergic reactions, as evidenced by the observations of contact dermatitis and — following inhalation of garlic powder — severe asthmatic attacks [43,44]. Garlic-sensitive animals and patients cross-react to onions and also to different garlic ingredients, of which the most active are allicin and diallyldisulfide [45]. Other authors observed a cross-reactivity to tulip but not to onions [37,38]. In garlic-sensitive patients epicutaneous testing proves the presence of specific antibodies and allergy to garlic and other Alliaceae [46].

Dermatological Reactions

Local irritating effects of garlic oil may occur after topical application to the skin or rectal mucosa, with some severe cases reported in infants [47]. See also the section on allergic reactions.

Endocrine Reactions

Hormone-like effects of garlic and garlic extracts have been reported in exper-imental studies, with rats and cats showing estrogenic and ACTH-like effects [48,49].

Gastrointestinal Reactions

Ingestion of fresh garlic bulbs, garlic extracts, or garlic oil may cause nausea, vomiting, and diarrhea [50–52]; the latter effect has been attributed to the content of adenosine as a secretomotor laxative [53].

Hematological Reactions

Although many pharmacological and clinical studies have demonstrated distinct effects of garlic on hemorheologic parameters (see the section on pharmacology and uses), no clinical reports on hematological adverse effects or drug interactions with antithrombotic drugs have been found in the literature. A theoretical risk, however, cannot be excluded.

Respiratory Reactions

See the section on allergic reactions.

Fertility, Pregnancy, and Lactation

One study described the effect of *Allium sativum* on regulation of fertility and concluded that aqueous, alcoholic, and petroleum ether extracts of *Allium sativum* showed no anti-implantation activity in the rat [54]. In guinea pigs garlic extract stimulated rhythmic contractions of the uterus [55]. Experimental or clinical data on adverse effects of garlic ingestion during pregnancy or lactation were not retrieved from the literature.

Mutagenicity and Carcinogenicity

Genotoxicity of fresh garlic juice and an alcoholic garlic extract has been tested in vivo [56] and in vitro [57]. No mutagenicity was observed in a bacterial test system (Ames test), and only cytotoxic but no mutagenic effects have been found in the micronucleus test in mice and the CHE test in the Chinese hamster embryo [56,57]. Only with garlic pyrolysis products were positive results obtained in the Ames test [58,59] and the *Drosophila* test [60]. Data on a carcinogenic or co-carcinogenic potential of *Allium sativum* have not been recovered from the literature.

References

1. Traub HL (1968) The subgenera, sections and subsections of Allium L. Plant Life 24:147
2. Shankaranarayana ML, Raghavan B, Abraham KO, Natarayan CP (1974) Volatile sulfur compounds in food flavors. CRC – Crit Rev Food Technol 4:395–435
3. Fenwick GR, Hanley AB (1985) The Genus Allium, Part 1–3, CRC Crit Rev Food Sci Nutrit. 22:199–271, 273–377 and 23:1–73
4. Block E (1985) The chemistry of garlic and onions. Scientific American 252:114–119
5. Koch HP, Jäger W (1988) Selen im Knoblauch und in Knoblauchpräparaten. Dtsch Apoth Ztg 128:993–995

6. Al-Delaimy KS, Ali SH (1970) Antibacterial action of vegetable extracts on the growth of pathogenic bacteria. J Sci Food Agric 21:110–112
7. Amer M, Taha M, Tosson Z (1980) The effect of aqueous garlic extract on the growth of dermatophytes. Int J Dermatol 19:285–287
8. Delaha EC, Garagusi VF (1985) Inhibition of mycobacteria by garlic extract (Allium sativum). Antimicrob Agents Chemother 27:485–486
9. Sharma VD, Sethi MS, Kumar A, Rarotra JR (1977) Antibacterial property of Allium sativum Linn.: In vivo and in vitro studies. Indian J exp Biol 15:466–468
10. Tsai Y, Cole LL, Davis LE, Lockwood SJ, Simmons V, Wild GC (1985) Antiviral properties of garlic: in vitro effects on influenza B, herpes simplex and coxsackie viruses. Planta Med pp 460–461
11. Appleton JA, Tansey MR (1975) Inhibition of growth of zoopathogenic fungi by garlic. Mycologia 67:882–885
12. Azzouz MA, Bullerman LB (1982) Comparative antimycotic effects of selected herbs, spices, plant components and commercial antifungal agents. J Food Protection 45:1298–1301
13. Caporaso N, Smith SM, Eng RHK (1983) Antifungal activity in human urine and serum after ingestion of garlic (Allium sativum). Antimicrob Agents Chemother 23:700–702
14. Moore GS, Atkins RD (1977) The fungicidal and fungistatic effects of an aqueous garlic extract on medically important yeast-like fungi. Mycologia 69:341–348
15. Yamada Y, Azuma K (1977) Evaluation of the in vitro antifungal activity of allicin. Antimicrob Agents Chemother 11:743–749
16. Yoshida S, Kasuga S, Hayashi N, Ushiroguchi T, Matsuura H, Nakagawa S (1987) Antifungal activity of ajoene derived from garlic. Appl Environm Microbiol 53:615–617
17. Arora RC, Arora S (1981) Comparative effect of clofibrate, garlic and onion on alimentary hyperlipemia. Atherosclerosis 39:447–52
18. Bordia A (1981) Effect of garlic on blood lipids in patients with coronary heart disease. Am J Clin Nutr 34:2100–2103
19. Mohammad SF, Woodward SC (1987) Characterization of a potent inhibitor of platelet aggregation and release reaction isolated from Allium sativum (garlic). Thrombosis Res 44:793–806
20. Sainani GS, Desai DB, Gorhe NH, Natu SM, Pise DV, Sainani PG (1979) Dietary garlic, onion, and some coagulation parameters in Jain community. J Assoc Phys India 27:707–712
21. Ogston D (1985) Nutritional influences on the fibrinolytic system. Proc Nutrition Soc 44:379–384
22. Ariga T, Shiba S, Tamada T (1981) Platelet aggregation inhibitor in garlic. Lancet 1:150–151
23. Bordia A (1978) Effect of garlic on human platelet aggregation in vitro. Atherosclerosis 30:335–360
24. Boullin DJ (1981) Garlic as a platelet inhibitor. Lancet 1:776–777
25. Makheja AN, Vanderhoek JY, Bailey JM (1979) Inhibition of platelet aggregation and thromboxane synthesis by onion and garlic. Lancet 1:781
26. Chutani SK, Bordia A (1981) The effect of fried versus raw garlic on fibrinolytic activity in man. Atherosclerosis 38:417–421
27. Jain RC (1977) Effect of garlic on serum lipids, coagulability and fibrinolytic activity of blood. Am J Clin Nutr 30:1380–1381
28. Morck H (1988) Knoblauch bei Hyperlipoproteinämie einsetzbar. Pharm Ztg 133:21
29. Cavallito CJ, Bailey JH (1944) Allicin, the antibacterial principle of Allium sativum I. Isolation, physical properties and antibacterial action. J Am Chem Soc 66:1950–1951
30. Ruffin J, Hunter SA (1983) An evaluation of the side effects of garlic as an antihypertensive agent. Cytobios 37:85–89
31. Nakagawa S, Masamoto K, Sumiyoshi H, Harada H (1984) Acute toxicity test of garlic extract. J Toxicol 9:57–60
32. Nakagawa S,. Koji M, Hiromichi S, Kazuo K, Tokru F (1980) Effect of feeding raw garlic juice and extracted aged garlic juice on the growth of young rats and their organs. J Toxicol Sci 5:91–98
33. Shashikanth KN, Basappa SC, Murthy VS (1986) Effect of feeding raw and boiled garlic (Allium sativum L.) extracts on the growth, cecal microflora and serum proteins of albino rats. Nutr Rep Int 33:313–319
34. Kanezawa A, Nakagawa S, Sumiyoshi H, Masamoto K, Harada H, Nakagami S, Date S, Yokota

A, Nishikawa M, Fiwa T (1984) General toxicity testing of a garlic extract preparation containing vitamins (KYOLEPIN). Oyo Yakuri 27:909–929

35. Farkas MC, Farkas JN (1974) Hemolytic anemia due to ingestion of onions in a dog. J Am Anim Hosp Ass 10:65
36. Bogin E, Abrams M, Earon Y (1984) Effect of garlic extract on red blood cells. J Food Protection 47:100–101
37. Bleumink E, Doeglas HMG, Klokke AH, Nater JP (1972) Allergic contact dermatitis to garlic. Brit J Dermatol 87:6–9
38. Bleumink E, Nater JP (1973) Contact dermatitis to garlic; crossreactivity between garlic, onion and tulip. Arch Derm Forsch 247:117–124
39. Campolmi P, Lombardi P, Lotti R, Sertoli A (1982) Immediate and delayed sensitization to garlic. Contact Dermatitis 8:352–353
40. Mitchell JC (1980) Contact sensitivity to garlic (Allium). Contact Dermatitis 6:356–357
41. Schulz KH, Hausen BM (1975) Kontaktekzeme durch Pflanzen und Hölzer. Hautarzt 26:92–96
42. Van Ketel WG, De Haan P (1978) Occupational eczema from garlic and onion. Contact Dermatitis 4:53–64
43. Falleroni AE, Zeiss CR, Levitz D (1981) Occupational asthma secondary to inhalation of garlic dust. J Allergol Clin Immunol 68:156–160
44. Lybarger JA, Gallagher JS, Pulver DW, Litwin A, Brooks S, Bernstein IL (1982) Occupational asthma induced by inhalation and ingestion of garlic. J Allergy Clin Immunol 69:448–454
45. Papageorgiou C, Corbet JP, Menezes-Brandao F, Peceguieiro M, Benezra C (1983) Allergic contact dermatitis to garlic (Allium sativum L.). Identification of the allergens: the role of mono-, di-, and trisulfides present to garlic. A comparative study in man and animal (guinea pig). Arch Dermatol Res 275:229–234
46. Sinha SM, Pasricha JS, Sharma RC, Kandhari KC (1977) Vegetables responsible for contact dermatitis of the hands. Arch Dermatol 113:776–779
47. Mayerhofer E (1934) Nutzen und Schaden der Knoblauchanwendung im Kindesalter mit besonderer Berücksichtigung der Coeliakie. Arch Kinderheilkunde 102:106–116
48. Velazquez BL, Rodriguez JMO (1955) Action of garlic, corticotropin and cortisone on vaginal estrus. Arch Inst Farmacol Exptl (Madrid) 8:5–9
49. Velazquez BL, Rodriguez JMO (1955) Elimination of 17-keto steroids following the action of garlic extract. Arch Inst Farmacol Exptl (Madrid) 8:10–22
50. Schwahn H (1928) Hypertonie und Knoblauch. Schweiz Med Wochenschr 58:104–106
51. Flamm S (1935) Wurmkuren bei Schwangeren. Knoblauch-, Rainfarn-, Kürbiskuren. Hippokrates, pp 867–868
52. Anonymous (1986) The effect of essential oil of garlic on hyperlipemia and platelet aggregation. J Trad Clin Med 6:117–120
53. Turnheim K (1985) Adenosin irritiert den Darm. Österreich Apoth Ztg 39:724
54. Kamboj VP, Dhawan BN (1982) Research on plants for fertility regulation in India. J Ethnopharmacol 6:191–226
55. Velazquez BL, Sanchez B, Murias F, Mijan CD (1958) Garlic extract as an oxytocic substance. Arch Inst Farmacol Exptl (Madrid) 10:10–14
56. Abraham SK, Kesavan PC (1984) Genotoxicity of garlic, turmeric and asafoetida in mice. Mutat Res 136:85–88
57. Yoshida S, Hirao Y, Nakagawa S (1984) Mutagenicity and cryotoxicity tests of garlic. J Toxicol Sci 9:77–86
58. Takemura N, Shimizu H (1978) Mutagenicity of pyrolysis products of alliin and vitamin B. Mutat Res 54:255–256
59. Kada T, Sadaie Y, Hara M (1978) Analysis of mutagen-antimutagen reactions in food and food additives by the rec-assay and reversion-assay procedures. Mutat Res 53:206–207
60. Abraham SK, Kesavan PC (1983) An analysis of genotoxicity of spices in Drosophila. Mutat Res 108:373–383

Aristolochia Species

P.A.G.M. De Smet

Botany

The principal members of the genus of *Aristolochia* (Aristolochiaceae) which have been traditionally used in Western medicine are *A. clematitis* L. and *A. serpentaria* L. The former plant is called (long) birthwort or aristolochy in English and Osterluzei or Wolfskraut in German; both the roots or rhizomes and the herb have been in use for medicinal purposes. The latter botanical is known as Virginian snakeroot, Texan snakeroot, or serpentary; its medicinal parts are the roots and rootstock [1-6].

According to Penso's *Index Plantarum Medicinalium* [7], at least 65 other *Aristolochia* species are or have been employed as medicinal plants in various parts of the world. Due to an expanding public interest in exotic herbal remedies such species may occasionally reach the Western drug market. For instance, a few years ago an oriental herbal pill called Chien Pu Wan was introduced in the Netherlands for the treatment of rheumatic disorders. One of its 21 declared ingredients was 10 mg *Aristolochia fang-chi* Wu per pill (recommended dosage: 6-10 pills per day). The pill had escaped premarket evaluation by the Dutch health authorities by posing as a food supplement [8].

Chemistry

The herb of *Aristolochia clematitis* contains 0.026%-0.4% essential oil, tannins, resin-like substances, the bitter principle clematitin, β-sitosterin, and flavonol glycosides. The roots or rhizomes provide 0.24%-0.4% essential oil, tannin, resin, β-sitosterin, and allantoin [1,2,9].

The roots yield a yellow, bitter, and acidic substance that has become known as aristolochic acid (AA). Chemically, AA is a mixture of several chemically related nitrophenanthrene derivatives. The main constituents are 3,4-methylenedioxy-8-methoxy-10-nitrophenanthrene-1-carboxylic acid (aristolochic acid I = AA-I) and its nor-derivative aristolochic acid II (= AA-II). Minor components are aristolochic acid III, aristolochic acid IIIa, aristolochic acid IV, and aristolochic acid IVa [10-13].

In a TLC study by Schunack et al. [14], the roots of *A. clematitis* yielded approximately 2–5 mg/g AA-I and 2–6 mg/g AA-II, depending on habitat and harvest time; leaves showed lower levels of 1–2 mg/g AA-I and ≤ 1 mg/g AA-II. Gracza and Ruff [13] analyzed, by means of HPLC, several commercially available samples of Tinctura Aristolochiae clematitis, and recovered 0.1 mg/ml AA-I and 0.03–0.04 mg/ml AA-II.

Mengs and coworkers [15,16] indicate that AA as its sodium salt contains 77.2% AA-I and 21.2% AA-II, while Schmeiser et al. [17] recovered 65% AA-I and 35% AA-II from a commercially purchased AA mixture.

The roots of *Aristolochia serpentaria* contain tannin, a bitter principle, and 1%–2% essential oil with borneol [2]. Coutts et al. [18] recovered 0.046% AA and a trace of the lactam derivative aristored from a sample of dried serpentary root and rhizome.

Aristolochic acids and their lactam derivatives (aristolactams) have been isolated from several *Aristolochia* species other than *A. clematitis* and *A. serpentaria* [19]. The chemistry of these other species is reviewed in Table 1, in so far as they have been listed as medicinal plants in Penso's *Index Plantarum Medicinalium* [7].

Pharmacology and Uses

AA showed antineoplastic activity in subclinical testing [20,21], but this effect has not been confirmed in human trial [22]. AA can increase the phagocytic activity of leukocytes in laboratory animals [23,24], and it has been reported to stimulate the defence mechanism against herpes simplex infections of the rabbit eye [25]. Stimulation of phagocytic activity has also been observed in human volunteers [26], but placebo-controlled double-blind studies to confirm that AA is useful in human patients with microbial infection and/or a compromised immunological system have not been recovered from the literature. Yet AA has been recommended as a supplementary therapy for immunologically weakened patients. It has also served as an antiphlogistic agent and for the treatment of chronic, inflammatory skin diseases [27].

Aristolochia extracts have been employed for similar purposes, such as the treatment of arthritis, gout, rheumatism, and festering wounds [28]. The herb and roots of *A. clematitis* have also been in use as ingredients of homeopathic preparations [2].

The roots of *A. serpentaria* have been employed as bitters recommended for dyspepsia [5,6].

Pharmacokinetics

Krumbiegel et al. [29] studied the metabolism of AA-I and AA-II following oral administration to rats. In the case of AA-I, 83% of the dose was recovered in the

Table 1. The occurrence of aristolochic acids and aristolactams in species of *Aristolochia* other than *A. clematitis* and *A. serpentaria* [19] in so far as they have been listed as medicinal plants in Penso's *Index Plantarum Medicinalium* [7]

Aristolochia species	Ethno-botany[a]	Chemistry[b]
A. argentina Hesse	Am, Eu	AA: I, II, III, IV, IVa AR: I, AII, AIII, BII, BIII
A. bracteata Retz.	Af, As	AA: I AR: aristored
A. debilis Sieb. et Zucc.	As	AA: I, II, IIIa, IVa, B, debilic acid, 7-hydroxy-aristolochic acid I, 7-methoxy-aristolochic acid I AR: I
A. esperanzae O.K.	Am	AA: I, II, III, IV, IVa
A. fang-chi Wu	As	AA: I, IIIa, B AR: I
A. indica L.	Am, As, Eu	AA: I, IVa, methyl aristolochate AR: I, AII, aristolochic acid IVa methyl ether lactam, aristolactam I N-β-D-glucoside, aristolactam-C N-β-glucoside
A. kaempferi Willd.	As	AA: I
A. longa L.	Am, As, Eu	AA: I, II
A. manshuriensis Kom.	As	AA: I, II, IV, IVa, debilic acid, aristoloside
A. maxima Jacq.	Am	AA: I
A. mollissima Hance	As	AA: I
A. reticulata Nutt.	Am, As, Eu	AA: I AR: aristored
A. rotunda L.	Am, As, Eu	AA: I, II, IIIa AR: I
A. taliscana sic	Am	AR: taliscanine

[a] Geographical areas use are indicated by the following abbreviations: Af = Africa; Am = America; As = Asia; Eu = Europe.
[b] AA — aristolochic acids; AR = aristolactams. The annotations I, IIIa, and IVa are synonymous with the annotations A, C, and D, respectively.

form of aristolactam Ia (46% in the urine and 37% in the feces). This metabolite was excreted by the kidney predominantly in conjugated form. Minor urinary and fecal metabolites of AA-I were aristolactam I, aristolochic acid Ia, aristolic acid I, and 3,4-methylenedioxy-8-hydroxy-1-phenanthrenecarboxylic acid. In the case of AA-II, aristolactam II accounted for 13.5% of the administered dose (4.6% in the urine and 8.9% in the feces), with aristolactam Ia and 3,4-methylenedioxy-1-phenanthrenecarboxylic acid as additional metabolites. An unidentified metabolite of AA-II with a lactam structure was also encountered.

Experiments in other species revealed similar metabolite patterns of AA-I and AA-II in the mouse, but urine samples of guinea pigs, rabbits, dogs, and man did not yield all the metabolites found in rats. When human subjects were treated with a daily dose of 0.9 mg AA (AA-I + AA-II) for three days, only aristolactam I and aristolactam II could be identified in the urine collected on the third day [29].

Schulz et al. [30] measured AA levels in bodily fluids of human patients, who were treated with 0.9–1.35 mg oral AA per day for 3–5 days. By means of semiquantitative TLC analysis, they found 1/9 to 1/6 of the daily administered dose in urine, 1/7 to almost 1/3 in bile, not more than 1/100 in saliva, and 1/40 to 1/20 in breast milk. In at least one patient, the daily urinary excretion of AA rose from 1/9 on day 1 to almost 1/5 on day 3, which was suggestive of accumulation of AA in the human body. Approximately 5 μg/ml of AA was demonstrated in cerebrospinal liquid, but the researchers were unable to recover AA from serum. This report has been rightly criticized, however, for its poor reproduction of results and for its lack of information on metabolites [29].

Adverse Reaction Profile

General Animal Data

Che et al. [31] found AA-I to be lethal to rats at an oral dose level of 40 mg/kg and to hamsters at an oral dose level of 25 mg/kg.

Mengs [32] tested AA in rodents of both sexes and reported oral LD_{50} values of 203.4 mg/kg for male rats, 183.9 mg/kg for female rats, 55.9 mg/kg for male mice, and 106.1 mg/kg for female mice. He obtained intravenous LD_{50} values of 82.5 mg/kg, 74.0 mg/kg, 38.4 mg/kg, and 70.1 mg/kg, respectively. Predominant histological features were severe necrosis of the renal tubules, atrophy of the lymphatic organs, and widespread superficial ulceration of the forestomach.

Pakrashi and Chakrabarty [33] studied chromatographic fractions of the chloroform extract of *Aristolochia indica* root in the mouse. One fraction resulted in degenerative changes of the kidney while another fraction produced hemorrhagic spots with dilated blood vessels in the liver. The same research group also tested isolated constituents of *Aristolochia indica* root in the mouse and saw no acute toxicity from single intragastric doses of 1000 mg/kg of p-coumaric acid [34], 100 mg/kg of a sesquiterpene [35] later identified as (12S)-7,12-secoish-waran-12-ol [31], or 60 mg/kg of methyl aristolate [36]. However, repeated administration of methyl aristolate at a dose level of 60 mg/kg/day for 4 weeks (5 days/week) increased liver alkaline phosphatase activity, depleted liver glycogen, and decreased kidney alkaline phosphatase activity [37].

In goats treated with 0.5–5.0 g/kg/day of *Aristolochia bracteata* leaves by stomach tube, the main signs of poisoning were diarrhea, dyspnea, tympany, arching of the back, and loss of condition and hair from the back. Prominent pathological findings were hemorrhages in lungs, heart, and kidneys, fatty change and congestion in the liver, mucoid abomasitis and enteritis, and straw-colored fluid in serous cavities. In the serum, increases in aspartate aminotransferase activity and in ammonia and urea concentrations were detected, together with decreases in the levels of total protein and magnesium [38].

General Human Data

See for data on the human toxicity of AA the section of renal reactions.

Endocrine Reactions

Siess and Seybold [39] studied the influence of a homeopathic mother tincture of *Aristolochia clematitis* on the onset of the estrus in infantile and castrated female mice, and observed no estrogenic activity from a daily oral dose of 0.05 ml/animal.

The research group of Pakrashi reported antiestrogenic activity of aristolic acid [40] and a sesquiterpene [41] later identified as (12S)-7,12-secoishwaran-12-ol [31]. Both compounds are constituents of the root of *Aristolochia indica*.

Gastrointestinal Reactions

According to a textbook on Chinese medicine, the alcohol extract of aristolochia fruit (*Aristolochia contorta* Bge. or *A. debilis* Sieb. et Zucc.) may cause nausea, gastric discomfort or mild diarrhea in individual patients [42].

Jackson et al. [22] observed nausea in cancer patients treated intravenously with AA (see the section on renal reactions for details), but this effect was not a major problem.

Hematological Reactions

Jackson et al. [22] performed complete blood counts in cancer patients treated intravenously with AA and noted no significant hematological toxicity (see the section on renal reactions for details).

Hepatic Reactions

See for information about hepatotoxicity in animals the section on general animal data.

Although initial toxicity studies of AA in dogs had shown predominately hepatotoxicity, Jackson et al. [22] did not observe such toxicity in cancer patients treated intravenously with AA (see the section on renal reactions for details).

Renal Reactions

It is well established that AA can produce nephrotoxic reactions in the rabbit, the mouse, and the rat [32,42–46]. High doses of AA also lead to kidney damage in human beings [22,47].

Jackson et al. [22] tested intravenous AA in a phase I study involving 20 cancer patients. Two patients were given 24-h infusions while the remaining 18 patients received AA by a rapid infusion of 5–15 minutes. Dosage regimens ranged from 0.1 mg/kg per day for 5 days to a single dose of 2 mg/kg. Eight of 10 patients who were treated with 1 mg/kg/day for 3 or more days developed elevated blood urea nitrogen levels that occurred as early as the fourth day of therapy and persisted for as long as 2 months after the end of the treatment. The glomerular filtration rate, which was measured in a few patients, decreased as early as the second day. Several patients died with acute toxic nephrosis. In contrast, no renal toxicity occurred in nine of 10 patients, who received a daily dose of less than 1 mg/kg.

Thiele et al. [47] have associated the use of AA in man with necrosis of proximal tubuli and massive vasopressin-resistant polyuria. These manifestations of renal toxicity are similar to those observed in the rabbit [44].

Fertility, Pregnancy, and Lactation

The roots of *Aristolochia indica*, which is commonly known as Indian birthwort, have a reputation in Indian folk medicine as an emmenagogue and abortifacient [31,48]. Pakrashi and coworkers have extensively investigated the antifertility effects of this traditional medicine and its isolated constituents in rodents [33–36,40,41,48–53]. This research group found that various extracts of the root (petroleum ether, benzene, alcohol, chloroform, and fractions of the chloroform extract) had interceptive activity in the mouse [33,48,49]. Subsequently, the group reported that the following root constituents showed antifertility effects in the mouse or rabbit: aristolic acid [40,51,53], methyl aristolate [36], aristolactam N-β-D-glucoside [52], p-coumaric acid [34,52], and an unspecified sesquiterpene [35,41] later identified as (12S)-7,12-secoishwaran-12-ol [31]. No teratogenic effects were observed when chromatographic fractions of the chloroform extract [33] or p-coumaric acid [34] were tested in the mouse, but the water soluble fraction of the chloroform extract was found to have antispermatogenic activity in this animal species [50].

The antifertility effects of *Aristolochia indica* in rodents have also been investigated by Che et al. [31]. These investigators found that an alcoholic extract of *Aristolochia indica* root decreased fertility when administered postcoitally to rats or hamsters, but attempts to obtain the compound(s) responsible for this activity were unsuccessful. Petroleum ether, chloroform and aqueous fractions as well as various isolates and pure compounds (aristolochic acid I, aristolic acid, methyl aristolate, savinin, (12S)-7,12-secoishwaran-12-ol, cis-p-coumaric acid and trans-p-coumaric acid) were all inactive and/or toxic at the doses employed.

According to Saha et al. [54] aqueous leaf, stem and root extracts of *Aristolochia bracteata* showed little stimulant effect on the isolated guinea pig uterus previously sensitized by diethylstilbestrol. Matsui et al. [55] reported that subcutaneous treatment with an aqueous extract of *Aristolochia mollis* for 5 days did not affect the fertility of female mice.

The passage of AA into human breast milk following oral maternal use has been studied by Schulze et al. [30]. These investigators treated three nursing mothers with 1.35 mg of AA for three days and found 1/40 to 1/20 of the daily maternal dose in the milk. Just as the urinary excretion of AA (see the section on pharmacokinetics), the daily excretion of AA into the milk increased during treatment. Unfortunately, no information was given about metabolites.

Mutagenicity and Carcinogenicity

Recent studies in rodents suggest that AA is one of the most effective carcinogens yet known [15,56,57].

In one of these studies, intragastric administration of 10 mg/kg per day for three months induced severe papillomatosis of the entire forestomach with occasional signs of malignancy. Three to six months later, without further treatment, 14 of 35 rats (40%) had developed squamous cell carcinomas and another 31% showed microcarcinomas in the forestomach. Metastases (in regional and peripheral lymp nodes, intestinal mesentery, small intestine, and diaphragm) were observed in 46% of the animals, and occasionally carcinomas were seen in the kidneys, renal pelvis, and urinary bladder. When only 0.1 mg/kg per day was given for three months, no abnormalities were detected at the end of the treatment period, but nine months later 4 of 13 rats (31%) showed papilloma, and 15% had microcarcinoma or carcinoma in the forestomach; occasional hyperplasia of the transitional epithelium of the renal pelvis was also noted. When the low dose of 0.1 mg/kg was administered daily for twelve months and evaluated after four additional months, carcinoma in the forestomach occurred in 5 of 9 rats (56%) with formation of metastases in one animal [15].

These findings prompted the manufacturer who had initiated the study to take his AA product from the market in 1981 [58]. Shortly thereafter, the FRG health authorities decided to withdraw the licence of all AA preparations, including all homeopathic *Aristolochia* dilutions up to D10 [59–61]. It was taken into consideration that AA affects plant cells in concentrations as low as 0.5–10 nmol/ml [62] and that AA may accumulate in the human body [30].

AA was later reported to exert a carcinogenic effect of similar strength in the mouse. It induced papillomatous changes and, at a later stage, squamous cell carcinomas in the forestomach of this species after treatment with 5.0 mg/kg per day for three weeks. Other findings were adenocarcinoma in the glandular stomach, malignant lymphomas, adenomas of the kidneys, carcinomas of the lungs, and hemangiomas of the uterus [57].

Since the first carcinogenicity data became known, AA has been reported to be a direct mutagen in the *Salmonella typhimurium* strains TA 100 and TA 1537 [63], to have genotoxic activity in *Drosophila* tests [28], and to induce structural chromosome aberrations and sister chromatid exchanges in human lymphocytes [27]. AA was also shown to increase the mutant frequencies in extrahepatic tissue after administration by oral gavage to rats [64] and to produce genotoxic effects in the mouse micronucleus test [16].

AA-I and AA-II were found to have almost equal mutagenic potency in *Salmonella* strains TA 100 and TA 1537 [17]. However, comparative mutagenicity studies of these acids in vivo (in a subcutaneous granulation tissue in rats) and in vitro (in the corresponding target cells) suggest that the genotoxic activity of AA in mammals may be mainly caused by AA-I [65]. Research on DNA adduct formation by AA-I and AA-II has not shown a direct correlation with the initiation of the carcinogenic process and subsequent tumor formation in target tissues in the rat [66].

The corresponding lactam derivatives of AA-I and AA-II (aristolactam I and aristolactam II) are mutagenic in *Salmonella* strains, provided that a metabolizing system is present, but their potency is distinctly lower than that of AA-I and AA-II. An even weaker response was observed with aristolochic acid Ia (the O-demethylated derivative of AA-I). This latter compound was only mutagenic without the metabolizing system [67].

Other structural relatives for which mutagenic potential has been demonstrated by *Salmonella* testing include the methyl ester of AA-I, aristolic acid, and methyl aristolate [68].

References

1. Pylarczyk W (1958) Aristolochia clematitis L., die Osterluzei. I. Mitteilung. Planta Med 6:258–299
2. List PH, Hörhammer L (1972) Hagers Handbuch der Pharmazeutischen Praxis, 4th edn, vol 3: Chemikalien und Drogen (Am-Ch). Berlin: Springer-Verlag
3. Lust JB (1974) The Herb Book. New York: Bantam Books
4. Gessner O, Orzechowski G (1974) Gift- und Arzneipflanzen von Mitteleuropa, 3rd edn. Heidelberg: Carl Winter Universitätsverlag
5. Spoerke Jr DG (1980) Herbal Medications. Santa Barbara: Woodbridge Press Publishing Co.
6. Reynolds JEF (ed) (1989) Martindale The Extra Pharmacopoeia. 29th edn. London: The Pharmaceutical Press
7. Penso G (1983) Index Plantarum Medicinalium Totius Mundi Eorumque Synonymorum. Milano: Organizzazione Editoriale Medico Farmaceutica
8. De Smet PAGM (1986) 'Chien Pu Wan' pillen. Pharm Weekbl 121:437–442
9. Hoppe HA (1975) Drogenkunde, vol 1: Angiospermen. 8th edn. Berlin: Walter de Gruyter
10. Pailer M, Belohlav L, Simonitsch E (1955) Zur Konstitution der Aristolochiasäuren. Monatsh Chem 86:676–680
11. Pailer M, Bergthaller P, Schaden G (1965) Über die Isolierung und Charakterisierung von vier neuen Aristolochiasäuren (aus Aristolochia clematitis L.). Monatsh Chem 96:863–883
12. Pailer M, Bergthaller P (1966) Die Konstitution der Aristolochiasäuren III und IIIa. Monatsh Chem 97:484–493

13. Gracza L, Ruff P (1981) Einfache Methode zur Bestimmung der Aristolochiasäuren durch HPLC. Dtsch Apoth Ztg 121:2817-2818
14. Schunack W, Mutschler E, Rochelmeyer H (1967) Über das Vorkommen der Aristolochiasäuren I und II in *Aristolochia clematitis* L. in Abhängigkeit von Jahreszeit und Standort. Pharmazie 22:118-120
15. Mengs U, Lang W, Poch J-A (1982) The carcinogenic action of aristolochic acid in rats. Arch Toxicol 51:107-119
16. Mengs U, Klein M (1988) Genotoxic effects of aristolochic acid in the mouse micronucleus test. Planta Med 54:502-503
17. Schmeiser HH, Pool BL, Wiessler M (1984) Mutagenicity of the two main components of commercially available carcinogenic aristolochic acid in *Salmonella typhimurium*. Cancer Lett 23:97-101
18. Coutts RT, Stenlake JB, Williams WD (1959) The chemistry of the *Aristolochia* species. V. A comparative study of acidic and basic constituents of *A. reticulata* Linn., *A. serpentaria* Linn., *A. longa* Linn. and *A. indica* Linn. J Pharm Pharmacol 11:607-17
19. Mix DB, Guinaudeau H, Shamma M (1982) The aristolochic acids and aristolactams. J Nat Prod 45:657-666
20. Filitis LN, Massagetov PS (1962) Anticancer property of aristolochic acid. Chem Ab 56:4060b
21. Kupchan SM, Doskotch RW (1962) Tumor inhibitors. I. Aristolochic acid, the active principle of *Aristolochia indica*. J Med Pharm Chem 5:657-659
22. Jackson L, Kofman S, Weiss A, Brodovsky H (1964) Aristolochic acid (NSC-50413): phase I clinical study. Cancer Chemother Rep 42:35-37
23. Möse JR (1966) Weitere Untersuchungen über die wirkung der *Aristolochia*-säure. Arzneim Forsch 16:118-122
24. Bartfeld H (1977) Immunologische Untersuchungen zum Nachweis der abwehrsteigernden Wirkung von Aristolochiasäure. Arzneim Forsch 27:2297-2298
25. Möse JR, Stünzner D, Zirm M, Egger-Büssing C, Schmalzl F (1980) Experimentelle Beeinflussung der Herpes-simplex-Infektion des Kaninchen-Auges durch Aristolochiasäure. Arzneim Forsch 30:1571-1573
26. Kluthe R, Vogt A, Batsford S (1982) Doppelblindstudie zur Beeinflussung der Phagozytosefähigkeit von Granulozyten. Arzneim Forsch 32:443-445
27. Abel G, Schimmer O (1983) Induction of structural chromosome aberrations and sister chromatid exchanges in human lymphocytes in vitro by aristolochic acid. Hum Genet 64:131-133
28. Frei H, Würgler FE, Juon H, Hall CB, Graf U (1985) Aristolochic acid is mutagenic and recombinogenic in *Drosophila* genotoxicity tests. Arch Toxicol 56:158-166
29. Krumbiegel G, Hallensleben J, Mennicke WH, Rittmann N, Roth HJ (1987) Studies on the metabolism of aristolochic acids I and II. Xenobiotica 17:981-991
30. Schulz M, Weist F, Gemählich M (1971) Dünnschichtchromatographischer Nachweis der *Aristolochia*-Säure in verschiedenen Körperflüssigkeiten. Arzneim Forsch 21:934-936
31. Che CT, Ahmed MS, Kang SS et al. (1984) Studies on *Aristolochia*. III. Isolation and biological evaluation of constituents of *Aristolochia indica* roots for fertility-regulating activity. J Nat Prod 47:331-341
32. Mengs U (1987) Acute toxicity of aristolochic acid in rodents. Arch Toxicol 59:328-331
33. Pakrashi A, Chakrabarty B (1977) Biological properties of interceptive agents from Aristolochia indica Linn. Indian J Med Res 66:991-998
34. Pakrashi A, Pakrasi P (1978) Biological profile of p-coumaric acid isolated from *Aristolochia indica* Linn. Indian J Exp Biol 16:1285-1287
35. Pakrashi A, Shaha C (1977) Effect of a sesquiterpene from *Aristolochia indica* Linn. on fertility in female mice. Experientia 33:1498-1499
36. Pakrashi A, Shaha C (1978) Effect of methyl ester of aristolic acid from *Aristolochia indica* Linn. on fertility of female mice. Experientia 34:1192-1193
37. Pakrashi A, Shaha C (1979) Short term toxicity study with methyl ester of aristolic acid from *Aristolochia indica* Linn. in mice. Indian J Exp Biol 17:437-439
38. Barakat SE, Wasfi IA, Adam SE (1983) The toxicity of *Aristolochia bracteata* in goats. Vet Pathol 20:611-616

39. Siess M, Seybold G (1960) Untersuchungen über die Wirkung von *Pulsatilla pratensis*, *Cimicifuga racemosa* und *Aristolochia clematitis* auf den Östrus infantiler und kastrierter weißer Mäuse. Arzneim Forsch 10:514–520

40. Pakrashi A, Chakrabarty B (1978) Anti-oestrogenic & anti-implantation effect of aristolic acid from *Aristolochia indica* (Linn.). Indian J Exp Biol 16:1283–1285

41. Pakrashi A, Shaha C (1977) Anti-implantation & anti-oestrogenic activity of a sesquiterpene from the roots of *Aristolochia indica* Linn. Indian J Exp Biol 15:1197–1198

42. Shiying G (1986) Madouling. In: Chang H-M, But PP-H (eds) Pharmacology and applications of Chinese materia medica. Singapore: World Scientific Publishing, pp 157–159

43. Decsi L, Méhes G, Varga F (1958) The role of the proximal tubular cells of the kidney in antidiuretic hormone action in the rabbit. Acta Physiol Sci Hung 13:21–26

44. Méhes J, Decsi L, Varga F, Kovács S (1958) Selektive chemische Ausschaltung der Harnkanälchen. I. Ordnung bei Kaninchen. Naunyn-Schmiedeberg's Arch Exp Pathol Pharmakol 234:548–565

45. Hedwall PR (1961) Einfluß der Aristolochiasäure auf die Nierenfunktionen von Ratten. Naunyn-Schmiedeberg's Arch Exp Pathol 24:550–551

46. Peters G, Hedwall PR (1963) Aristolochic acid intoxication: a new type of impairment of urinary concentrating ability. Arch Int Pharmacodyn 145:334–355

47. Thiele KG, Muercke RC, Berning H (1967) Nierenerkrankungen durch Medikamente. Dtsch Med Wschr 92:1632–1635

48. Pakrashi A, Pakrashi PL (1977) Interceptive & abortifacient activity of *Aristolochia indica* L. & possible mode of action. Indian J Exp Biol 15:428–430

49. Pakrashi A, Chakrabarty B, Dasgupta A (1976) Effect of the extracts from *Aristolochia indica* Linn. on interception in female mice. Experientia 32:394–395

50. Pakrashi A, Pakrashi PL (1977) Antispermatogenic effect of the extract of *Aristolochia indica* Linn on male mice. Indian J Exp Biol 15:256–259

51. Pakrashi A, Chakrabarty B (1978) Antifertility effect of aristolic acid from *Aristolochia indica* (Linn) in female albino rabbits. Experientia 34:1377

52. Pakrashi A, Pakrasi P (1979) Antifertility efficacy of the plant *Aristolochia indica* Linn on mouse. Contraception 20:49–54

53. Ganguly T, Pakrashi A, Pal AK (1986) Disruption of pregnancy in mouse by aristolic acid. I. Plausible explanation in relation to early pregnancy events. Contraception 34:625–637

54. Saha JC, Savini EC, Kasinathan S (1961) Ecbolic properties of Indian medicinal plants. I. Indian J Med Res 49:130–151

55. Matsui AS, Rogers J, Woo YK, Cutting WC (1967) Effects of some natural products on fertility in mice. Med Pharmacol Exp Int J Exp Med 16:414–424

56. Mengs U (1983) On the histopathogenesis of rat forestomach carcinoma caused by aristolochic acid. Arch Toxicol 52:209–220

57. Mengs U (1988) Tumour induction in mice following exposure to aristolochic acid. Arch Toxicol 61:504–505

58. Anonymous (1981) Tardolyt-Dragées zurückgezogen. Österreich Apoth Ztg 35:317

59. Anonymous (1981) Zum Zulassungswiderruf Aristolochiasäure-haltiger Fertigarzneimittel. Pharm Ztg 126:1373–1374

60. Anonymous (1982) BGA hält am Verbot für Aristolochiasäure-haltige Arzneimittel fest. Dtsch Apoth Ztg 122:2487

61. Hagemann U, Grase R, Thiele A, Bass R, Schönhöfer PS (1982) Probleme der Arzneimittelsicherheit: Aristolochiasäure. Münch Med Wschr 124:611–612

62. Moretti C, Rideau M, Chénieux JC, Viel C (1979) Isolement de l'acide aristolochique de deux aristoloches malgaches. Détermination de sa cytotoxicité sur cellules végétales. Comparaison avec les cellules animales. Planta Med 35:360–365

63. Robisch G, Schimmer O, Göggelmann W (1982) Aristolochic acid is a direct mutagen in *Salmonella typhimurium*. Mutat Res 105:201–204

64. Maier P, Schawalder HP, Weibel B, Zbinden G (1985) Aristolochic acid induces 6-thioguanine-resistant mutants in an extra-hepatic tissue in rats after oral application. Mutat Res 143:143–148

65. Maier P, Schawalder H, Weibel B (1987) Low oxygen tension, as found in tissues in vivo, alters the mutagenic activity of aristolochic acid I and II in primary fibroblast-like rat cells in vitro. Environ Mol Mutagen 10:275–284
66. Schmeiser HH, Schoepe KB, Wiessler M (1988) DNA adduct formation of aristolochic acid I and II in vitro and in vivo. Carcinogenesis 9:297–303
67. Schmeiser HH, Pool BL, Wiessler M (1986) Identification and mutagenicity of metabolites of aristolochic acid formed by rat liver. Carcinogenesis 7:59–63
68. Pezzuto JM, Swanson SM, Mar W, Che C-T, Cordell GA, Fong HHS (1988) Evaluation of the mutagenic and cytostatic potential of aristolochic acid (3,4-methylenedioxy-8-meth-oxy-10-nitrophenanthrene-1-carboxylic acid) and several of its derivatives. Mutat Res 206:447–454

Asafetida

P.A.G.M. De Smet

Botany

Asafetida is an oleo-gum resin obtained by incising the living rhizome and roots of *Ferula assa-foetida* L., *F. rubricaulis* Boiss., *F. foetida* (Bunge) Regel, and other species of *Ferula* (Umbelliferae). Vernacular names include asafetida, asant, devil's dung, and gum asafetida [1-4].

Contamination of asafetida with other materials, such as sand and other gum resins, has been common [1,3,5].

Chemistry

Asafetida contains 10-65% of resin, 25-30% of bassorin-like gum, and 6-20% of essential oil [6-8]. The resin was initially considered to consist primarily of the ferulic acid ester of asaresinotannol [4]. Caglioti et al. [9] later reported the presence of three sesquiterpene-umbelliferone complexes, which they named farnesiferols A, B, and C. Kajimoto et al. [10] recently isolated two other sesquiterpene-umbelliferone complexes, called asacoumarin A and asacoumarin B, from the root or rhizome of *Ferula assa-foetida* purchased on the Chinese market. They noted that the previously described farnesiferols might be artifacts derived from asacoumarin A.

The essential oil contains 17%-37% of disulfides [6,7], such as 1-methylpropyl 1-propenyl disulfide, 1-(methylthio)-propyl 1-propenyl disulfide, and 1-methylpropyl 3-(methylthio)-2-propenyl disulfide [11,12]. Recently the isolation of asadisulfide from *F. assa-foetida* was described [10].

Samimi and Unger [5] analyzed Afghan samples of *Ferula foetida* roots and found 0.15-0.68% of essential oil containing 0.15-1.97% of sulfur. They also purchased commercial samples of asafetida in Afghan bazars and recovered 2.4-37.1% of ash (a measure for mineral admixtures). The ash-free part of these samples contained 7.3-24.7% of essential oil with a sulfur content of 0.91-4.54%.

An Indian research group [3,13] studied commercial asafetida samples called hing and hingra. Hing asafetida, which is used for flavoring purposes, is derived chiefly from *Ferula alliacea* and also to a limited extent from *F. narthex* and *F.*

assa-foetida. Samples of this type yielded 6.7–19.6% of essential oil with a sulfur content of 3.3–12.3%. A sample of hingra asafetida, which is obtained from *F. foetida* and is used for medicinal purposes, was found to contain 10.2% of essential oil with 6.6% of sulfur.

Pharmacology and Uses

Asafetida has been employed as a carminative and as an expectorant. It was formerly used in psychiatric disorders, but any effect it may have had in these conditions should in all probability be attributed to the psychological response to its objectionable odor and taste [1,2,14]. Asafetida has also been applied in topical preparations for breaking children of the habit of sucking their thumb [15].

Asafetida is used to give Worcestershire sauce its distinctive aroma [1].

Adverse Reaction Profile

General Human Data

Asafetida has a bitter acrid taste and a disagreeable, garlic-like odor, which is due chiefly to its volatile oil [1,2]. It imparts its odor to excretions and eructations [14,16]. Lewin [16] mentions that swollen lips, gastric burning, belching, flatulence, and diarrhea have sometimes been observed following the medical use of asafetida. A burning feeling during urination, headaches, and dizziness are also said to be possible. Unfortunately, Lewin does not provide an original reference to back up these claims.

Bordia and Arora [17] observed no overt side effects in ten healthy volunteers, who received a large oral dose of 3 g asafetida together with 100 g butter on bread slices. According to American textbooks [1,14], half an ounce (approximately 15 g) has been taken as one dose with no noticeable effects other than a local action, but these statements are not supported by a primary reference.

Gastrointestinal Reactions

Desai and Kalro [18] studied the effects of intragastric instillation of asafetida in doses of 0.1, 0.2, and 0.4 g/h in 14 human volunteers. Infusion of 0.2 and 0.4 g/h significantly increased the deoxyribonucleic acid content of gastric aspirate, suggesting increased exfoliation of gastric surface epithelial cells. The lower dose rate of 0.1 g/h did not produce a significant change. In view of such experimental damage to the gastric mucosa, it would seem prudent to avoid the use of large doses of asafetida in patients with a peptic ulcer. It should perhaps be added, however, that even though red chilli powder causes similar experimental gastric damage, a daily regimen of 3 g red chilly powder (1 g with each meal) was reported not to influence the healing of duodenal ulcer [19].

See also the general human data of the adverse reaction profile.

Hematological Reactions

Kelly et al. [20] observed a case of methemoglobinemia in a 5-week-old male infant who had been given glycerited asafetida by his mother for treatment of colic. Besides cyanosis, the infant showed tachypnea, grunting, lethargy, a distended abdomen without bowel sounds, and bloody stools with mucus. The cyanosis did not disappear spontaneously but cleared within minutes when the child was given an intravenous infusion of methylene blue. The level of methemoglobin drawn prior to this infusion was 34.7% compared to 2.1% after the administration of methylene blue. To determine whether the glycerited asafetida had played a role, its oxidative effects on purified adult and fetal hemoglobin were studied in vitro. Incubation with adult hemoglobin for 2.5 h produced a minimal degree of methemoglobin formation, but when fetal hemoglobin was tested under the same experimental conditions, almost 90% was converted to the methemoglobin form by the end of 2.5 h. The known ingredients of glycerited asafetida other than asafetida (glycerol, propylene glycol, calcium carbonate) had no demonstrable oxidative effect on adult or fetal hemoglobin.

Fertility, Pregnancy, and Lactation

A brief entry from India in *Chemical Abstracts* stated that a mixture containing asafetida as one of its ingredients prevents conception for at least one year when 22 daily doses are taken while abstaining from intercourse. The powdered constituents for a course were said to be 4 drams of the active principle of *Embelia ribes*, 4 drams of *Piper longum*, 2 drams of purified asafetida, and 4 drams of purified borax, to give 22 doses [21]. It goes without saying that such an undetailed claim cannot be accepted as evidence. Even if there is some truth in it, this would not prove that asafetida has contraceptive activity since the other two vegetal ingredients of the mixture, *Embelia ribes* and *Piper longum*, are both listed as Indian plants investigated for fertility regulation [22].

Walia [23] studied the effect of asafetida on mouse spermatocytes in vivo. Male mice received a single dose of 10–5000 mg/kg bw by intragastric tube or were given this dose once daily for 32 days. The findings in animals treated with one dose were similar to those in controls. In the chronic experiment, however, three types of chromosomal aberrations (namely fragments, translocations, and detached X and Y) were observed in animals treated with 50 mg/kg bw or more. It should be noted that human intake is normally substantially lower than these experimental dose levels.

The literature has yielded no references on the use of asafetida during pregnancy and lactation.

Mutagenicity and Carcinogenicity

Shashikanti and Hosono [24] reported a weak mutagenic effect of asafetida towards streptomycin-dependent strains of *Salmonella typhimurium* TA 98.

Clastogenic effects of asafetida on chromosomes have been detected in plant cells of *Vicia faba* [25] and in mouse spermatocytes (see the section on fertility, pregnancy, and lactation). Abraham and Kesavan [26] studied asafetida (as a hot water extract) in *Drosophila melanogaster* and did not find a significant increase in the frequency of sex chromosome loss and sex-linked recessive lethal mutations. These researchers also evaluated the capacity of asafetida to induce sister-chromatid exchanges (SCEs) in spermatogonia of mice [27]. An intragastric dose of 0.5 g/kg bw did not produce a significant increase in the number of SCEs per diploid genome, but such an increase was detected following the administration of 1 g/kg bw. This test dose was very high, however, and its effect was weaker than that of the positive control (0.005 g/kg bw cyclophosphamide).

Studies on the carcinogenicity of asafetida have not been recovered from the literature.

References

1. Osol A, Farrar GE (1955) The dispensatory of the United States of America. 25th edn. Philadelphia: J.B. Lippincott Company
2. Wade A, Reynolds JEF (eds) (1977) Martindale the extra pharmacopoeia. 27th edn. London: The Pharmaceutical Press
3. Raghavan B, Abraham KO, Shankaranarayana ML, Sastry LVL, Natarajan CP (1974) Asafoetida. II. Chemical composition and physicochemical properties. Flavour Industry 5:179–181
4. Martinetz D, Kohs KH (1987) Der Asant, ein vergessenes Heilmittel und Gewürz. Naturwiss Rundsch 40:85–91
5. Samimi MN, Unger W (1979) Die Gummiharze Afghanischer "Asa foetida"- liefernder Ferula-Arten. Beobachtungen zur Herkunft und Qualität Afghanischer "Asa foetida". Planta Med 36:128–133
6. List PH, Hörhammer L (1973) Hagers Handbuch der Pharmazeutischen Praxis. 4th edn Vol 4: Chemikalien und Drogen (CI-G). Berlin: Springer-Verlag
7. Hoppe HA (1975) Drogenkunde. vol 1. Angiospermen. 8th edn. Berlin: Walter de Gruyter
8. Martinetz D, Kohs KH (1988) Asa foetida — Heilmittel der asiatischen Volksmedizin. Pharmazie 43:720–722
9. Caglioti L, Naef H, Arigoni D, Jeger O (1958) Zur Kenntnis der Sesquiterpene und Azulene. 126. Mitteilung Über die Inhaltsstoffe der *Asa foetida*. I. Farnesiferol A. Helv Chim Acta 41:2278–2292
10. Kajimoto T, Yahiro K, Nohara T (1989) Sesquiterpenoid and disulphide derivatives from *Ferula assa-foetida*. Phytochemistry 28:1761–1763
11. Shankaranarayana ML, Raghavan B, Abraham KO, Natarajan CP (1974) Volatile sulfur compounds in food flavors. CRC Crit Rev Food Technol 4:395–435

12. Budavari S (ed) (1989) The Merck index. An encyclopedia of chemicals, drugs, and biologicals. Rahway: Merck & Co, Inc.
13. Abraham KO, Shankaranarayana ML, Sastry LVL, Natarajan CP (1973) Asafoetida. I. Oxidimetric determination of the volatile oil. Flavour Industry 4:301–302
14. Sollmann T (1957) A manual of pharmacology and its applications to therapeutics and toxicology. 8th edn. Philadelphia: W.B. Saunders Company
15. Anonymous (1982) Rote Liste 1982. Aulendorf: Editio Cantor, no. 38 009
16. Lewin L (1962) Gifte und Vergiftungen. Lehrbuch der Toxikologie. 5th edn. Ulm/Donau: Karl F. Haug Verlag
17. Bordia A, Arora SK (1975) The effect of essential oil (active principle) of asafoetida on alimentary lipemia. Indian J Med Res 63:707–711
18. Desai HG, Kalro RH (1985) Effect of black pepper & asafoetida on the DNA content of gastric aspirates. Indian J Med Res 81:325–329
19. Kumar N, Vij JC, Sarin SK, Anand BS (1984) Do chillies influence healing of duodenal ulcer? Br Med J 288:1803–1804
20. Kelly KJ, Neu J, Camitta BM, Honig GR (1984) Methemoglobinemia in an infant treated with the folk remedy glycerited asafoetida. Pediatrics 73:717–719
21. Das PC (1966) Oral contraceptive. Chem Abstracts 64:19328–19329
22. Kamboj VP, Dhawan BN (1982) Research on plants for fertility regulation in India. J Ethnopharmacol 6:191–226
23. Walia K (1973) Effect of asafoetida (7-hydroxycoumarin) on mouse spermatocytes. Cytologia (Tokyo) 38:719–724
24. Shashikanth KN, Hosono A (1986) In vitro mutagenicity of tropical spices to streptomycin-dependent strains of *Salmonella typhimurium* TA 98. Agric Biol Chem 50:2947–2948
25. Das TN, Raj AS, Rao BVR (1968) Cytological studies in *Vicia faba* L. treated with asafoetida. Cytologia 33:100–111
26. Abraham SK, Kesavan PC (1978) Evaluation of possible mutagenicity of ginger, turmeric, asafoetida, clove and cinnamon administered alone and in combination with caffeine or theophylline in *Drosophila melanogaster*. Mutat Res 53:142
27. Abraham SK, Kesavan PC (1984) Genotoxicity of garlic, turmeric and asafoetida in mice. Mutat Res 136:85–88

Berberine

K.F. Lampe

Botany

The alkaloid berberine is present in 23 genera spanning 7 plant families. The most important berberine-containing herbal medications are derived from *Berberis aristata* DC. (India), *B. vulgaris* L. (Europe), *Mahonia aquifolium* (Pursh) Nutt. (N Am), *M. nervosa* (Pursh) Nutt. (N Am), *M. repens* (Lindl.) G. Don f. (N Am) of the Berberidaceae, *Hydrastis canadensis* L. (N Am), *Coptis chinensis* Wils. (China), *C. trifolia* (L.) Salisb. (NE Asia, Alaska), *C. teeta* Wallich, syn. *C. teetoides* C.Y. Cheng (Himalaya), *Xanthorrhiza simplicissima* Marshall (N Am) of the Ranunculaceae, *Sanguinaria canadensis* L. (N Am) of the Papaveraceae, and *Phellodendron amurense* Rupr. (Japan, E Asia) of the Rutaceae. In some of these plants berberine does not constitute the only physiologically dominant alkaloid, for example in *Hydrastis canadensis* or *Sanguinaria canadensis*. A number of additional berberine-containing plants of restricted geographical application in herbal medicine have been described for India [1] and China [2,3].

Unless otherwise specified, only extracts of plants in the genera *Mahonia* or *Berberis* or the alkaloid berberine and its salts will be considered. The major crude drug sources for berberine in commerce are *M. aquifolium* and *M. nervosa* [4]. The taxonomy of *Mahonia* and *Berberis* was revised most recently by Ahrendt [5].

Berberis vulgaris may be selected as a representative of that genus. Its vernacular name is barberry in English (occasionally it is called pipperidge bush or sowberry in Great Britain), Berberitze or Sauerdorn in Germany, epine-vinette in France, crespino in Italy, agrecejo or alvo in Spain, and uva-espin in Portugal. *Mahonia aquifolium* is known as Oregon or mountain grape, holly-mahonia, holly-barberry, or holly-grape, and as blue barberry in the United States and Canada. Where it has been introduced elsewhere it generally is known as mahonia or by some variant spelling of the generic name.

Chemistry

Berberine is found in highest concentration, about 6.1%, in the root bark of *B. vulgaris*, with lesser amounts in the above-ground stem bark and just 0.4% in the woody portion of the root [6]. Only traces of berberine are present in the leaves, and the alkaloid is absent from the flowers, fruit pulp, and seeds [7]. It is present, however, in the seeds of some other species in this genus. Other alkaloids in *B. vulgaris* include berbamine, berberrubine, bervulcine, columbamine, isotetrandine, jatrorrhizine, oxycanthine, palmatine, and vulcracine [8]. Alkaloids contained in other species of *Berberis* have been tabulated [9–11].

Similarly, medicinal collections of *Mahonia* are made from the rhizomes and roots. In addition to berberine, *M. aquifolium* has been reported to contain the alkaloids aromoline, berbamine, columbamine, corytuberine, isoboldine, isocorydine, isotentrandine, jatrorrhizine, magnoflorine, obanegine, oxyberberine, oxycanthine, and palmatine [12–14]. Berberine is absent from the leaves and seeds in this species. Magnoflorine is the predominant alkaloid in the above-ground stem bark. Alkaloids contained in other species of *Mahonia* have been reviewed [15].

Pharmacology and Uses

Except in China and in ayurvedic medicine in India, the therapeutic application of galenical preparations of berberine-containing plants or of berberine itself is considered obsolete [4]. A historical survey of such preparations and their associated health claims is given in numerous compendia [16–20].

Most animal and clinical studies in the 20th century have focused on berberine or one of its salts.

Little attention has been given to the potential pharmacological influence of the alkaloids other than berberine in *Berberis* and *Mahonia*. One study in which both the berberine and total alkaloid content of *Berberis* and *Mahonia* extracts were determined showed no correlation between the oral LD_{50} and the amount of berberine present [21]. The rather limited studies of the pharmacology of individual nonberberine alkaloids have been summarized elsewhere [2,11,22–26].

Berberis aristata and other berberine-containing plants have been used for millenia in China and India, primarily as antidiarrheal medications. During the 20th century the use of berberine salts has attracted particular attention for the management of diarrhea associated with cholera [27] in addition to the use of berberine salts for diarrhea of other etiology. Despite the rather large body of published open clinical observations [28,29] only two controlled studies have examined the effect of berberine alone, in combination with tetracycline, and by tetracycline alone on fluid loss by diarrhea in patients with cholera or in non-cholera diarrhea. In the first study, in which berberine chloride was employed in a dose of 100 mg four times daily, the alkaloid did not exhibit a significant vibriostatic effect, exhibited only a slight effect on stool volume, and possibly reduced the vibriostatic effect of tetracycline. Neither tetracycline nor berberine demonstrated any benefit over placebo in patients with noncholera diarrhea of unspecified etiologies [28]. In a later study, different dosage regimens were studied: 400 mg berberine sulfate as a single-bolus dose for enterotoxigenic *Escherichia coli*-induced diarrhea and either 400 mg as a single-bolus dose or 1200 mg berberine sulfate in 400 mg doses every 8 h for 24 h for cholera. These doses of berberine produced a significant reduction of mean stool volume during enterotoxigenic *E. coli*-diarrhea regardless of strain (ST or LT). Although berberine produced a modest antisecretory effect in cholera patients, this was overshadowed by the far more powerful and specific activity of tetracycline [29].

The antibacterial [3,30,31] and antiamebic [32] activity of berberine-containing plant extract or of berberine salts have been examined in vitro and in animal models. There are case reports purporting value of oral berberine medication as an antigiardial drug [33] and in visceral leishmaniasis [34].

The other traditional application of berberine-containing plants is as a cholagogue [16]. A clinical study supporting this activity in patients with chronic cholecystitis using an oral dose of 5 to 20 mg berberine sulfate or chloride administered before meals three times a day for one or two days has been reported [35].

The nonoral use of berberine (IV infusion, intradermal injection) is not discussed here. Other claims made for the efficacy of berberine in malaria, arthritis, dysmenorrhea, gout, renal disease, and a number of other conditions have not been substantiated [20].

Pharmacokinetics

Attempts at distribution studies in rats after oral administration of berberine sulfate were unsuccessful since, even with doses as high as 1 g/kg, only traces of berberine were found in a few tissues. This is as would be anticipated for a quaternary compound. Examination of the intestines of these animals revealed that the drug was neither being absorbed nor destroyed [36].

The oral administration of 500 mg/kg berberine sulfate to infant rabbits (10 days; 100 to 150 g) did result in absorption, producing a maximum whole blood concentration of 0.8 μg/ml at 8 h. The distribution of berberine in the heart, pancreas, liver, kidney, lung, and spleen at 12 h and the elimination in the urine and stool at 12, 24, and 48 h were reported [37].

Following parenteral administration to rats, only small quantities (less than 1%) are excreted in unchanged form in the urine [36]. The remaining berberine undergoes hepatic biotransformation. The elimination half-life of berberine chloride in rats following intraperitoneal or oral administration is between 5 and 6 h [25].

No human pharmacokinetic data for berberine is available, although a qualitative observation has been made that, unlike animals, a considerable quantity of berberine is excreted unchanged in the urine of man [1].

Adverse Reaction Profile

General Animal Data

The oral LD_{50} in mice of berberine, with a 24-h observation period, is 3.29 mg/10 g [21].

An oral dose of 2.75 g berberine to dogs (weight unspecified) produced severe gastrointestinal irritation, profuse, watery diarrhea, salivation, muscular tremors, and paralysis. Respiration was not affected. After death the intestines were found to be contracted, generally empty or containing mucous and watery fluid, and inflamed [38].

Oral doses of 100 mg/kg berberine sulfate were reported to be well tolerated by rats, with the comment that "no marked CNS effects were seen" [32].

An oral dose of 25 mg/kg the sulfate to cats induced depression in about 1 h lasting for 6 to 8 h; 50 mg/kg caused salivation and sporadic emesis but with recovery within 24 h. A dose of 100 mg/kg induced persistent emesis for 6 to 8 h and the death of all animals 8 to 10 days later [39].

The chronic oral administration of 25 mg/kg berberine sulfate for 10 days to cats was not associated with any gross or microscopic changes. Doses of 50 or 100 mg/kg induced serous hemorrhagic inflammation of the small and large intestine [39].

The intraperitoneal administration of 5, 20, or 40 mg/kg berberine chloride to cats produced sedation at all doses beginning within 3 to 5 min and persisting for less than 2 h. A single cat exhibited a transient rage reaction. These authors also reported that the intraperitoneal administration of 5 mg/kg berberine chloride markedly reduced amphetamine-induced motor hyperactivity in mice [40].

An oral dose of 25 mg/kg berberine sulfate in cats induced sedation in about 1 h, lasting for 6 to 8 h. Lethal intravenous doses of berberine sulfate in the dog or cat cause central respiratory failure prior to cardiac arrest. These doses are associated also with pulmonary edema and hemorrhage [1].

General Human Data[1]

Berberine has been reported to be well tolerated in therapeutic doses of 0.5 g; serious intoxications in man being unknown [41]. It should be noted carefully, however, that no systematic studies have been conducted during which contemporary laboratory methods have been employed to assess organ function during either the acute or chronic administration of berberine salts or of berberine-containing plant extracts. *Hagers Handbuch* lists a number of berberine-related side effects, but without reference [42]. Many of these could not be verified, nor is it clear if some of the stated adverse effects were found only in

---

[1] See also the note added in proof on p. 261.

animal studies utilizing parenteral rather than oral administration. A short general review of the safety of herbal medications lists berberine as possibly hepatotoxic, but also without reference [43]. The unreferenced symptoms of toxicity given by Roth et al. [41], "nausea, emesis, diarrhea, renal irritation, nephritis," appear to be a composite of effects elicited following the oral administration of 2.75 g berberine (base or salt not stated) to unanesthetized dogs, weight not stated [38], and the observation by Mezey [44] that two out of ten unanesthetized dogs developed hematuria at an intravenous dose of 8–10 mg/kg; this author reported the lethal dose in dogs by this route to be 10–20 mg/kg [44].

The Department of National Health and Welfare of Canada has restricted access to *Berberis vulgaris*, *Hydrastis canadensis*, and *Mahonia aquifolium* by adding these plants, or any part or derivative of these plants, to a list of food adulterants that may not be sold in food stores. The regulation does not affect the use of such products in medicines, the practice of herbology (which falls under Provincial jurisdiction), nor does it affect individuals growing such products for their own use [45].

Cardiovascular Reactions

No side effects related to cardiovascular activity have been noted with oral preparations containing berberine or its salts in animal studies or for the treatment of diarrhea in man.

Berberine has been shown to lower peripheral vascular resistance and to increase the inotropic activity of the canine heart, with or without preexisting myocardial failure. Berberine was given by intravenous infusion at rates of 0.02 and 0.2 mg/kg/min for 30 min to 12 patients with failure refractory to digitalis and diuretics. Despite the salutory effect, significant untoward effects appeared in 4 of these patients as repetitive episodes of ventricular tachycardia with a torsades de pointes morphology 1 to 20 h after the infusion. No predisposing factors for the adverse outcome could be identified [46].

Gastrointestinal Reactions

In reports of the therapeutic use of berberine salts for diarrhea in children there are occasionally children who do not tolerate the medication because it induces emesis. The interpretation of these reports is complicated, however, because of the underlying pathophysiological process and the fact that the berberine salt was often part of a mixture of agents, e.g., in combination with an anticholinergic compound and an antihistamine [47].

Fertility, Pregnancy, and Lactation

Decoctions of certain berberine-containing plants have been employed in folk medicine as abortifacients, oxytocics, or as antifertility agents [48]. These applications have not received extensive investigation. Berberine causes a strong contraction of the isolated mouse uterus [22]. This effect, employing berberine chloride, is more pronounced in the pregnant mouse uterus [49]. Crude plant extracts containing berberine with other alkaloids give a plant-specific response on the isolated uterus, either stimulant or antispasmodic depending on the plant [21]. The safety of berberine or extracts of berberine-containing plants has not been established in respect to fertility, pregnancy, and lactation.

Mutagenicity, Cytotoxicity, and Carcinogenicity

Berberine is a mitochondrial mutagen in yeast [50]. It can be shown that berberine binds to DNA by intercalation [30,51]. Berberine inhibits the synthesis of DNA, RNA, protein, and lipids, and the oxidation of glucose when incubated in vitro with sarcoma 180 tumor from ascitic fluid of mice [52]. This effect on S 180 was marginal in vivo; it is postulated that it its uptake into the tumor cell is blocked competitively by glucose since both undergo active transport into the cell by the same pathway. The safety of berberine or extracts from berberine-containing plants has not been established in respect to potential mutagenic or carcinogenic effects.

References

1. Chopra RN, Dikshit BB, Chowhan JS (1932) Pharmacological action of berberine. Ind J Med Res 19:1193–1203
2. Chang H-M, But PP-H (1986) Pharmacology and applications of Chinese materia medica. World Scientific, Singapore, I:62–71
3. Chang H-M, But PP-H (1987) Pharmacology and applications of Chinese materia medica. World Scientific, Singapore, II:1029–1040
4. Tyler VE (1987) The new honest herbal. George F. Stickley, Philadelphia, pp 28–29
5. Ahrendt LWA (1961) *Berberis* and *Mahonia*. A taxonomic revision. J Linnean Soc London 57:1–410
6. Supek Z, Tomić D (1946) Farmakološko-kemijsko istraživanje žutike (*Berberis vulgaris* L.) Liječnički Vjesnik 68:16–18
7. Petcu P, Goina T (1970) Neue Methoden zur Extrahierung der Alkaloide aus *Berberis vulgaris*. Planta Medica 18:372–375
8. Döpke W (1963) Neue Alkaloide aus *Berberis vulgaris* L. Naturwissenschaften 50:595
9. Manske RHF, Ashford WR (1954) Protoberberine alkaloids. In: Manske RHF, Holmes HL (eds) The Alkaloids; vol 4. New York, Academic Press, pp 77–118
10. Jeffs PW (1967) Protoberberine alkaloids. In: Manske RHF (ed) The Alkaloids; vol 9. New York, Academic Press, pp 41–115
11. Drost K, Szaufer M, Kowalski Z (1974) Alkaloidy rodzaju *Berberis* L. i ich działanie farmakologiczne. Herba Polonica 20:301–307

12. Košťálová D, Brázdoviačová B, Tomko J (1981) Isolation of quaternary alkaloids from *Mahonia aquifolium* (Pursh) Nutt. I. Chem Zvesti 35:279–283

13. Slavik J, Bochořáková J, Košťálová D, Hrochová V (1985) Alkaloids of *Mahonia aquifolium* (Pursh) Nutt. II. Chem Papers 39:537–542

14. Košťálová D, Hrochová V, Tomko J (1986) Tertiary alkaloids of *Mahonia aquifolium* (Pursh) Nutt. III. Chem Papers 40:389–394

15. Suess TR, Stermitz FR (1981) Alkaloids of *Mahonia repens* with a brief review of previous work in the genus *Mahonia*. J Nat Prod 44:680–687

16. British Herbal Medicine Association (1976) British herbal pharmacopoeia. London, pp 31, 33

17. Duke JA (1985) CRC handbook of medicinal herbs. CRC Press, Boca Raton, Florida pp 78, 287–288, 585–586

18. Grieve M (1931) A modern herbal. Harcourt, Brace & Company, New York, I:82–84

19. Moore M (1979) Medicinal plants of the mountain west. Museum of New Mexico Press, Santa Fe, New Mexico, pp 32–33, 117–119

20. Shideman FE (1950) A review of the pharmacology and therapeutics of *Hydrastis* and its alkaloids, hydrastine, berberine and canadine. Bull National Formulary Committee 18(1–2):3–19

21. Haginawa J, Harada M (1962) Pharmacological studies on crude drugs. V. Comparison of berberine type alkaloid-containing plants on their components and several pharmacological actions. Yakugaku Zasshi 82:726–731

22. Imaseki I, Kitabatake Y, Taguchi T (1961) Studies on effect of berberine alkaloids on intestine and uterus in mice. Yakugaku Zasshi 81:1281–1284

23. Preiniger V (1975) The pharmacology and toxicology of the Papaveraceae alkaloids. In: Manske RHF (ed) The alkaloids, chemistry and physiology. Academic Press, New York, 15:207–261

24. Kondo Y (1976) Organic and biological aspects of berberine alkaloids. Heterocycles 4:197–219

25. Schiff PL Jr (1987) The *Thalictrum* alkaloids: chemistry and pharmacology. In: Pelletier SW (ed) Alkaloids: chemical and biological perspectives. John Wiley & Sons, New York, 5:271–637

26. Mrozikiewicz A, Kowalewski Z, Drost-Karwoska K, Bobkiewicz T, Klimaszewska O (1980) Badania farmakokinetyczne chlorku berberyny. Herba Polonica 26:123–127

27. Lahiri SC, Dutta NK (1967) Berberine and chloramphenicol in the treatment of cholera and severe diarrhea. J Ind Med Assoc 48:1–11

28. Khin-Maung-U, Myo-Khin, Nyunt-Nyunt-Wai, Aye-Kyaw, Tin-U (1986) Clinical trial of berberine in acute watery diarrhoea. Br Med J 291:1601–1605

29. Rabbani GH, Butler T, Knight J, Sanyal SC, Alam K (1987) Randomized controlled trial of berberine sulfate therapy for diarrhea due to enterotoxigenic *Escherichia coli* and *Vibrio cholerae*. J Infect Dis 155:979–984

30. Amin AH, Subbaiah TV, Abbasi KM (1969) Berberine sulfate: antimicrobial activity, bioassay, and mode of action. Can J Microbiol 15:1067–1076

31. Hahn FE, Ciak J (1975) Berberine. In: Corcoran JW, Han FE (eds) Antibiotics; vol 3. Mechanism of action of antimicrobial and antitumor agents. New York, Springer-Verlag, pp 577–584

32. Kulkarni SK, Dandiya PC, Varandani NL (1972) Pharmacological investigations of berberine sulfate. Jap J Pharmacol 22:11–16

33. Gupte S (1975) Use of berberine in treatment of giardiasis. Am J Dis Child 129:866

34. Munshi CP, Vaidya PM, Buranpuri JJ, Gulati OD (1972) Kala-azar in Gujarat. J Ind Med Assoc 59:287–293

35. Turova AD, Konovalov MN, Leskov AI (1964) Berberine, an effective cholagogue. Med Prom SSSR 18(6):59–60

36. Schein FT, Hanna C (1960) Absorption, distribution and excretion of berberine. Arch Int Pharmacodyn 124:317–325

37. Bhide MB, Chavan SR, Dutta NK (1969) Absorption, distribution and excretion of berberine. Ind J Med Res 57:2128–2131

38. Phillips CDF (1895) Pharmacological actions of berberine. Brit Med J ii:1551–1552

39. Turova AD, Leskov AI, Bichevina VI (1962) Berberine. Lekarstv Sredstva iz Rast pp 303–307

40. Shanbhag SM, Kulkarni HJ, Gaitonde BB (1970) Pharmacological actions of berberine on the central nervous system. Jap J Pharmacol 20:482–487

41. Roth L, Daunderer M, Kormann K (1988) Giftpflanzen. Pflanzengifte, ed. 3. Ecomed, Landsberg, pp 145–146, 810
42. List PH, Hörhammer L (1967–1980) Hagers Handbuch der pharmazeutischen Praxis, ed 4. Springer Verlag, Berlin, III:415–419
43. Anonymous (1986) Herbal medicines — safe and effective? Drug Ther Bull 24:97–100
44. Mezey K (1945) Plantas medicinales colombianas; *Berberis rigidifolia*; primer estudio quimico, farmacodinámico y toxicológico. Med y Cir, Bogotá 9:331–341
45. Department of National Health and Welfare (1989) Food and drug regulations — amendment (Schedule No. 705). Canada Gazette Part 1 (March 11), pp 1350–1359
46. Marin-Neto JA, Maciel BC, Secches AL, Gallo L, Jr (1988) Cardiovascular effects of berberine in patients with severe congestive heart failure. Clin Cardiol 11:253–260
47. Sharda DC (1970) Berberine in the treatment of diarrhea of infancy and childhood. J Ind Med Assoc 54:22–24
48. Farnsworth NR, Bingel AS, Cordell GA, Crane FA, Fong HHS (1975) Potential value of plants as sources of new antifertility agents I. J Pharm Sci 64:535–598
49. Furuya T (1957) Pharmacological action, including toxicity and excretion of berberine hydrochloride and its oxidation product. Bull Osaka Med School 3:62–67
50. Meisel MN, Sokolova TS (1960) Inherited cytoplasmic changes induced in yeast by acriflavine and berberine. Doklady Akad Nauk SSSR 131:436–439
51. Rungsitiyakorn A, Wilairat P, Pamojpan B (1981) On the pH dependence of binding of berberine to DNA. J Pharm Pharmacol 33:125–127
52. Creasey WA (1979) Biochemical effects of berberine. Biochem Pharmacol 28:1081–1084

Cinnamomum Species

K. Keller

Botany

Cinnamon consists of the dried bark of different species of the genus *Cinnamomum* (family Lauraceae). For pharmaceutical purposes the following species are used:

Cinnamomum verum J.S. Presl (*Cinnamomum zeylanicum* Blume, *Cinnamomum ceylanicum* Nees), Ceylon cinnamon

Cinnamomum aromaticum Nees (*Cinnamomum cassia* Blume), Cassia cinnamon and on smaller scale:

Cinnamomum burmanii (Nees) Blume, Batavia cassia
Cinnamomum loureirii Nees, Saigon cinnamon.

Beside the bark, the flowers of *Cinnamomum aromaticum* Nees are also used [1].

Chemistry

The most important constituent of cinnamon is 0.5%–2.5% (Saigon cinnamon up to 6%) of essential oil. According to US NF XVI, cinnamon oil is the volatile oil distilled with steam from the twigs and leaves of *Cinnamomum aromaticum* Nees (cassia oil).

The principal component of all cinnamon oils is cinnamaldehyde. There are some differences in the composition of the volatile oil depending on the species and the part of plant used (see Table 1).

Further constituents are presented in the monographs published by Lawrence [5] and Wijesekara [3]. These components, however, have no importance in the risk evaluation of cinnamon.

It is important to note that in the Lauraceae family the occurrence of different chemotypes is rather common [4]. For the risk evaluation the occurrence of a safrole chemotype of *Cinnamomum verum* is of interest. Usually cinnamon oils contain up to 2% safrole. The essential oil from the bark of that chemotype

Table 1. Components of cinnamon oils

C. verum	Cinnamaldehyde	Eugenol	Coumarin
Bark	55–75%	5–18%	< 0.0008%
Leaves	1–8%	65–95%	
C. aromaticum			
Bark and leaves	70–95%	traces	> 0.03%

Characteristic constituents:
1.5–3.8% o-methoxycinnamaldehyde [2,3]
8–11.5% mucilage [4]

contains 10.8% safrole, 10.9% eugenol, and 52.5% cinnamaldehyde. The volatile oil distilled from the leaves contains 52.3% safrole [3].

Pharmacology and Uses

The antimicrobial activity of cinnamon, the volatile oil, and cinnamaldehyde has been investigated in different studies. In agar diffusion and serial dilution tests all substances showed pronounced antimicrobial effects against different bacteria and fungi [6–8]. Cinnamon inhibited growth and mycotoxin production of mycotoxin-producing *Aspergillus* species [6,7]. Kellner reported antimicrobial activities of cinnamon oil and cinnamaldehyde in the vapor phase [9–11]. Besides the antimicrobial properties, Deininger reported in vitro antiviral effects of cassia flower oil and cinnamaldehyde against herpes- and adenovirus. The range of activity was rather narrow. In rabbits the feeding of cinnamaldehyde before and after infection had a protective effect against Ps.R. virus infection [12]. These results require further confirmation.

Cinnamaldehyde is reported to have a hypotensive effect in anesthetized dogs and guinea pigs, apparently by causing a peripheral vasodilatation. Cinnamaldehyde caused positive inotropic and chronotropic effects in isolated guinea pig heart preparations. Repeated application resulted in a cardiac inhibition. Doses of 5–10 mg/kg i.v. and concentrations of 10^{-4} to 10^{-5} g/ml in organ preparations were used. In the experiments concerning vascular effects 10 mg cinnamaldehyde i.v. were equivalent to 10 μg glyceryltrinitrate [13].

As for many other essential oils a papaverin-like spasmolytic effect of cinnamon oil and cinnamaldehyde has been reported [13,14]. Furthermore an inhibition of the stomach movement in rats and dogs, an inhibition of intestinal propulsion in mice, and a reduction of gastric erosions in stressed mice were found [13,15,16]. In contrast to Harada, Akira also described a reduction of the ulcus index in stressed mice and in serotonin-induced ulcers by an aqueous extract of Chinese cinnamon [17].

The doses of cinnamaldehyde or essential oil in the experiments were rather high: for example 5–10 mg/kg i.v. and 250–500 mg/kg i.p. A dose of 100 mg/kg of the aqueous extract of cassia bark was given, but the corresponding amount of the bark and the composition of the extract were not reported. Only the experiments published by Plant [15,16] concern the normal dose range (5–25 ml water of cinnamon).

In mice 125–500 mg/kg i.p. and 250–1000 mg/kg p.o. led to a decrease in spontaneous motor activity, antagonism to methamphetamin-induced hyperactivity, and prolongation of hexobarbital-induced anesthesia; hypothermic and antipyretic effects in mice have also been reported [18]. In rabbits the influence of cinnamaldehyde on the EEG was studied in gallamine-paralyzed preparations with intact brains. A dose of 10–20 mg/kg cinnamaldehyde i.v. or i.a. produced a centrally originating EEG activation through a direct or indirect excitatory action on the brainstem reticular structure [19].

Fundaro reported a depressive effect of 500 mg/kg Ceylon cinnamon oil p.o. on the operant conditioning behavior in rats. With doses ranging from 25 to 150 mg/kg no effects were seen [20].

Inhibition of complement-depending immune reactions by water extracts from cassia bark has been reported. Type IV reaction, contact dermatitis, was not inhibited by the extract [21,22]. The effects have been attributed to diterpenes present in cassia bark [23,23a].

Cinnamon is officially approved in France [24] and the Federal Republic of Germany [25] as a carminative. The use as a carminative and mild astringent is mentioned in Martindale [26] and other textbooks [27]. Dosage is 0.3 to 2 g of the powdered bark or 0.05 to 0.2 ml of the volatile oil.

Pharmacokinetics

Cinnamaldehyde is reported to be poorly absorbed through the skin [28]. Following i.p. injection of cinnamaldehyde, benzoic acid, hippuric acid, and cinnamic acid were found in urine [29]. After rats had received 0.23 and 0.3 mmol cinnamaldehyde i.p., 29.3% of the compound was found in urine as hippuric acid [30]. A relatively low absorption might be explained by partial "tanning" of mucous membranes by cinnamaldehyde and inhibition of further absorption. The hyperkeratosis observed by Skramlik [31] and Hagan [34] in toxicity experiments may support this interpretation.

Adverse Reaction Profile

General Animal Data

The acute toxicity of cinnamaldehyde depends strongly on the mode of application. Harada reported LD_{50} values in mice of 132 mg/kg i.v., 610 mg/kg i.p., and 2225 mg/kg p.o. An aqueous extract was virtually nontoxic (LD_{50} 4980 mg/kg i.p.) [18]. The LD_{50} value reported by Skramlik for the volatile oil of Ceylon cinnamon was 4160 mg/kg and that for cassia oil was 5200 mg/kg (rat, p.o.) [31]. In the monographs published by Opdyke oral LD_{50} values between 2.2 ml/kg and 3.4 ml/kg are reported [30,32,33]. Although Meyer [28] has reported that cinnamon oil is poorly absorbed through the skin, other researchers have found relatively low dermal LD_{50} values of 0.59 mg/kg for cinnamaldehyde, 0.69 mg/kg for Ceylon cinnamon oil and 0.32 mg/kg for cassia oil [30,32,33].

Rats tolerated 70 mg cinnamaldehyde p.o. for 8 weeks without any symptoms of toxicity [31]. When 1000, 2500, and 10 000 ppm cinnamaldehyde was added to the diet of rats over a 16-week period, slight swelling of the hepatic cells and slight hyperkeratosis of the squamous portion of the stomach were observed in the 10 000 ppm group [34]. No macroscopic effects were seen at levels of 1000 ppm and 2500 ppm. Similar symptoms were found by Skramlik, who also reported the occurrence of nephritis [31].

General Human Data

Risks of cinnamon use are determined mainly by the essential oil and cinnamaldehyde, which reacts as an α-β-unsaturated aldehyde with amino and sulfhydryl groups and is responsible for the cytotoxic, irritant, and sensitizing properties of cinnamon.

The pharmacological and toxicological investigations do not demonstrate a special risk for man. The observation by Plant [15,16] in his experiments with dogs that in higher doses vomiting occurred, corresponds with reported side effects in humans [35].

The Council of Europe in 1973 included different cinnamon species in its list of substances, spices and seasonings commonly added to foodstuffs in small quantities the use of which is admissible with the possible limitation of the active principle in the final product. For cinnamaldehyde an ADI value was set at 1.25 mg/kg [36].[1]

Allergic Reactions

See the section on dermatological reactions.

Dermatological Reactions

Cinnamaldehyde 5% in petrolatum is a skin irritant [30,37]. Cinnamon oil caused, after 48 h of contact, a second-degree burn on the posterior thigh of an 11-year-old boy [37a].

---

[1]See also the note added in proof on p. 262

Hausen stated in 1988 that cinnamaldehyde is the leading substance responsible for allergic reactions caused by cosmetics or perfumes [38]. Already in 1920 urticaria caused by cinnamon was described [35]. Although numerous cases are documented in the literature, the real number of complications seems to be underestimated. People accept side effects of "natural" substances in a different way than those of "chemical" substances. In some reports it is mentioned that the patient was aware of slight allergic reactions a long time before the more severe signs appeared. Those symptoms were accepted, however, as a sign of the "medicinal" action of the preparation or as a common disease such as herpes labialis or aphthes. Allergic reactions occurred after contact with cinnamon oil or cinnamaldehyde in ointments, toothpaste, mouthwash, or foods [37,39–44]. Symptoms were mainly the swelling of lips and tongue, itching, burning sensation, blistering of the oral mucosa, and urticaria. Some cases of orofacial granulomatosis were reported after contact with cinnamon oil in toothpaste [43]. The lowest concentration causing positive reactions in patch tests was 0.01% [42].

Severe reactions such as anaphylaxis have not been reported. All cases recovered when the cinnamon-containing preparation was withdrawn. In most cases authors stated that an atopic disposition was present in the patient or members of his family. Cross-reactions occur in persons allergic to Peru balsam. In a group of 117 patients, allergic to Peru balsam, 14.5% reacted positively to Chinese cinnamon, in contrast of 1 of 220 patients not allergic to Peru balsam [45]. Cross-reactions were more pronounced, however, with cloves [*Syzygium aromaticum* (L.) Merr. et L.M. Perry]: 46.2% of the former group presented positive reactions. Nater found that cinnamaldehyde (0.3–3 mg/ml) is a histamine liberator in human leukocytes in vitro. This author attributes the skin reactions partly to this effect [37].

A "quenching effect" described by Opdyke [30,39] consists in the reduction or prevention of allergic skin reactions by other substances like limonene or eugenol present in volatile oils. The clinical relevance of these experiments is not well established. One can speculate that eugenol, which is an inhibitor of prostaglandin biosynthesis [46], could have some influence on inflammation. If this is true, a different allergological risk should be expected for Ceylon cinnamon oil and cinnamaldehyde. There are no clinical data confirming this speculation, however.

To conclude, the opinion of Mathias [42] can be accepted that preparations with more than 0.01% cinnamaldehyde are suspect. People with atopic disposition should not use cinnamon-containing products.

Gastrointestinal Reactions

See the section on general human data.

Oropharyngeal Reactions

See the section on dermatological reactions.

Drug Interactions

Cassia bark (2 g in 100 ml) markedly retarded the in vitro dissolution of tetracycline hydrochloride and methacycline hydrochloride from gelatine capsules [47]. In the presence of cassia bark about 20% of tetracycline hydrochloride was in solution after 30 min in contrast to 97% when only water was used. The effect was comparable to that of the antacid magnesium trisilicate. It was attributed to the adsorption of the antibiotic on the particles. There are no further investigations to establish which individual constituents of cassia bark (volatile oil, cinnamaldehyde or mucilage) are responsible for this effect. As a dose of 1 to 2 g cinnamon is not uncommon, care should be taken not to use tetracycline and related substances together with cinnamon at that dose level.

As a reaction between free primary amines with cinnamaldehyde must be expected, the essential oil should not be taken together with corresponding drugs with narrow therapeutic range.

Fertility, Pregnancy, and Lactation

Lewin reports that cinnamon was used in antiquity and the middle ages as abortifacient [48]. It must be taken into account that in old sources cinnamon (cassia) was confused with *Cassia fistulosa*, which contains anthraquinones [49]. An unspecified "large amount of cinnamon" was reported to have caused methemoglobinemia, hematinuria, albuminuria, and cylindruria in a pregnant woman. Abortion was not reported [48]. The daily intake of 100 drops of tincture of cinnamon did not result in abortion. In another book Lewin has stated, however, that cinnamon can cause abortion [50]. Cases are not mentioned. In one case report of successful self-induced abortion an insufficiently identified substance was used [51]. The author stated that the black to brown colored liquid was cinnamon tincture; the dosage was not given. The fact that a single dose of cinnamon might cause abortion seems to be doubtful, especially if one considers the widespread use of cinnamon.

The reports cited by Roth [52] and *Hagers Handbuch* [53] concerning the action of cinnamon on the uterus are based on the reports by Lewin [50,48] and Madaus [54], who quotes Clarus' *Handbook* from 1860. It seems that there are no concrete case reports concerning self-induced abortion with cinnamon.

Abramovici found teratogenic effects with cinnamaldehyde in chick embryos [55]. In these experiments malformations were closely related to toxic effects of cinnamaldehyde. The maximum teratogenic effect was seen at a dose of 0.5 mmol/embryo with 58.2% malformations and 49% lethality. Experiments with chick embryos are of limited value for the risk assessment for humans.

Further data on toxic effects of cinnamon or cinnamon oil during pregnancy were not found. To conclude, it can be stated that cinnamon does not present any special risk in pregnancy. As there are still insufficient data concerning the mutagenic effects, prolonged use of the essential oil should be restricted during pregnancy.

Mutagenicity and Carcinogenicity[1]

Cinnamaldehyde or extracts from cinnamon were investigated for mutagenic effects in *Salmonella* (Ames assay). In most of the experiments negative results were obtained [56–65]. Lutz et al. correlated these negative results with the chemical structure of different α,β-unsaturated aldehydes [56–58]. Nevertheless, positive results were also reported for alcoholic extracts from cinnamon and for cinnamaldehyde [66,67]. In one experiment, o-methoxycinnamaldehyde gave positive results in the Ames test, whereas cinnamaldehyde was negative [62]. Further investigations with botanically and chemically well-characterized cinnamon preparations are necessary.

In contrast to the tests with *Salmonella* strains, cinnamon and cassia oil were positive in *B. subtilis* DNA repair tests [65,68–70].

Cinnamon oil and cinnamaldehyde gave positive results in chromosomal aberration tests using Chinese hamster cell cultures [59,66] and in *Drosophila* test systems [71,72]. An aqueous extract from cinnamon was negative in a *Drosophila* test system [73]. Negative results were reported with the micronucleus test in the mouse (125–500 mg/kg i.p.) [74].

The results of the in vitro bacterial mutagenicity tests must be interpreted with care because the concentrations used were within the dose range where antimicrobial effects of cinnamaldehyde or cinnamon oil have been proven. Growth retardation due to an antimicrobial effect is the reason for the reported "antimutagenic" effect [75] of cinnamaldehyde [76,77].

With respect to the in vitro systems with mammalian cell cultures it must be taken into account that cinnamon extracts and cinnamaldehyde exhibit cytotoxic effects with an ED_{50} of 50–60 μg/ml in KB cells (monolayer cell line from a human mouth carcinoma) and 20–24 μg/ml [78] or 4.8 μg/ml [79] in mouse L 1210 cell cultures. The cytotoxic effect is correlated with a decrease in protein synthesis and is attributed to the reaction of cinnamaldehyde with amino and sulfhydryl groups. These rather unspecific effects are strongly influenced by the culture medium and other experimental conditions.

There are insufficient data for the evaluation of the carcinogenic risk of cinnamon. Further investigations should use chemically and botanically defined preparations because of the amounts of the carcinogenic safrole, of coumarin, and of o-methoxycinnamaldehyde can be expected to influence the results.

---

[1]See also the note added in proof on p. 262

References

1. Berger F (1949) Handbuch der Drogenkunde. Vienna
2. Wichtl M (1988) In: Hartke K (ed) DAB 9-Kommentar. Stuttgart, pp 368–370
3. Wijesekera RO (1978) The chemistry and technology of cinnamon. CRC Crit Rev Food Sci Nutr 10:1–30
4. Hegnauer R (1966) Chemotaxonomie der Pflanzen vol 4. Basel, pp 350–381
5. Lawrence BM (1969) Can Inst Food Technol J 2:178
6. Bullerman LB, Lieu FY, Seier SA (1977) Inhibition of growth and aflatoxin production by cinnamon and clove oils, cinnamic aldehyde and eugenole. J Food Sci 42:1107–1109
7. Hitokoto H, Morozumi S et al. (1978) Inhibitory effects of condiments and herbal drugs on the growth and toxin production of toxigenic fungi. Mycopathologia 66:161–167
8. Yousef RT, Tawil GG (1980) Antimicrobial activity of volatile oils. Pharmazie 35:698–701
9. Kellner W, Kober W (1954) Möglichkeiten der Verwendung ätherischer Öle zur Raumdesinfektion. Arzneim Forsch 4:319–325
10. Kellner W, Kober W (1955) Möglichkeiten der Verwendung ätherischer Öle zur Raumdesinfektion. Arzneim Forsch 5:224–229
11. Kellner W, Kober W (1956) Möglichkeiten der Verwendung ätherischer Öle zur Raumdesinfektion. Arzneim Forsch 6:768–772
12. Deininger R (1985) Neues aus der Terpenforschung. Der Kassenarzt 7:47–55
13. Harada M, Yano S (1975) Pharmacological studies on Chinese cinnamon. II. Effects of cinnamaldehyde on the cardiovascular and digestive systems. Chem Pharm Bull 23:941–947
14. Reiter M, Brandt W (1985) Relaxant effects on tracheal and ileal smooth muscles of the guinea pig. Arzneim Forsch 35:408–414
15. Plant OH, Miller GH (1926) Effects of carminative volatile oils on the muscular activity of the stomach and colon. J Pharmacol Exp Ther 27:149–164
16. Plant OH (1921) Effects of carminative volatile oils on the muscular movements of the intestine. J Pharmacol Exp Ther 22:311–324
17. Akira T, Tanaka S, Tabata M (1986) Pharmacological studies on the antiulcerogenic activity of Chinese cinnamon. Planta Med 52:440–443
18. Harada M, Ozaki Y (1972) Pharmacological studies on Chinese cinnamon. I. Central effects of cinnamaldehyde. Yakugaku Zasshi 92:135–140
19. Harada M, Fujii Y, Kamiya J (1976) Pharmacological studies on Chinese cinnamon. III. Electroencephalographic studies of cinnamaldehyde in the rabbit. Chem Pharm Bull 24:1784–1788
20. Fundaro A, Cassone MC (1980) Azione degli olii essenziale di camomilla, canella, assenzio, macis e origano su un comportamento operativo nel ratto. Boll Soc Ital Biol Sper 56:2375–2380
21. Nagai H, Shimazawa T et al. (1982) Immunopharmacological studies of the aqueous extract of Cinnamomum cassia (CCAq). I. Anti-allergic action. Japan J Pharmacol 32:813–822
22. Nagai H, Shimazawa T et al. (1982) Immunopharmacological studies of the aqueous extract of Cinnamomum cassia (CCAq). II. Effect of CCAq on experimental glomerulonephritis. Japan J Pharmacol 32:823–831
23. Nohara T, Kashiwada Y et al. (1981) Constituents of cinnamomi cortex. V. Chem Pharm Bull 29:2451–2459
23a. Nohara T, Kashiwada Y, Tomimatsu T, Nishioka I (1982) Two novel diterpenes from bark of Cinnamomum cassia. Phytochemistry 21:2130–2132
24. Ministère des Affaires Sociales et de l'Emploi: Spécialités Pharmaceutiques à Base de Plantes: Bull Off No 86 bis/20 August 1986
25. Bundesgesetzblatt (Anlage) I, No. 12 of 4.4.1986
26. Reynolds JEF, Prasad AB (1982) Martindale: the extra pharmacopoeia, 28th edn. London: The Pharmaceutical Press
27. Tyler VE (1988) Pharmacognosy. 9th edn. Lea & Febiger, Philadelphia
28. Meyer FR, Meyer E (1959) Perkutane Resorption von ätherischen Ölen und ihren Inhaltsstoffen. Arzneim Forsch 8:516–519
29. Friedmann E, Mai H (1931) Verhalten der Cinnamalessigsäure und des Zimtaldehyds im Tierkörper. Biochem Z 242:282–287

30. Opdyke DLJ (1979) Monographs on fragrance raw materials: Cinnamic aldehyde. Fd Cosm Toxicol 17:253-258
31. Skramlik EV (1959) Über die Giftigkeit und Verträglichkeit von ätherischen Ölen. Pharmazie 14:435-445
32. Opdyke DLJ (1975) Monographs on fragrance raw materials. Fd Cosm Toxicol 13:109-110
33. Opdyke DLJ (1975) Monographs on fragrance raw materials. Fd Cosm Toxicol 13:111-112
34. Hagan EL, Hausen WH, Fitzhugh OG, Jenner PM, Jones WI (1967) Food flavourings and compounds of related structure. II. Subacute and chronic toxicity. Fd Chem Toxicol 5:141-157
35. Noorden-Salomon (1920) Handbuch der Ernährungslehre. Berlin [cited in: Heupke W, Holländer E (1932) Die Wirkung der Gewürze auf die Abscheidung des Magensaftes. Dtsch Arch Klin Med 173:241-255]
36. Council of Europe (1973) Natural flavouring substances, their sources and added artificial flavouring substances. Strasbourg
37. Nater JP, De Jong JM et al. (1977) Contact urticarial skin responses to cinnamaldehyde. Contact Dermatitis 3:151-154
37a. Sparks T (1985) Cinnamon oil burn. West J Med 142:835
38. Hausen BJM (1988) Allergiepflanzen-Pflanzenallergene. Landsberg, pp 95-96
39. Allenby CF, Goodwin BF, Safford RJ (1984) Diminution of immediate reactions to cinnamic aldehyde by eugenole. Contact Dermatitis 11:322-323
40. Calnan CD (1976) Cinnamon dermatitis from an ointment. Contact Dermatitis 2:167-170
41. Drake TE, Maibach HI (1976) Allergic contact dermatitis and stomatitis caused by a cinnamic aldehyde-flavored toothpaste. Arch Dermatol 112:202-203
42. Mathias CGT, Chappler RR, Maibach HI (1980) Contact urticaria from cinnamic aldehyde. Arch Dermatol 116:74-76
43. Patton DW, Ferguson MM et al. (1985) Oro-facial granulomatosis: a possible allergic basis. Brit J Oral Maxillofac Surg 23:235-242
44. Roberts MJ (1976) New-product pruritus. Brit Med J 2:47
45. Niinimäki A (1984) Delayed-type allergy to spices. Contact Dermatitis 11:34-40
46. Wagner H, Wierer M, Bauer R (1986) In vitro inhibition of prostaglandin biosynthesis by essential oils and phenolic compounds. Planta med 52:184-187
47. Miyazaki S, Inoue H, Nadai T (1977) Effect of antacids on the dissolution behavior of tetracycline and methacycline. Chem Pharm Bull 27:2523-2527
48. Lewin L (1925) Die Fruchtabtreibung durch Gifte und andere Mittel. Georg Stilke, Berlin
49. Karsten G, Weber U, Stahl E (1962) Lehrbuch der Pharmakognosie. Stuttgart, pp 196-200
50. Lewin L (1929) Gifte und Vergiftungen. Georg Stilke, Berlin
51. Bichlmeier J (1941) Über Abtreibungen im Landgerichtsbezirk Nordhausen in den Jahren 1935-1939 und ihre Bekämpfung. Dtsch Z Ges Gerichtl Med 35:125-163
52. Roth L, Daunderer M, Kormann K (1988) Giftpflanzen-Pflanzengifte. 3rd edn. Landsberg, p 210
53. List PH, Hörhammer L (1973) Hagers Handbuch der Pharmazeutischen Praxis, 4th edn, vol 4: Chemikalien und Drogen (CI-G). Berlin: Springer-Verlag
54. Madaus G (1938) Lehrbuch der biologischen Heilmittel. Leipzig: Georg Thieme Verlag, pp 998-1002
55. Abramovici A, Rachmuth-Roizman P (1983) Molecular structure-teratogenicity relationships of some fragrance additives. Toxicology 29:143-156
56. Eder E, Henschler D, Neudecker T (1982) Mutagenic properties of allylic and α,β-unsaturated compounds: consideration of alkylating mechanisms. Xenobiotica 12:831-848
57. Eder E, Neudecker T, Lutz D, Henschler D (1980) Mutagenic potential of allyl and allylic compounds. Structure-activity relationship as determined by alkylating and direct in vitro mutagenic properties. Biochem Pharmacol 29:993-998
58. Eder E, Neudecker T, Lutz D, Henschler D (1982) Correlation of alkylating and mutagenic activities of allyl and allylic compounds: standard alkylation test vs kinetic investigations. Chem Biol Interact 38:303-315
59. Kasamaki A, Takahashi H, Tsumura N, Niwa J, Fujita T (1982) Genotoxicity of flavouring agents. Mutat Res 105:387-392
60. Lijinsky W, Andrews AW (1980) Mutagenicity of vinyl compounds in Salmonella typhimurium. Teratog Carcinog Mutagen 1:259-267

61. Marnett LJ, Hurd HK, Hollstein MC, Levin DE, Esterbauer H (1985) Naturally occurring carbonyl compounds are mutagens in Salmonella tester strain TA104. Mutat Res 148:25-34
62. Mortelmans K, Haworth S, Lawlor T, Speck W, Tainer B (1986) Salmonella mutagenicity tests. II. Results from the testing of 270 chemicals. Environ Mutagenesis 8 Suppl: 1
63. Prival MJ, Sheldon AT, Popkin D (1982) Evaluation, using Salmonella typhimurium, of the mutagenicity of seven chemicals found in cosmetics. Fd Chem Toxicol 20:427-432
64. Sasaki Y, Endo R (1978) Mutagenicity of aldehydes in Salmonella. Mutat Res 54:251
65. Sekizawa J, Shibamoto T (1982) Genotoxicity of safrole-related chemicals in microbial test systems. Mutat Res 101:127-140
66. Ishidate M, Sofuni T, Yoshikawa K, Hayashi M, Nohmi T (1984) Primary mutagenicity screening of food additives currently used in Japan. Fd Chem Toxicol 22:623-636
67. Shashikanth KN, Hosono A (1987) Screening of streptomycin-dependent strains of Salmonella typhimurium and Escherichia coli for in vitro detection of spice-induced mutagenicity. Lebensmittel-Wiss Technol 20:91-94
68. Paovalo C, Chulasiri MU (1986) Bacterial mutagenicity of fractions from chloroform extracts of ceylon cinnamon Cinnamomum zeylanicum. J Food Prot 49:12-13
69. Ungsurungsie M, Suthienkul O (1982) Mutagenicity screening of popular Thai spices. Fd Chem Toxicol 20:527-530
70. Ungsurungsie M, Paovalo C, Noonai A (1984) Mutagenicity of extracts from Ceylon cinnamon in the rec assay. Fd Chem Toxicol 22:109-112
71. Venkatasetty R (1972) Genetic variation induced by radiation and chemical agents in Drosophila melanogaster. Diss Abstr Int B 32:5047-5048
72. Woodruff RC, Manson JM, Valencia R, Zimmering S (1985) Chemical mutagenesis testing in Drosophila. V. Results of 53 coded compounds tested for the National Toxicology Program. Environ Mutagenesis 7:677-702
73. Abraham SK, Kesavan PC (1985) A preliminary analysis of the genotoxicity of a few spices in Drosophila. Mutat Res 143:219-224
74. Hayashi M, Sofuni T, Ishidate M (1984) A pilot experiment for the micro nucleus test. The multi-sampling at multi-dose levels method. Mutat Res 141:165-169
75. Ohta T, Watanabe M, Moriya M, Shirasu Y, Kada T (1983) Analysis of the antimutagenic effect of cinnamaldehyde on chemical mutagenesis in E. coli. Mutat Res 107:219-227
76. De Silva HV, Shankel DM (1987) Effects on the antimutagen cinnamaldehyde on reversion and survival of selected Salmonella tester strains. Mutat Res 187:11-19
77. Rutten B, Gocke E (1988) The "antimutagenic" effect of cinnamaldehyde is due to a transient growth inhibition. Mutat Res 201:97-105
78. Chulasiri MU, Picha P, Rienkijkan M, Preechanukool K (1984) Cytotoxic effect of petroleum ether and chloroform extracts from Ceylon cinnamon (Cinnamomum zeylanicum Nees) barks on tumor cells in vitro. Int J Crude Drug Res 22:177-180
79. Moon KH, Pack MY (1983) Cytotoxicity of cinnamic aldehyde on leukemia L1210 cells. Drug Chem Toxicol 6:521-535

Cymbopogon Species

D. Corrigan

Botany

There are up to 60 species of *Cymbopogon* (family Poaceae or Graminae) native to tropical and subtropical regions of Africa and Asia. Several species are extensively cultivated in Central and South America, Africa, the East and West Indies, and Asia for the distillation of essential oils from their leaves. Taxonomic classification is complicated by hybridization, polyploidy, and synonymy with the related genus *Andropogon* [1].

The most significant species include *Cymbopogon citratus* (D.C.) Stapf. which gives West Indian lemongrass oil; *C. flexuosus* Stapf. (syn. *Andropogon nardus* var. *flexuosus*) is the source of East Indian lemongrass oil; *C. Nardus* (L) W. Watson (syn. *Andropogon nardus*) is the source of Ceylon citronella oil; *C. winterianus* Jowitt is used to produce Java citronella oil; palmarosa oil, which is also known as East Indian geranium oil, is distilled from the leaves of *C. Martini* (Roxb.) Stapf. var *motia*. *C. proximus* (A. Rich.) Stapf. is an important species from Egypt and the Sudan which is used in folk medicine.

Chemistry

More attention has been paid to the constituents of the essential oils than to other constituents of the various species. The oils fall into two main types, a "geraniol" type containing acyclic monoterpenes such as geraniol, citral, and citronellal or a "menthane" group containing predominantly monocyclic monoterpenes such as limonene, piperitone, or menthone but no geraniol. Most of the commercially available oils fall into the geraniol group.

Oil of citronella from both Ceylon and Java contains citronellal, geraniol, and citronellol as major components. The *Pharmaceutical Codex* [2] states that Ceylon citronella oil (ex *C. nardus*) contains 10% citronellal and 18% geraniol while the Javanese oil (ex *C. winterianus*) contains 35% citronellal and 21% geraniol. The Java-type oils are characterized by low concentrations of monoterpenes (2.9–3.8%) compared to the Ceylon oils which contain 23.8% monoterpenes, chiefly tricyclene, α-pinene, camphene, limonene, and cis- and trans-β-ocimene.

The Java oil has a higher content of sesquiterpenes while the higher monoterpene content of the Ceylon type makes it less stable to oxidation than the Java
type [3].

West Indian lemongrass (*C. citratus*) contains 0.2–3% of volatile oil from the
fresh grass. Citral is the major component of the oil, constituting between 65% and
85%. Citral is a mixture of geranial (α-citral) and neral (β-citral). The other major
component is myrcene (12–20%). Minor components include dipentene, meth-
ylheptenone, linalool, methylheptenol, α-terpineol, geraniol, nerol, citronellol,
citronellal, and volatile acids [4].

East Indian lemongrass oil (*C. flexuosus*) contains slightly more citral (70–85%)
than the West Indian product. Some strains rich in geraniol (35–50%) have been
reported in which citral is a minor component (10–20%), and which contain
significant amounts of methyleugenol (20%) [4]. Such geraniol-rich oils resemble
palmarosa oil (*C. Martini* var. *motia*) which, according to *Martindale*, contains
75–95% geraniol together with geranyl acetate [5]. A recent report has shown that
palmarosa oil contains over 100 compounds, many related to geraniol, while some
40 pyrazine and pyridine derivatives were also identified as the components
responsible for the similarity between the odour of palmarosa oil and the odor of
freshly baked rye bread [8]. Other varieties of *C. martini* as well as *C. nervatus*, *C.
commutatis*, and *C. densiflorus* are reported to contain unusual menthadienols.
The oil from *C. proximus* from the Sudan was reported to be an excellent source
of piperitone by Banthorpe et al. [1], who also reported that in certain habitats a
high proportion (up to 70%) of the *C. proximus* oil comprised sesquiterpenes of
the elemane and eudesmane types.

The nonvolatile constituents have been studied to a limited extent. Among the
few compounds of note which have been characterized is a dicyclic sesquiter-
penoid-diol which was isolated from the unsaponifiable fraction of the petrol
ether extract of the leaves of *C. proximus* and called proximadiol [7]. It was
subsequently shown that the structure of this compound had previously been
assigned to a sesquiterpene cryptomeridiol (CAS Registry number 4666–84–6)
isolated from *Cryptomeria japonica* [8]. β-Sitosterol, hexacosanol, and triacon-
tanol were isolated from Nigerian *C. citratus* aerial parts as well as an unidentified
non-crystalline alkaloid and a saponin glucoside possibly based on fucosterol [9].

Pharmacology and Uses

Lemongrass has widespread uses in folk medicine. People from all parts of the
world use the leaves to prepare an infusion or decoction which is taken to treat
gastrointestinal ailments, nervous disturbances, feverish conditions and as a
diuretic, antiemetic and antirheumatic, according to references cited by Carlini
et al. [10]. The roots of *C. citratus* are used in West Africa as chewing sticks or are
rubbed on the teeth to clean them [11]. Commercial lemongrass oil is extensively
used for its fragrance in soaps, detergents, creams and perfumes. *Martindale*
includes a report that it has only 10–15% of the repellant activity of dimeth-

ylphthalate [12]. *Martindale* also mentions that lemongrass oil was formerly used as a carminative.

Citronella oil is used in perfumery, as a fragrance in soaps and household cleaning products, and in antimating preparations applied to dogs in estrus. It is also used as an active constituent in certain insect repellants. In Europe the oil is used in doses of 0.1 g in sedative dragees, as an embrocation containing typically 1% of the oil, and as a sedative bath additive [13].

Samaan investigated the effects of the essential oil of *C. schoenanthus* in the intact dog at doses of 0.25–0.1 ml/kg body weight and found that it depressed the heart and stimulated respiration; isolated toad heart was depressed at dilutions of 1 in 100 000, while dilutions of 1 in 10 000 caused relaxation of plain muscle in rabbit intestine, guinea pig and rabbit uteri, dog bladder, and bull urether [14].

Dilutions of *C. citratus* oil of 1 in 10 000 in horse serum to which acetylcholine had been added inhibited serum cholinesterase by 34% compared to a 60% inhibition produced by peppermint oil [15]. Tests of the antibacterial activity of the oils showed that lemongrass oil was consistently the most active, whether in the Rideal-Walker test (phenol coefficient 20) or in Garrod's test (coefficients lemongrass 17.5, citronella 10.0, and eucalyptus 3.0). Lemongrass oil was effective against a range of gram-negative and gram-positive organisms [16]. Onawunmi et al. showed that the antibacterial properties are largely due to the presence of α-citral (geranial) and β-citral (neral) while the presence in the oil of myrcene enhanced the activity of the other two compounds [11].

The pharmacological effects of the oleoresin from *C. proximus* have been extensively studied [17]. When injected into a 10 kg dog, 2 ml of a 1% alcoholic solution of the oleo-resin caused an immediate fall in blood pressure. The fall in blood pressure was equivalent to that produced by 2 ml 0.1% acetylcholine solution in the same animal. Low concentrations of the oleo resin caused a rapid, prolonged relaxation of the isolated ileum of rabbits and guinea pigs. The extract had 1.78 times the activity of papaverine when barium chloride was used as spasmogen. When given orally to guinea pigs, a protective action against bronchial spasm produced by histamine sprays gradually developed. An antiasthmatic effect was also reported for *C. distans* of Chinese origin by Huang [18].

The sesquiterpene cryptomeridiol was found to be a potent coronary dilator in the rabbit heart at a dose level of 2.5 mg. A dose of 5 mg caused inhibition of the myocardium, and the drug was capable of antagonizing the coronary constrictor effect of vasopressin. Doses of 50 mg/ml in Tyrode's solution decreased tone without affecting rhythmic contractions in rabbit jejunum [7]. Abdel-Moneim et al. [7] reported that the compound had unique antispasmodic properties as it produced relaxation of the smooth muscle fibers without abolishing the propulsive movement of the tissue. The authors comment on the value of this principle in the propulsion of renal and uretric calculi.

Carlini's group investigated lemongrass leaf tea, which is a popular folk treatment for nervous and gastrointestinal disturbances in Brazil [10]. The aqueous infusion (called abafado in Portuguese) was tested in rats and mice and compared to citral. Although the citral content of the essential oil of the plant material ranged from 46.6% to 70.9%, no information on the actual citral content of the various teas was reported. Doses up to 208 times the estimated human dosage of lemongrass tea were used and the animals subjected to a battery of 14 different pharmacological tests designed to test any possible CNS depressant effect as well as antipyretic activity and gastrointestinal effects. Oral doses of up to 40 times the human dose or of 200 mg/kg citral did not decrease the body temperature or increase transit time of a charcoal meal. In general there was no experimental support for any of the alleged folk uses of the plant. The only demonstrable effects were those obtained when the intraperitoneal route was used which resulted in a decrease in the body temperature of rats and of charcoal intestinal transit of mice. No CNS effects were noted.

Carbajal et al. [19] also tested decoctions of C. citratus in rats. They found dose-related hypotensive effects on i.v. administration, but only weak diuretic and anti-inflammatory effects after oral dosing. No cardiac depressant effect or direct relaxant effect on vascular smooth muscle was found.

Carlini's group also investigated the hypnotic effect of lemongrass leaf tea in 50 human volunteers using a double-blind placebo-controlled trial [20]. Lemongrass had no effect compared to the placebo on sleep induction, sleep quality, dream recall, and reawakening. Eighteen subjects with high anxiety scores were submitted to an anxiety-inducing test under double-blind conditions. No anxiolytic effects were noted, and the authors concluded that their data do not lend support to the popular use of lemongrass to treat nervous, intestinal, or feverish conditions [20].

Adverse Reaction Profile

Both types of lemongrass oil were granted GRAS (generally recognized as safe) status in 1965, are approved for food use by the United States Food and Drug Administration (FDA), and are also deemed admissible by the Council of Europe [21]. An acceptable daily intake of 500 µg/kg body weight has been established for citral, citronellal, and geranyl acetate, all calculated as citral [22]. Citronella oil also has GRAS status, as well as FDA and Council of Europe approval [23].

General Animal Data

The acute oral LD_{50} in rats was calculated as 7.3 g/kg body weight by Von Skramlik for lemongrass oil [24]. According to Opdyke the acute oral LD_{50} for both the West and East Indian lemongrass oils was over 5 g/kg body weight. The acute dermal LD_{50} in rabbits was over 2 g/kg body weight for East Indian oil while it exceeded 5 g/kg in the West Indian variety [21]. The corresponding value for citronella oil was more than 5 g/kg body weight for rats dosed orally and 4.7 ml/kg for the dermal LD_{50} in rabbits [23]. The oil from C. schoenanthus appears to be more toxic in that for the rabbit. Samaan reported an LD_{50} of 0.6 ml/kg body weight, and he also reported that the LD_{50} in the toad was 0.75 ml/kg body weight. A single i.v. injection of 0.25 ml/kg body weight was fatal in the dog within a few minutes. Lethality was reduced when the oil was injected in fractions over 2.5 h [14]. The sesquiteprene cryptomeridiol from *C. proximus* was subjected to a 24-h acute toxicity test and gave an LD_{50} in mice dosed i.p. of 500 mg/kg body weight [7].

An aqueous infusion prepared from lemongrass leaves was administered orally to adult rats for 2 months in doses up to 20 times larger than the estimated corresponding human dosage [10]. No effect was induced which could be taken as evidence of toxicity. The paper by Carbahal et al. [19] refers to toxicological studies on *C. citratus* carried out in Cuba and notes that the decoction prepared from the plant lacks significant toxic, teratogenic, and mutagenic effects.

General Human Data

Mant has reported a case of accidental poisoning when a 21-month-old child drank approximately 10 ml of Antimate of which citronella oil is the active constituent [25]. Despite rapidly initiated emesis followed by gastric lavage and intensive therapy using adrenaline and coramine, the child died several hours later. Postmortem examination revealed intense cyanosis, numerous punctate hemorrhages in the white matter of the brain, and early basal collapse of the lungs. In addition, the mucous membrane of the lower 2 inches of the esophagus had become detached. Information on the acute toxicity of plant material of any *Cymbopogon* species to humans has not been recovered from the literature.

A Brazilian group administered lemongrass tea to healthy human volunteers [20]. The testing was performed using 4 g of plant, which was double the normal amount used to prepare the tea in Brazil. Following a single dose or 2 weeks of daily oral administration, no changes in serum glucose, urea, creatinine, cholesterol, triglycerides, lipids, total bilirubin, indirect bilirubin, GOT, GPT, alkaline phosphatase, total protein, albumin, LDH, or CPK were noted. Six of the 11 volunteers presented direct bilirubin values slightly above normal (up to 0.25 μg/l), and four had increased amylase. These increases were not accompanied by any clinical sign which could be interpreted as a toxic effect, particularly as the GOT and GPT levels were normal.

Central Nervous System Reactions

Five of Carlini's volunteers reported sleepiness 4 h after drinking lemongrass tea, as did one patient in the 14-day study. These reported side effects are in contrast to the lack of sedative action in the clinical trial reported by this group in the same paper [20].

Dermatological Reactions

Opdyke [23] cites a report that citronella oil applied at full strength to intact or abraded rabbit skin caused irritation but also notes that three different samples of oil (Formosan, Sri Lankan, and Javanese) produced no irritation in a 48-h closed patch test in 25 human subjects at a concentration of 8%. No sensitization reactions were reported from the same test. Because of its rarity, Lane commented on a case of acneform type folliculitis induced by citronella oil [26]. He believed that this was a case of individual sensitivity to the oil. Keil reported three cases of eczematous contact-type hypersensitivity to oil of citronella [27]. In two of the cases he established that the essential allergen was citronellal. Geraniol gave only a weakly positive reaction in one case and a negative reaction in another. Geranyl acetate gave relatively mild papular reactions, but citronellol elicited far more intense reactions than geraniol, while citral gave moderately positive reactions. Keil also refers to probable cross-sensitivity, in persons sensitive to citronella oil, to oil from other species of the family. He makes the point that dermatitis due to citronella is probably far more common than has been suspected and may be wrongly attributed to poison ivy. Mitchell and Rook include a report on cross-sensitivity between palmarosa oil and oil of citronella [28]. Rudzki and Grzywa suggested using a mixture of citronella and cassia oils for testing of patients with dermatitis because the probability of detecting hypersensitivity to essential oils is increased. They found that among 750 patients with dermatitis, 11 were sensitive to citronella and standard sensitivity tests using Peru balsam indicated sensitivity in 30% of the cases [29].

Mitchell and Rook include several reports of vesicular dermatitis due to lemongrass oil in dockers handling a cargo of the oil [28]. Citral was implicated as the harmful chemical. Opdyke [21], reporting on both East and West Indian lemongrass oil, notes that both were mildly irritating when the full-strength oils were applied to the backs of hairless mice and swine and under occlusion to intact or abraded rabbit skin. No evidence of irritation or sensitization was found in human patch tests. Tests on hairless mice and swine showed no phototoxicity.

Gastrointestinal Reactions

In Carlini's study of lemongrass tea, three different strengths were prepared from 2, 4 and 10 g of leaves [20]. Volunteers who ingested the 10 g tea complained of a slight stomach upset. One of the eight volunteers who drank the 4 g tea daily for 14 days complained of diarrhea.

Ocular Reactions

Samaan reported that pure oil from *C. schoenanthus* caused a slight inflammatory reaction in the eye or when injected intraperitoneally into the rabbit [14].

Renal Reactions

Four volunteers in the Brazilian study of lemongrass reported polyuria 4 h after a single dose of tea made from 4 g of leaves. In the 14 day test one of the eight participants complained of polyuria [20].

Respiratory Reactions

Jarikre and Bazuaye recorded two cases of acute pulmonary edema or toxic alveolitis associated with the use of a traditional Nigerian fever therapy for malaria consisting of a concoction of the leaves of *Carica papaya*, *Citrus sinensis* and *Cymbopogon citratus* [30]. This mixture was consumed twice daily for 2–3 days by steam inhalation, bathing, and drinking. The pulmonary edema was secondary to increased capillary permeability resulting in transudation of fluids across the membrane into the lung interstitium. The toxic effect could undoubtedly have been due to the inhalation of firewood smoke and steam during the inhalation stage of the therapy, but a case could be made implicating lemongrass on the basis of the work of Samaan with *C. schoenanthus* essential oil in rabbits [14]. Postmortem examination showed the presence of a large amount of hemorrhagic congestion of the lungs which the author suggested could be explained by the rapid excretion of the oil by the lungs. These effects do, however, stand in contrast with the antiasthmatic and antihistamine properties reported for *C. distans* and *C. proximus*, respectively [17,18].

Fertility, Pregnancy, and Lactation

Carlini and coworkers report an absence of effects in male and female rats and in their offspring when an aqueous tea made from *C. citratus* leaves was administered prior to mating or during pregnancy [31]. Carbajal [19] also reported no teratogenic effects from a decoction of the leaves of lemongrass. No data on the effect of any of the *Cymbopogon* oils during pregnancy or lactation have been recovered from the literature.

Mutagenicity and Carcinogenicity

Lewis and Elvin-Lewis state (without any literature citation) that *C. citratus*, *C. nardus* and *C. flexuosus* are mutagenic because of the presence of citronellal [32]. Information on the carcinogenicity of any *Cymbopogon* species or their oils has not been recovered from the literature.

References

1. Banthorpe DV, Duprey RJH, Hassan M, Janes JF, Modawi BM (1976) Chemistry of the Sudanese flora. I. Essential oils of some *Cymbopogon* species. Planta Med 29:10–19
2. Anonymous (1979) The pharmaceutical codex. 11th ed. The Pharmaceutical Press, p 198
3. Carlin JT, Kramer S, Chi-Tang H (1988) Comparison of commercial citronella oils from various origins. In: Lawrence BM, Mookherjee BD, Willis BJ (eds) Flavors and fragrances: a world perspective. Proceedings of the 10th International Congress of Essential Oils, Fragrances and Flavors, Washington, DC, USA, 1986; Elsevier Science Publications. Amsterdam, pp 495–504
4. Leung AY (1980) Encyclopaedia of common natural ingredients used in food, drugs and cosmetics. New York: Wiley-Interscience, pp 218–219
5. Reynolds JEF (ed) (1982) Martindale the extra phamacopoeia, 28th edn. London: The Pharmaceutical Press, pp 680–681
6. Surburg H (1988) Minor components of palmarosa oil. In: Lawrence BM, Mookherjee BD, Willis BJ (eds). Flavors and fragrances: a world perspective. Proceedings of the 10th International Congress of Essential Oils, Fragrances and Flavors, Washington, DC, USA, 1986; Elsevier Science Publications. Amsterdam, pp 505–515
7. Abdel-Moneim FM, Ahmed ZF, Fayez MBE, Ghaleb H (1979) Constituents of local plants. XIV. The antispasmodic principle in *Cymbopogon proximus*. Planta Med 17:209–216
8. Locksley HD, Fayez MBE, Radwan AS, Chari VM, Cordell GA, Wagner H (1982) Constituents of local plants. XXV. Constitution of the antispasmodic principle of *Cymbopogon proximus*. Planta Med 45:20–22
9. Olaniyi AA, Sofowora EA, Oguntimehin BO (1975) Phytochemical investigation of some Nigerian plants used against fevers. II. *Cymbopogon citratus*. Planta Med 28:187–189
10. Carlini EA, Contar JDP, Silva-Filho AR, Siliveira-Filho NG, Frochtengarten ML, Bueno OFA (1986) Pharmacology of lemongrass (*Cymbopogon citratus* Stapf.) I. Effects of teas prepared from the leaves on laboratory animals. J Ethnopharmacol, 17:37–64
11. Onawunmi GO, Yisak W, Ogunlana EO (1984) Antibacterial constituents in the essential oil of *Cymbopogon citratus* (DC.) Stapf. J Ethnopharmacol 12:279–286
12. Tiwari BK (1966) Indian J Exp Biol 4:128 (cited in [5] p 677)
13. Arzneibüro der Bundesvereinigung Deutscher Apothekerverbände Pharmazeutische Stoffliste (1990) 7th edn. Frankfurt Am Main: Werbe- und Vertriebsgesellschaft Deutscher Apotheker
14. Samaan K (1934) Pharmacological action of the oil of *Cymbopogon schoenanthus*. Quart J Pharm Pharmacol 7:215–221
15. Caujolle F, Vincent D, Franck C (1944) Action of essential oils on serum cholinesterase. Compt Rend Soc Biol 138:556–558
16. Bose SM, Bhima Rao CN, Subramanyan V (1949) Relationship between chemical composition and constituents of certain essential oils and their bactericidal properties. J Sci Ind Res 8B:157–162
17. Borolossy AW, El-Sayed HI (1960) Pharmacology of an oleoresin from *C. proximus*. Egypt Pharm Bull 42:425–430
18. Hunang TF, Li H-L, Chiao TF (1976) Vitamin K3 in experimental relaxation of ileum spasm and clinical treatment of biliary colic in biliary ascariosis. Biol Ab 62, abstract 9890 (cited in [10])
19. Carbajal D, Casaco A, Arruzazabala L, Gonzalez R, Tolon Z (1989) Pharmacological study of *Cymbopogon citratus* leaves. J Ethnopharmacol 25:103–107
20. Leite JR, Seabra MLV, Maluf E et al. (1986) Pharmacology of lemongrass (*Cymbopogon citratus* Stapf.). III. Assessment of eventual toxic, hypnotic and anxiolytic effect on humans. J Ethnopharmacol 17:75–83
21. Opdyke DLJ (1976) Lemongrass oil. Fd Cosmet Toxicol 14:455–457
22. Anonymous (1980) Evaluation of certain food additives and contaminants. 23rd Report of the Joint FAO/WHO Expert Committee on Food Additives. Technical Report Series 648. Geneva: World Health Organization
23. Opdyke DLJ (1973) Citronella oil. Fd Cosmet Toxicol 11:1067
24. Skramlik EV (1959) Über die Giftigkeit und Vertraglichkeit von ätherischen ölen. Pharmazie 14:435–445

25. Mant KA (1961) A case of poisoning by oil of citronella. Med Sci Law 1:170–171
26. Lane CG (1922) Dermatitis caused by oil of citronella. Arch Dermatol Syph 5:589–590
27. Keil H (1947) Contact dermatitis due to oil of citronella. J Invest Dermatol 8:327–334
28. Mitchell J, Rook A (1979) botanical dermatology. Greengrass, Vancouver, pp 332–334
29. Rudzki E, Grzywa Z (1985) The value of a mixture of cassia and citronella oils for detection of hypersensitivity to essential oils. Dermatosen 33:59–62
30. Jarikre LN, Bazuaye EA (1986) Acute pulmonary oedema (toxic alveolitis) associated with traditional fever therapy. East Afr Med J 63:656–659
31. Formigoni MLOS, Lodder HM, Tilho OG, Ferreira TMS, Carlini EA (1986) Pharmacology of lemongrass (*Cymbopogon citratus* Stapf.) II. Effects of daily two month administration in male and female rats and in offspring exposed "in utero". J Ethnopharmacol 17:65–74
32. Lewis WH, Elvin-Lewis MPF (1977) Medical botany. Wiley-Interscience New York, p 94

Eucalyptus Species

D. Corrigan

Botany

There are more than 500 species of *Eucalyptus* belonging to the family Myrtaceae. The major species of commercial interest are *E. globulus* Labill., *E. fruticetorum* F. von Muell. (*E. polybractea*), and *E. smithii* R.T. Baker which are used for the distillation of essential oil (eucalyptus oil). Vernacular names include fever tree leaves, blue gum leaves, and eucalyptus leaves. Other important species include *E. amygdalina*, *E. citriodora*, *E. rostrata*, and *E. viminalis*.

Chemistry

The most notable constituents of *Eucalyptus* are the essential oil and the tannins. The essential oil may be distilled from the fresh or dried leaves. According to Grieve [1], the eucalyptus oils may be divided into three types depending on their commercial uses: (a) medicinal oils usually distilled from *E. globulus* giving 1.5−3.5% of oil, of which 70−95% is, 1,δ-cineole (also known as eucalyptol); (b) industrial oils from species such as *E. viminalis* which are used for flotation purposes in the mining industry − such oils contain large quantities of phellandrene which MacPherson [2] reports as being irritating when inhaled; and (c) aromatic oils from *E. citriodora* containing chiefly citronellol. The point has been made that the large number of species plus the existence of chemical races means a great variety of oils and that the term "eucalyptus oil" is meaningless unless the species from which it is derived is stated [1]. The other significant components of *E. globulus* oil include α-pinene, d-limonene, and p-cymene with traces of β-pinene, α-phellandrene, camphene, and γ-terpinene. Small amounts of sesquiterpenes also occur.

Tannins occur in both the leaf and the bark of the trees. One sample of *E. globulus* leaf powder sold in capsule form had a tannin content of 11% (Booth and Corrigan 1989, unpublished observations). *E. cornea* had 25% of tannins, but the plant part tested was not specified [3]. Some species are the source of a kino e.g., eucalyptus kino or red gum is the dried exudate from the bark of *E. rostrata* Schlecht. Botany bay kino is a similar product from *E. globulus* and *E. resinifera* consisting of 28% kino tannin and 48% catechin [4].

In addition, eucalyptus has been reported to contain 2–4% of ursolic acid derivatives, polyphenolic acids, and flavonoids such as quercetin and rutin [5]. Morton [6] cites reports that *E. macrorryncha* F.V.M. contains 12–20% of rutin. Cyanogenetic glycosides have been detected in both fresh and dried leaves of several species, e.g., *E. corynocalyx* (0.179% HCN), *E. cladocalyx* (0.5% HCN), and also in *E. viminalis* [7,8]. Under certain conditions, e.g., drought, the cyanide content of *E. cladocalyx* can be sufficiently high to cause mortality in sheep and goats feeding on the leaves. [9]

Pharmacology and Uses

Three products from eucalyptus are used medicinally, namely the oil, the kino, and the dried leaves. The oil is used as an antiseptic, antispasmodic stimulant agent in bronchitis, asthma, and minor respiratory complaints. A 1% ointment has been used in rhinitis and a 25% liniment as a rubefacient. The vapors are often inhaled in asthma, pharyngitis, and related conditions. In aromatherapy the oil is used externally to soothe coughing, promote scar formation in burns and injuries, and as an antirheumatic. Internally it is recommended by aromatherapists for asthma, diabetes, measles, and rheumatism. Boyd and Pearson [10] stated in 1946 that the average recommended dose of oil of eucalyptus in humans is of the order of 10 mg/kg body weight. However, the 28th edition of *Martindale* gives 0.05–0.2 ml as the recommended dose range [10a]. Boyd and Pearson studied the expectorant effect of the oil in a variety of laboratory animals and found that the maximum expectorant effect was obtained with a dose of 50 mg/kg body weight [10]. Subsequent work by Boyd and Sheppard with rabbits [11] led them to conclude that the addition of eucalyptus oil to steam inhalation adds little to therapy. Burrow et al. [12] investigated the use of eucalyptus oil as a nasal decongestant in human volunteers and found that while the oil had a stimulant or sensitizing effect on nasal cold receptors, thus giving a sensation of increased airflow, no decongestant effect was demonstrated. The oil does have slight antibacterial action as measured by the Rideal-Walker test (*E. globulus* 3.0, *E. australiana* 5.8, and *E. cinearifolia* 4.8) [13]. The oil from *E. viminalis* reportedly has activity against influenza viruses A2 and A in chickens [14].

The dried leaf is sold as a treatment for respiratory tract conditions. Older texts recommended the use of a fluid extract (28 g plant to 465 ml of H_2O) in scarlet, typhoid and intermittent fevers, ulcers, and local infections [15].

The tannin-rich kino was formerly included in the *British Pharmaceutical Codex* (1949) as an astringent for the throat in the form of a gargle, and internally it was used to treat diarrhea and dysentery. Read et al. [16] reported on a tannin fraction from 29 different *Eucalyptus* species. While this tannin was a potent histamine liberator when administered i.v. or i.p., it was ineffective orally. *E. robusta* was the most and *E. smithii* the least active of the species tested.

Pharmacokinetics

While no pharmacokinetic data directly relating to eucalyptus oil have been recovered from the literature, Kovar and colleagues [17] have reported blood levels of the major constituent of the oil, eucalyptol (1,8-cineole) after inhalation and oral administration of the essential oil of rosemary (*Rosmarinus officinalis* L.). When 0.5 ml of oil was allowed to evaporate the concentrations of eucalyptol in the breathing air and in the blood were in the ratio of 1.0:0.83. After oral dosing the blood level reached a peak after 5 min. The elimination of the eucalyptol from the blood after inhalation was biphasic with a short half-life of 6 min during the first 10 min and a half-life of about 45 min during a second phase, reflecting possible different elimination rates from a central and from a peripheral compartment.

In relation to the use of eucalyptus oil in aromatherapy, it is noteworthy that Meyer and Meyer [18] found that the oil was rapidly absorbed across the intact shaved skin of mice.

Adverse Reaction Profile

Both eucalyptus oil and eucalyptol were granted GRAS (generally recognized as safe) status in 1965 and both are approved for food use by the United States Food and Drug Administration. The Council of Europe permits the use of the oil as a spice or seasoning. Eucalyptol is included in the Council list of admissible artificial flavoring substances at a level of 15 ppm [19,20].

In France an infusion of *E. globulus* leaf is accepted for product registration purposes as being "traditionally used during benign acute bronchial disorders" and as such no toxicological study is required. However, when the powdered leaf is supplied, a reduced toxicological study is required [21].

General Animal Data

Reported LD_{50} values for the oil are quite high. For instance, Von Skramlik [22] found the LD_{50} in the rat to be 4.44 g/kg body weight. Ohsumi et al. [23] determined the oral LD_{50} of the oil in mice and calculated it as 3.32 g/kg body weight, which they compared with a value of 1.82 g/kg body weight for oil of clove. The acute oral LD_{50} of eucalyptol was reported [19] as 2.48 g/kg in the rat while the acute dermal LD_{50} in rabbits exceeded 5 g/kg.

Puztai et al. [24] reported a study of the chronic toxicity of a mixture of oil of eucalyptus, fennel, and turpentine administered to 50 rats over a period of 10–16 weeks. They found a slight reduction in diuresis after 10 weeks, but liver function was unchanged. There was no evidence of histological damage to either the liver or kidney. A decrease in body weight was noted in the latter part of the 16-week treatment. Lysenko [25] injected eucalyptus oil i.m. into rabbits daily for 5 days. He found that inflammatory edema after burns was reduced. In addition, blood coagulation was retarded, leukocytosis was increased, but there was no effect on hemoglobin content or on erythrocyte count.

General Human Data

It is difficult to reconcile animal values with the literature reports of deaths and other acute toxic reactions in humans who had taken the oil orally. Withauer [26] for example refers to 17 fatal poisonings due to eucalyptus oil reported in the medical literature between 1889 and 1922. MacPherson [2] reports that death has occurred in adults after ingesting as little as 4–5 ml oil, and that death is usual after doses of 30 ml. On the other hand, Gurr and Scroggie [27] report that recovery occurred in some patients who had taken between 120 and 220 ml oil. MacPherson does however comment that idiosyncratic reactions are quite noticeable. The toxic effects are rapid in onset and include epigastric burning, abdominal pain, and spontaneous vomiting which may be delayed up to 4 h after ingestion, respiratory problems, bronchospasm, and tachypnea with severe respiratory depression. CNS involvement includes diminution or loss of reflexes and depression of consciousness which may progress to coma. Convulsions may occur, particularly in children.

Central Nervous System Reactions

The toxicity of eucalyptus oil appears to be underestimated by some authorities. For example, O'Mullane [28] attributed the adverse CNS effects found in a 13-year-old boy who swallowed 5 ml of a commercial product called Olbas Oil to the menthol content of the oil. The composition of the product was menthol 4.1%, oil of cajuput 15.5%, clove oil 0.1%, eucalyptus 35.5%, juniper berry 2.7%, peppermint 35.5%, and wintergreen 3.7%. He apparently did not consider the possibility that the effects might have been due wholly or in part to the eucalyptus oil which, according to MacPherson [2], may profoundly affect the nervous system. Steinmetz et al. [29] have reported that eucalyptol at a concentration of 2 ml per liter has an inhibitory action on the oxygen consumption and on Na^+/K^+ gradients in rat brain cortical slices. They suggest that these effects may explain the CNS effects reported for a number of essential oils containing eucalyptol.

Dermatological Reactions

Opdyke [19,20] concludes that eucalyptus oil and eucalyptol are generally nonirritating, nonsensitizing, and nonphototoxic both in animal tests and in patch tests with human volunteers. However, Mitchell and Rook [30] include several reports of urticaria (from handling foliage), dermatitis, and skin irritation relating to a number of *Eucalyptus* species.

Rudzki et al. [31] report that eucalyptus oil causes contact allergy. It is worth noting that in 1912 Oppenheim [32] recorded the case of a 36-year-old patient who became ill after consuming 20 cough drops containing eucalyptus oil. Initially he developed spots on the back of the hand, but on the following day both hands and feet were covered with erythematous efflorescences resembling those produced by balsam of Copaiba.

Gastrointestinal Reactions

Dzhanashiya and Startsev [33] found that teas made from *E. viminalis*, *E. cinerea*, *E. macarthuri*, and *E. dalrympeana* given to monkeys reduced the digestive ability of gastric juice but did not affect the ability to degrade protein.

The tannin content of the leaf drug might be expected to cause mild constipation with frequent use, but information on the long-term effects of frequent use of the leaf material is scarce. Two cases of rectal bleeding were reported after the use of suppositories containing eucalyptol and other terpenes [34]. In one of the cases it was claimed that a further episode of bleeding was precipitated three weeks later when the patient (a 4-year-old boy) was given a pastille containing terpenes, although it is debatable whether the concentration of terpenes being eliminated would be high enough to cause such an effect.

Metabolic Reactions

Revoredo [35] found that an extract of *E. citriodora* leaves administered orally caused temporary hypoglycemia in alloxan-diabetic rabbits but did not lead to normal values. Administration of the extract preceding a glucose tolerance test produced a flat blood sugar curve. An unidentified compound named myrtilin was believed to be responsible. Boukef [36] isolated a phenolic heteroside called calyptoside which showed hypoglycemic activity in rabbits.

In 1922 John [37] as a result of reports from medical practitioners in Scotland, Tenerife, and Algeria outlining the benefits of a eucalyptus infusion in reducing glucosuria, administered from 1 to 3 liters of an infusion of eucalyptus daily for two to three months, to 20 patients representing the full range of types and stages of diabetes, but there was no noticeable effect on the progress of the disease. He also noted that there was no sign of injury to the treated patients in the form of albuminuria, gastrointestinal disturbances, or subjective feelings.

Respiratory Reactions

Patel and Wiggins [38] reported a case of accidental poisoning in a 3-year-old boy who swallowed 10 ml of oil. On admission he was comatose, with constricted pupils, markedly reduced muscle tone, and undetectable tender reflexes. Respiration was shallow and irregular with BP 75/40 mmHg. Recovery was rapid after careful gastric lavage with sodium bicarbonate solution, and the boy was discharged 48 h after admission. They warn that attempts to induce vomiting should be avoided in such cases because of the risk of aspiration of oil. Gastric lavage should be performed with great care using, where possible, a cuffed endotracheal tube. Urinary output should be monitored, and in severe cases peritoneal or hemodialysis is claimed to be of value.

The cooling effect of the oil on the respiratory tract has already been noted [12]. This effect is similar to that produced by both camphor and menthol and strongly suggests that ointments containing either eucalyptus oil or eucalyptol should not be applied to or near the nostrils in infants and small children because of the risk of spasm of the glottis.

Drug Interactions

A number of studies have demonstrated that eucalyptus leaves, the oil, and eucalyptol can all induce microsomal enzyme activity in both in vitro and in vivo tests [39–42]. While there have been no recorded interactions between eucalyptus and other drugs at a clinical level, a number of animal studies indicate possible areas of concern.

Jori [39] reported that the metabolism of pentobarbitone was increased when eucalyptol (1,8-cineole) was administered subcutaneously or by aerosol to female rats using doses of 500 mg/kg. The sleeping time was approximately 50% less than in control rats.

A similar effect on Hexenal sleeping time in mice was noted by Nemirovskii [43] using eucalyptus oil. Seawright et al. [40] found that E. caleyi foliage induced mixed-function oxidases in rats, and they further observed that these leaves were consumed by sheep on overgrazed pasture and increased their susceptibility to overdosing from carbon tetrachloride used as an anthelminthic. In 1982 Noble et al. [41] also reported that the oil from E. caleyi enhanced the activity of liver detoxification enzymes of livestock grazing on eucalyptus and suggested that it might increase their susceptibility to mortality from carbon tetrachloride drenches. White and coworkers [42] evaluated the effect of microsomal enzyme induction by E. globulus foliage on the toxicity of a mixture of pyrrolizidine alkaloids (extracted from Senecio longilobus) in rats. Induction of mixed-function oxidase activity by eucalyptus (10% by weight in the diet) resulted in a reduction in the oral LD_{50} of the alkaloid mixture from 320 mg/kg to 127 mg/kg at 72 h post administration. White et al. were uncertain as to whether the reduction was due to increased metabolic production of pyrroles from the alkaloids, associated with the enzyme induction, or due to the average decrease in body weight of 30 g per rat which occurred prior to the administration of the alkaloids. This weight loss in rats fed eucalyptus leaves had previously been noted by Seawright [40].

Fertility, Pregnancy, and Lactation[1]

No data on teratogenicity have been recovered from the literature. Studies in rats showed that eucalyptol probably cannot cross the blood-milk barrier in amounts sufficient to affect hepatic microsomal enzymes in the offspring, but it is able to penetrate the placental tissue and to reach a concentration in fetal blood adequate for stimulating hepatic enzyme activity after a dose of 500 mg/kg given s.c. [44].

Mutagenicity and Carcinogenicity

E. citriodora is included by Lewis and Elvin-Lewis in a list of plants which are mutagenic due to the presence of citronellal [45]. Field and Roe [46] stated that eucalyptus oil was a weak promotor of papilloma formation by 9,-10-dimethyl-12-benzanthracene in mice. Phellandrene, one of the constituents of the oil also had a weak promoting effect when applied to mice at a concentration of 40% in acetone.

References

1. Leyel CF (1931) A modern herbal by Mrs Grieve. London: Jonathan Cape
2. MacPherson J (1925) The toxicology of eucalyptus oil. Med J Aust 2:108–110
3. Swamy M, Theresa YM, Nauydanma Y (1981) Screening of eucalyptus trees of Gudular for tannins. Leather Sci (Madras) 28:366–368, through Chem Abstr 96:17265
4. Dukes JA (1985) A handbook of medicinal herbs. Boca Raton: CRC Press, pp 185–186
5. Leung AY (1980) Encyclopedia of common natural ingredients used in food, drugs and cosmetics. New York: Wiley-Interscience, pp 166–167
6. Morton JF (1977) Major medicinal plants. Springfield: Thomas, p 367
7. Finnemore H, Cox CB (1929) Cyanogenetic glycosides in Australian plants. J Proc Roy Soc NS Wales 62:369–378
8. Finnemore H, Reichard SK, Large DK (1936) Cyanogenetic glycosides in Australian plants. III. *E. cladocalyx*. J Proc Roy Soc N S Wales 69:209–214
9. Webber JJ, Roycroft CR, Callinan JD (1985) Cyanide poisoning of goats from sugar gums (*Eucalyptus cladocalyx*). Aust Vet J 62:28
10. Boyd EM, Pearson GL (1946) On the expectorant action of volatile oils. Am J Med Sci 211:602–610
10a. Reynolds JEF, Prasad AB (eds) (1982) Martindale the extra pharmacopoeia, 28t edn. London: The Pharmaceutical Press
11. Boyd EM, Sheppard EP (1968) The effect of steam inhalation of volatile oils on the output and composition of respiratory tract fluid. J Pharmac Exp Therap 163:250–256
12. Burrow A, Eccles R, Jones AS (1983) The effects of camphor, eucalyptus and menthol vapour on nasal resistance to airflow and nasal sensation. Acta Otolaryngol 96:157–161
13. Greig-Smith R (1919) The germicidal activity of the eucalyptus oils. I. Proc Linn Soc NSW 44:72–92, through Chem Abstr 13:3208

---

[1]See also the note added in proof on p. 262

14. Vichkanova SA, Goryunova LV (1973) Antiviral activity displayed by the essential oil of *E. viminalis*. Farmakol Toksikol (Moscow) 36:339–341, through Chem Abstr 79:38916
15. Potter H, Wren RW (1941) Potters cyclopedia of botanical drugs and preparations. 5th ed. London: Potter and Clarke, pp 131–132
16. Read GW, Naguwa GS, Wigington JJ, Lenney JF (1970) A histamine liberator in the tannin fraction of the eucalyptus. Lloydia 33:461–471
17. Kovar KA, Gropper B, Friess D, Ammon HPT (1987) Blood levels of 1,8-cineole and locomotor activity of mice after inhalation and oral administration of rosemary oil. Planta Medica 53:315–318
18. Meyer FR, Meyer E (1959) Percutaneous absorption of essential oils and their constituents. Arzneim Forsch 9:516–519
19. Opdyke DLJ (1975) Eucalyptol. Fd Cosmet Toxicol 13:105–106
20. Opdyke DLJ (1975) Eucalyptus Oil. Fd Cosmet Toxicol 13:107–108
21. Ministere des Affaires Sociales de France (1986) Avis aux Fabricants concernant les demandes d'autorisation de mise sur le marche de specialites pharmaceutiques a base de plantes. Bulletin Officiel No 86/20 bis, August
22. Von Skramlik E (1959) Über die Giftigkeit und vertraglichkeit von ätherischen Ölen. Pharmazie 14:435–445
23. Ohsumi T et al. (1984) Study on acute toxicities of essential oils used in endodontic treatment. Kyusha Shika Gakkai Zasshi 38:1064–1071, through Chem Abstr 102:179007
24. Puztai F, Kelentey B, Szucs L, Soltesz J (1983) Chronic toxicity of a mixture of volatile oils in rats. Pharmazie 18:238–241
25. Lysenko LV (1967) Antiphlogistic action of eucalyptus oil azulene. Farmakol Toksikol 30:341–343
26. Withauer W (1922) Über Vergiftung mit Eucalyptusöl. Klin Wschr 1:1460–1461
27. Gurr FW, Scroggie JG (1965) Eucalyptus oil poisoning treated by dialysis and mannitol infusion with an appendix on the analysis of biological fluids for alcohol and eucalyptol. Australas Ann Med 14:238–249
28. O'Mullane NM, Joyce P, Kamath SV, Tham MK, Knass D (1982) Adverse CNS effects of menthol containing Olbas oil. Lancet 1:1121
29. Steinmetz MD, Vial M, Millet Y (1987) Actions de l'huile essentielle de Romarin et de certaines de ses constituants (eucalyptol et camphre) sur le cortex cerebral de rat in vitro. J Toxicol Clin Exp 7:259–271
30. Mitchell J, Rook A (1979) Botanical Dermatology. Vancouver: Greengrass, pp 484–486
31. Rudzki E, Grzywa Z, Bruno WS (1976) Sensitivity to 35 essential oils. Contact Dermatitis 2:196
32. Oppenheim M (1912) Exanthema produced by eucalyptus cough drops. Dermat Wochensch. No. 8, through Chem Abstr 6:3288
33. Dzhanashiya NM, Startsev VG (1970) Comparative evaluation of the influence of some species of Eucalyptus and antibiotics on the peptic activity of the gastric juice of monkeys. Antibiotiki (Moscow) 15:547–548, through Chem Abstr 73:64659
34. Vincens M, Lagier G, Medernach C, Wierdiki C, Leperchey F (1982) Rectites terpeniques, 2 cas cliniques. Therapie 37:328–330
35. Revoredo NL (1958) Hypoglycaemic activity of *E. citriodora*. Monit Farm y Terap 64:37–38, through Chem Abstr 52:10414
36. Boukef K (1976) Study of a phenolic heteroside isolated from the leaves of *E. globulus* Labill. Plant Med Phytother 10:119–127
37. John HL (1922) A trial of eucalyptus infusion in diabetes. J Metabol Res 1:489–495
38. Patel S, Wiggins J (1980) Eucalyptus oil poisoning. Arch Dis Child 55:405–406
39. Jori A, Bianchetti A, Prestini PE (1969) Effect of essential oils on drug metabolism. Biochem Pharmacal 18:2081–2085
40. Seawright AA, Steele DP, Menrath RE (1972) Seasonal variation in hepatic microsomal oxidation metabolism in vitro and susceptibility to carbon tetrachloride in a flock of sheep. Aust Vet J 48:488–494
41. Noble RM et al. (1982) Induction of hepatic microsomal oxidative metabolism in mice by essential oil components from some *Eucalyptus* species. Queensl J Agric Animal Sci 39:9–14, through Chem Abst 100:46572

42. White RD, Swick RA, Cheeke PR (1983) Effects of microsomal enzyme induction on the toxicity of pyrrolizidine (*Senecio*) alkaloids. J Toxicol Env Health 12:633–640
43. Nemirovskii ON (1975) Toxicological characteristics of some essential oils according to the results of single and repeated exposures. Tr Lening Sanit-gig-Med Inst 111:61–65, through Chem Abstr 89:85417
44. Jori A, Briatico G (1973) Effect of eucalyptol on microsomal enzyme activity of foetal and newborn rats. Biochem Pharmacol 22:543–544
45. Lewis WH, Elvin-Lewis MPF (1977) Medical botany. New York: Wiley-Interscience, p 94
46. Roe FCJ, Field WEH (1965) Chronic toxicity of essential oils and certain other products of natural origin. Fd Cosmet Toxicol 3:311–342

Foeniculum vulgare

K. Keller

Botany

Fennel consists of the ripe dried fruits of *Foeniculum vulgare* Miller ssp. *capillaceum* (Gilibert) Holmboe var. *dulce* (Miller) Thellung (= sweet fennel) or of *Foeniculum vulgare* Miller ssp. *capillaceum* (Gilibert) Holmboe var. *vulgare* (Thellung) Miller (= bitter fennel) [1,2].

In popular medicine the root of fennel is also used.

Chemistry

The most important constituent of fennel is 2–6% of essential oil. The composition of the essential oil depends on the variety (see Table 1).

In the risk evaluation, the existence of a chemotype with estragole as main component of the essential oil must be considered [3].

The different fennel varieties are rather difficult to separate, mainly due to their tendency to hybridization [1,3 9]. The bitter taste of the var. *vulgare* is caused by the monoterpene ketone fenchone. Cis-anethol is present in fennel oil only as a trace component. Di-p-methoxystilbene, which is said to be formed by dimerization of anethole could not be identified by Kraus and Hammerschmidt, even in a sample, which was stored under extreme conditions [8].

Tóth found that the root of the var. *vulgare* contained 0.5–0.7% of essential oil, consisting mainly of dill-apiole [9].

Table 1.

Variety	trans-Anethole	Fenchone	Estragole
Sweet fennel	75–95%	< 1–8%	3–8%
Bitter fennel	60–75%	12–30%	2–7%
Bitter fennel "Anethole free"	traces	15%	80%

Pharmacology and Uses[1]

Investigations in animals and isolated organs have shown an inhibition of stomach movement and an increase in tonus and motility of small intestine [10,11,12,13].

The application of water extracts from fennel resulted in an increase in the mucociliar activity in the isolated ciliated epithelium of the frog esophagus [14]. Boyd described an increase in the output volume of respiratory tract fluid in urethanized rabbits caused by the inhalation of low doses of anethole and fenchone. This effect, especially that of anethole, was more evident in the autumn months of the year [15].

Fennel has been considered to possess estrogenic activity [16,17]. The estrogenic activity has been attributed to the dimers of anethole such as p-methoxystilbene (dianethole). Considering the fact that this compound was not found in fennel oil even after storage under extreme conditions [8], and that p-methoxystilbene as well as trans-anethole have weak estrogenic activity, these speculations do not seem to be substantiated. Also, there are no new systematic investigations on the postulated estrogenic activity of fennel oil.

In hepatectomized rats high doses of 100 mg/kg fennel oil s.c. over a 10-day period led to an increase in liver regeneration expressed as an increase in dry weight of liver tissue. The effect was attributed to the phenolethers present in fennel oil [18].

Preparations of fennel are used as carminative and expectorant. The use is approved in the Federal Republic of Germany [19] and in France [20]. Fennel is mentioned in many handbooks [1,2,21–23]. The dosage is 2–3 g fennel for infusions or 0.05 to 0.2 ml of the essential oil.

Adverse Reaction Profile

General Animal Data

The oral LD_{50} of bitter fennel oil in rats is reported by Opdyke to be 4.5 ml/kg compared to 3.8 g/kg for (sweet?) fennel oil [24,25]. Skramlik found an oral LD_{50} of 3.12 g/kg [26]. These LD_{50} values are within the range reported for anethole (LD_{50} p.o. in mice 3 g/kg, in rats 2 g/kg, in guinea pigs 2.2 g/kg) and for fenchone (in rats 6.2 g/kg) [26–28]. The acute toxicity of cis-anethole in rats and mice is about 20 times higher than that of trans-anethole [29]. The acute dermal LD_{50} of fennel oil in rabbits exceeded 5 ml/kg [24,25]. According to Lewin, 21 g fennel oil p.o. is lethal to rabbits [30].

In a feeding study, 10 000 ppm anethole fed to rats in the diet for 15 weeks produced slight hydropic changes in the liver of the male animals. In other feeding

[1]For pharmacokinetic data, see the section on mutagenicity, cytotoxicity, and carcinogenicity.

studies in rats neither 2500 ppm fed in the diet for 1 year nor 10 000 ppm in the diet for 15 weeks produced any effects [31]. The level causing no effect in the rat was 2500 ppm in the diet or 125 mg/kg body weight per day. In a feeding study in which dietary levels of 1000, 3000, 10 000, and 30 000 ppm anethole were fed to rats over 90 days, death occurred at the highest level, and survival was affected at the 10 000 ppm level. Hepatocellular edema, degeneration, and regeneration of the liver cells were found, proportional to the level of treatment, at levels ≥ 3000 ppm. No effect was seen at 1000 ppm [27,32].

General Human Data[1]

There are no data proving that the use of fennel presents any special human health risk. Acute or chronic poisoning with fennel oil in humans has not been reported. The Council of Europe included fennel (fruit) in its 1973 list of substances, spices, and seasonings commonly added to foodstuffs in small quantities, the use of which is deemed admissible, with the possible limitation of the active principle in the final product. An ADI value was not fixed [33].

Allergic Reactions

Even though fennel is mentioned by Steinegger and Hänsel [1] as a spice allergen, there are practically no case reports of allergic reactions to fennel. Some publications report a cross-reaction with fennel in the so called "celery-mugwort-spice" syndrome, but even in this context positive reactions to fennel are rare [34,35]. Considering the widespread use of fennel and the fact that case reports of allergic reactions are practically absent, fennel represents a low allergenic risk. See also the section on respiratory reactions.

Dermatological Reactions

Allergic skin reactions are rare (see the section on allergic reactions). Fennel is presented in a list of plants claimed to be responsible for photodermatitis in man [36]. It seems very doubtful that the fruits of fennel could produce phototoxic effects, because furocoumarins or similar compounds are lacking. Opdyke [24] states that no phototoxic effects were observed with fennel oil.

The dermal application of an infusion of fennel in man results in an aggravation of the inflammation caused by mustard oil, UV irradiation, or s.c. injection of tuberculin [37].

---

[1]See also the note added in proof on p. 262

Respiratory Reactions

There is one case report of asthma in a 9-year-old boy with atopic disposition caused by fennel [as vegetable; *Foeniculum vulgare* var. *azoricum* (Mill.) Thell.] and fennel seeds [37a]. Positive skin tests, the reproduction of asthma after eating fennel, and the relief from asthma by the elimination of fennel from the diet make a correlation between fennel and allergic asthma probable.

Drug Interactions

The i.p. injection of 50 mg/kg fennel oil resulted in an increase of the pentobarbital sleeping time in mice when it was injected simultaneously with pentobarbital [38]. Considering the dose level of fennel oil and the mode of application, interactions of fennel oil with other drugs in humans are not to be expected.

Fertility, Pregnancy, and Lactation

According to Madaus, fennel oil produces, like all essential oils, an excitation of the gravid uterus and can lead to abortion [39]. This effect has not been verified and is not likely when therapeutic doses of fennel or fennel oil are used. There are no case reports of successfully self-induced abortions with fennel or fennel oil. Even Lewin does not mention fennel oil in his book on criminal abortions [40].

Fennel has been used as a lactagogue since antiquity. Side effects have not been reported. In conclusion, fennel (especially infusions of fennel) does not seem to represent any special risk in pregnancy and lactation.

Mutagenicity, Cytotoxicity, and Carcinogenicity

Fennel oil and anethole were tested in HeLa cell cultures for their cytotoxic actions [41–43]. Fenchone led to negative results in the dose range of 1, 10, and 100 μg/ml. With fennel oil cytotoxic effects were found at a dose of 1 μg/ml and with anethole at a dose of 10 μg/ml. The results reported from these authors demand further confirmation because several data in the text are inconsistent with the data presented in the tables of the publication. Furthermore, the effects are attributed to anethole, but the data reported do not correlate with the amount of anethole in the different essential oils.

Aqueous or methanolic extracts from fennel did not show any mutagenicity in *Salmonella typhimurium* TA 98 and TA 100 with and without metabolic activation (Ames test) or in *Bacillus subtilis* rec assay [44,45]. Positive results were reported by Marcus and Lichtenstein [38] for fennel oil (2.5 mg/plate) in *Salmonella* TA 100 with a liver-activating system (Ames test).

Positive results were also reported for sweet fennel oil in the *Bacillus subtilis* DNA repair test [46]. Negative results were obtained with fennel oil in an in vitro chromosomal aberration test using a Chinese hamster fibroblast cell line [47].

Anethole was positive in Salmonella TA 100 whereas highly purified estragole was negative [46]. The authors pointed out that the results of mutagenicity testing were strongly influenced by the purity of the compounds used. Estragole with 96% purity was positive in *Salmonella typhimurium* TA100, TA 1535, TA 98, and TA 1537 (Ames test).

There are insufficient data to evaluate the carcinogenic risk of fennel. Anethole and estragole have been, like many other phenylpropanes, the subject of studies on carcinogenesis. In a 15-month study total doses of 4.4 μmol and 5.2 μmol estragole produced carcinomas of the liver after s.c. injection in mice [48]. The sulfuric ester of 1'-hydroxyestragole is considered to be the ultimate carcinogen. It must be taken into account that animals of the control group developed carcinomas of the liver. In the group of animals receiving estragole the incidence of tumors was approximately twice, or even three times as high, as in the control group. The authors concluded that estragole is a relatively weak carcinogen, and that the human health risk resulting from the use of estragole is probably small because of the limited use at low levels in spices or foods. In mice the i.p. injection of anethole did not induce primary lung tumors. Considering the fact that the known carcinogen safrole resulted in negative results as well, the model seems to be inappropriate for the evaluation of that substance group [49]. No carcinogenic effects were seen with cis-anethol (0.25 μmol/g) in mice [50]. Trans-anethole did not show any significant carcinogenic activity, either when fed for a year in the diet of female mice nor when injected i.p. in infant male mice [51].

These experiments correlate well with the fact that in mice experiments the binding of the carcinogens estragole and safrole to liver DNA was relatively high, whereas only low levels of adducts were detected with anethole [52,53]. The problems of the final risk evaluation of these compounds are still complicated by the fact that the metabolism in rats and mice depends upon the dose given to the animals [54–56]. In low dose levels O-demethylation dominates the bio-transformation, whereas in higher doses that have been used in the tests for carcinogenicity, mostly side chain oxidation takes place. The latter biotrans-formation results in the formation of the potent carcinogen 1'-hydroxyestragole. In view of these results it has been stated that the animal experiments should not be overinterpreted when the carcinogenic risk of phenylpropanes is to be evaluated. However, in 1988 it was reported that no dose-dependent differences in metabolism occurred in human volunteers treated with doses ranging from 1 to 250 mg/day [57]. In contrast to the results in rodents, anethole was mostly biotransformed in man by oxidation of the side chain. Furthermore, there are no investigations on the influence of a large amount of anethole on the mode of biotransformation of estragole.

It seems reasonable to conclude that the carcinogenic risk of fennel, especially when it is used occasionally as an infusion containing about 0.4 mg per 100 ml estragole [58] is relatively low. But when given to children, the amount of estragole in fennel should be as low as possible, and the estragole-rich chemotypes should preferably be excluded from use. Furthermore, it seems reasonable not to give fennel oil to children until further studies have proven that fennel has no carcinogenic risk.

References

1. Steinegger E, Hänsel R (1988) Lehrbuch der Pharmakognosie und Phytopharmazie. Berlin: Springer Verlag
2. Wichtl M (1988) In: Hartke K (ed) DAB 9-Kommentar. Stuttgart, pp 1689-1694
3. Shah CS, Qadry JS, Chauhan MG (1970) Chemical races in fennel. Planta med 12:285-290
4. Akgül A (1986) In: Brunke E-J (ed) Progress in essential oil research. Berlin: Walter De Gruyter, pp 487-489
5. Betts TJ (1968) Anethole and fenchone in the developing fruits of Foeniculum vulgare Mill. J Pharm Pharmac 20:469-472
6. Betts TJ (1968) Examination of fennel fruits by gas chromatography without preliminary distillation. J Pharm Pharmac 20 Suppl:61S-64S
7. Hegnauer R (1966) Chemotaxonomie der Pflanzen. vol 4. Basel: Birkhäuser
8. Kraus A, Hammerschmidt FJ (1980) Untersuchungen an Fenchelölen. Dragoco Report 27:31-40
9. Tóth L (1967) Untersuchungen über das ätherische Öl von Foeniculum vulgare. I. Die Zusammensetzung des Frucht- und Wurzelöles. Planta med 15:157-172
10. Plant OH, Miller GH (1926) Effects of carminative volatile oils on the muscular activity of the stomach and colon. J Pharmacol Exp Ther 27:149-164
11. Reiter M, Brandt W (1985) Relaxant effects on tracheal and ileal smooth muscles of the guinea pig. Arzneim Forsch 35:408-414
12. Niiho Y, Takayanagi I, Takagi K (1977) Effects of a combined stomachic and its ingredients on rabbit stomach motility in situ. Japan J Pharmacol 27:177-179
13. Imaseki I, Kitabatake Y (1962) Studies on effect of essential oils and their components on the isolated intestines of mice. Yakugaku Zasshi 82:1326-1329
14. Müller-Limroth W, Fröhlich HH (1980) Wirkungsnachweis einiger phytotherapeutischer Expektorantien auf den mukoziliären Transport. Fortschr Med 98:95-101
15. Boyd EM, Sheppard EP (1971) An autumn-enhanced mucotropic action of inhaled terpenes and related volatile agents. Pharmacology 6:65-80
16. Albert-Puleo M (1980) Fennel and anise as estrogenic agents. J Ethnopharmacol 2:337-344
17. Zondek B, Bergmann E (1938) Phenol methyl ethers as oestrogenic agents. Biochem J 32:641-645
18. Gershbein LL (1977) Regeneration of rat liver in the presence of essential oils and their components. Fd Cosm Toxic 15:173-181
19. Bundesgesetzblatt I (Anlage) No. 12; 4.4.1986
20. Ministère des Affaires Sociales et de l'Emploi: Spécialités Pharmaceutiques à Base de Plantes: Bull Off No 86 bis/20 Aout 1986
21. List PH, Hörhammer L (1973) Hagers Handbuch der pharmazeutischen Praxis. 4th edn vol 4: Chemikalien und Drogen (CI-G). Berlin: Springer-Verlag
22. Reynolds JEF, Prasad AB (1982) Martindale; the extra pharmacopoeia. 28th edn. London: The Pharmaceutical Press
23. Tyler VE (1988) Pharmacognosy. 9th edn. Philadelphia: Lea & Febiger
24. Opdyke DLJ (1976) Monographs on fragrance raw materials: fennel oil, bitter. Fd Cosm Toxicol 14:309
25. Opdyke DLJ (1974) Monographs on fragrance raw materials. fennel oil. Fd Cosm Toxicol 12:879-880
26. Skramlik EV (1959) Über die Giftigkeit und Verträglichkeit von ätherischen Ölen. Pharmazie 14:435-445
27. Opdyke DLJ (1973) Monographs on fragrance raw materials: anethole. Fd Cosm Toxicol 11:863-864
28. Opdyke DLJ (1976) Monographs on fragrance raw materials: fenchone. Fd Cosm Toxicol 14:769-771

29. Caujolle MF, Meynier D (1958) Toxicité de l'estragole et des anétholes (cis et trans). CR Hebd Séances Acad Sci 246:1465–1468
30. Lewin L (1929) Gifte und Vergiftungen. Berlin: Georg Stilke, p 839
31. Bär F, Griepentrog F (1967) Die Situation in der gesundheitlichen Beurteilung der Aromatisierungsmittel für Lebensmittel. Medizin Ernähr 8:244–251
32. Hagan EC, Hansen WH, Fitzhugh OG, Jenner PM et al. (1967) Food flavourings and compounds of related structure. II. Subacute and chronic toxicity. Fd Cosmet Toxicol 5:141–157
33. Council of Europe (1973) Natural flavouring substances, their sources and added artificial flavouring substances Strasbourg, p 67
34. Wüthrich B, Hofer T (1984) Nahrungsmittelallergie: das "Sellerie-Beifuß-Gewürz-Syndrom". Dtsch Med Wschr 109:981–986
35. Wüthrich B, Dietschi R (1985) Das "Sellerie-Karotten-Beifuss-Gewürz-Syndrom": Hauttest- und RAST-Ergebnisse. Schweiz med Wschr 115:358–364
36. Lewis WH, Elvin-Lewis MPF (1977) Medical Botany. New York: John Wiley & Sons, p 81
37. Arnold W (1927) Über Kamille, Pfefferminze und Fenchel. I. Mitteilung: Über die Beeinflussung von Entzündungsprozessen. Naunyn-Schmiedeberg's Arch Exp Pathol Pharmakol 123:129–159
37a. Levy SB (1948) Bronchial asthma due to ingestion of fennel and fennel seed. Ann Allergy 6:415–416
38. Marcus C, Lichtenstein EP (1982) Interactions of naturally occurring food plant components with insecticides and pentobarbital in rats and mice. J Agric Food Chem 30:563–568
39. Madaus G (1938) Lehrbuch der biologischen Heilmittel. Leipzig: Georg Thieme
40. Lewin L (1925) Die Fruchtabtreibung durch Gifte und andere Mittel, Berlin: Georg Stilke
41. Nachev C, Zolotovitch G, Siljanowska K, Stojcev S (1968) Untersuchungen über den cytotoxischen Effekt einiger ätherischer Öle und einzelner ihrer Bestandteile. I. Terpenkohlenwassertoffe und -alkohole. Parfumerie und Kosmetik 49:104–108
42. Siljanowska K, Stojcev S, Zolotovitch G, Nachev C (1969) Untersuchungen über den cytotoxischen Effekt einiger ätherischer Öle und einzelner ihrer Bestandteile. III. Ätherische Öle. Parfümerie und Kosmetik 50:293–296
43. Zolotovitch G, Siljanowska K, Stojcev S, Nachev C (1969) Untersuchungen über den cytotoxischen Effekt einiger ätherischer Öle und einzelner ihrer Bestandteile. II. Sauerstoffhaltige Verbindungen (ohne Alkohole). Parfümerie und Kosmetik 50:257–260
44. Morimoto I, Watanabe F, Osawa T, Okitsu T, Kada T (1982) Mutagenicity screening of crude drugs with Bacillus subtilis rec-assay and Salmonella/microsome assay. Mutat Res 97:81–102
45. Yamamoto H, Mizutani T, Nomukra H (1982) Studies on the mutagenicity of crude drug extracts. Yakugaku Zasshi 102:596–601
46. Sekizawa J, Shibamoto T (1982) Genotoxicity of safrole-related chemicals in microbial test systems. Mutat Res 101:127–140
47. Ishidate M, Sofuni T, Yoshikawa K, Hayashi M, Nohmi T, Sawada M, Matsuoka A (1984) Primary mutagenicity screening of food additives currently used in Japan. Fd Chem Toxicol 22:623–636
48. Drinkwater NR, Miller EC, Miller JA, Pitot HC (1976) Hepatocarcinogenicity of estragole (1-allyl-4-methoxybenzene) and 1'-hydroxyestragole in the mouse and mutagenicity of 1'-acetoxyestragole in bacteria. J Natl Cancer Inst 57:1323–1330
49. Stoner GD, Shimkin MB, Kniazeff AJ, Weisburger JH, Weisburger EK, Gori GB (1973) Test for carcinogenicity of food additives and chemotherapeutic agents by the pulmonary tumor response in strain A mice. Cancer Res 33:3069–3085
50. Wiseman RW, Miller EC, Miller JA, Liem A (1987) Structure-activity studies of the hepatocarcinogenicities of alkenylbenzene derivatives related to estragole and safrole on administration to preweanling male C57BL/6J × C3H/HeJF$_1$ mice. Cancer Res 47:2275–2283
51. Miller JA, Miller EC, Phillips D (1982) The metabolic activation and carcinogenicity of alkenylbenzenes that occur naturally in many spices. In: Stich HF (ed) Carcinogens and mutagens in the environment. Vol I. Boca Raton: CRC, pp 83–96
52. Philips DH, Reddy MV, Randerath K (1984) ^{32}P-post-labelling analysis of DNA adducts formed in the livers of animals treated with safrole, estragole and other naturally occurring alkenylbenzenes. II. Newborn male B6C3F$_1$ mice. Carcinogenesis 5:1623–1628
53. Randerath K, Haglund RE, Philips DH, Reddy MV (1984) ^{32}P-post-labelling analysis of DNA

adducts formed in the livers of animals treated with safrole, estragole and other naturally occurring alkenylbenzenes. I. Adult female CD-1 mice. Carcinogenesis 5:1613

54. Sangster SA, Caldwell J, Smith RL (1984) Metabolism of anethole. I. Pathways of metabolism in the rat and mouse. Fd Chem Toxic 22:695–706
55. Sangster SA, Caldwell J, Smith RL (1984) Metabolism of anethole. II. Influence of dose size on the route of metabolism of trans-anethole in the rat and mouse. Fd Chem Toxic 22:707
56. Zangouras A, Caldwell J, Hutt AJ, Smith RL (1981) Dose dependent conversion of estragole in the rat and mouse to the carcinogenic metabolite 1′-hydroxyestragole. Biochem Pharmacol 30:1383–1386
57. Caldwell J, Sutton JD (1988) Influence of dose size on the disposition of trans-(methoxy-^{14}C)anethole in human volunteers. Fd Chem Toxic 26:87–91
58. Fehr D (1982) Bestimmung flüchtiger Inhaltsstoffe in Teezubereitungen. 1. Mitteilung: Freisetzung des ätherischen Öls aus Fenchelfrüchten. Pharm Ztg 127:2520–2522

Gaultheria procumbens

E.L. Boyd

Botany

Gaultheria procumbens L. belongs to the Ericaceae family [1]. Vernacular names include wintergreen, teaberry, checkerberry, creeping wintergreen, partridge berry, boxberry, spiceberry, mountain tea, ground holly, grouse berry, dewberry, redberry, and hillberry [2]. Natural oils containing methyl salicylate were formerly obtained from the leaves of *Gaultheria procumbens* but are now distilled from the bark of *Betula lenta* L. of the Betulaceae family [3].

Chemistry

The oils known as gaultheria oil, wintergreen oil, betula oil, or sweet birch oil, contain not less than 98% ester calculated as methyl salicylate [1,3,4]. Although wintergreen oil contains methyl salicylate as the chief constituent, it also contains arbutin, ericolin, gallic acid, gaultheric acid, mucilage, tannin, wax, an ester, triacontane, and a secondary alcohol has also been reported [2,5]. Methyl salicylate can also be produced synthetically by distilling a mixture of salicylic acid and methyl alcohol [1,6].

Pharmacology and Uses

Methyl salicylate's pharmacological action is similar to that of other salicylates, but unlike most salicylates that are used orally for their analgesic, antipyretic, and anti-inflammatory effects methyl salicylate (sweet birch oil, wintergreen oil, gaultheria oil, and betula oil) is employed only for cutaneous counterirritation in the form of salves, liniments, and other preparations [7]. Methyl salicylate is also currently used as a flavoring agent for candies, soft drinks, dental preparations, cough drops, and chewing gum [5,6]. It is still listed as a flavoring agent for Aromatic Cascara Sagrada Fluidextract [8]. Past uses of methyl salicylate include its use as baths, liniments, and ointments for the treatment of gout, lumbago, rheumatism, and sciatica [5]. The berries have been used to make pies.

The leaves have been used to make a herbal tea (mountain tea). They have also been used as a condiment [5], and children have chewed the roots each spring to help prevent tooth decay [9]. The tea has been recommended as a gargle for sore throat and stomatosis, as a douche for leucorrhea, and as a collyrium for conjunctivitis [5]. There currently are more than forty topical preparations available on the U.S. market containing 2–55% methyl salicylate [10].

Pharmacokinetics

Although some references [7,11] indicate that methyl salicylate appears to be absorbed very rapidly from the gastrointestinal tract (GI) tract, and its onset of action may be sooner than from aspirin preparations, Levine et al. [12] state that its GI absorption is erratic and slow while cutaneous absorption is more rapid. Davison et al. [13] observed that in rats the conversion of methyl salicylate to salicylate occurred predominantly in the liver, and that very little hydrolysis of methyl salicylate occurred in human blood. They administered 0.42 ml methyl salicylate orally to 6 human volunteers and found that 39% was unhydrolyzed at 0.25 h, and 21% was detected in the plasma after 1.5 h. The peak total salicylate concentrations averaged 12.8 and 13.3 mg/l respectively. Danon et al. [14] used methyl salicylate as a model to test the hypothesis that exercise and environmental heat exposure could, by increasing skin temperature, cutaneous blood flow and sweating, enhance the absorption of certain drugs through the skin. The study was carried out under four experimental conditions: at rest and 22°C; at rest and 40°C; with exercise to 30% of VO_{2max} at 22°C; and with exercise to 30% of VO_{2max} at 40°C. The sequence of experiments was assigned at random with 1–2 week intervals between phases using 6 noninstitutionalized adult males. The researchers found that exercise, heat exposure, or both increased systemic availability of salicylate as indicated by levels of plasma concentrations of total salicylate and urinary salicyluric acid.

Plasma salicylate peaked at 2 h and was significantly higher than in controls after 1, 3, and 5 h of heat exposure. Under the most extreme conditions, namely heat exposure and exercise, plasma levels at all times were more than threefold higher than in the controls.

Adverse Reaction Profile

General Human Data

The clinical manifestations of oil of wintergreen poisoning are identical to those observed with other salicylates and include acid-base imbalance, altered glucose metabolism, and central nervous system toxicity [15–17]. The specific findings and their magnitude depends upon the dose of the salicylate consumed, the patient's age, and whether the ingestion was acute or chronic. Children under 5 years of age seem especially susceptible to the toxic effects of the salicylates and easily develop the severe acid-base and neurological disturbances characteristic of advanced toxicity [18].

Oil of wintergreen is classified as "very toxic" by Gleason [19] which means that the lethal dose for a 70-kg man is considered to be between 5 ml and 30 ml. Stevenson's [15] review of 43 cases of oil of wintergreen poisoning in the literature and three of his own cases revealed a 59% mortality rate, 41% of which occurred in infants. He reported two cases in which as little as 4 ml was lethal in infants, and 6 ml was lethal in a 21-year-old adult. He also reviewed a case in which 5 ml was lethal in a patient of his who was 1-month-old. Howrie et al. [16] reported a case in which a 21-month-old infant consumed 7.5 ml of wintergreen intended for use as homemade candy flavoring. The child presented with the clinical manifestations of salicylate poisoning.

Paynter and Alexander [20] reported a case of a 21-month-old admitted to the hospital with salicylate toxicity caused by a teething ointment containing choline salicylate. They calculated that the child ingested the equivalent of over 2.5 g acetylsalicylic acid from the ointment within a 48-h period. Johnson et al. [21] reviewed the range of equivalence values given for methyl salicylate, that is, the equivalence of a certain volume of methyl salicylate to some number of aspirin tablets, or to so many milligrams of aspirin, or "salicylate". According to their calculation, errors in published references ranged from approximately 2% to 61% with the mean error being 26%. They concluded that a satisfactory methyl salicylate equivalence is 1 ml 98% methyl salicylate to 1.4 g acetylsalicylic acid in salicylate potency.

An indication of the toxicity of oil of wintergreen is the requirement by the United States Poison Prevention Packaging Act of 1970 that liquid preparations containing more than 5 ml methyl salicylate by weight must be packaged in child-resistant containers [22]. Canadian pharmacists recently adopted a resolution that methyl salicylate should be removed as a single entity from the Canadian market [23].

Allergic Reactions

Intolerance to analgesics is common in patients with bronchial asthma, nasal polyps, and urticaria. In 8%–20% of adult asthmatics, acetylsalicylic acid and several other analgesics provoke asthmatic attacks probably through inhibition of cyclo-oxygenase [24]. In this group of patients cross-sensitivity between acetylsalicylic acid and nonsteroidal anti-inflammatory agents has been reported but does not appear to be a major problem between acetylsalicylic acid and other salicylates products, e.g., sodium salicylate, choline salicylate [24]. However, Hindson [25] reported a case in which a patient who had a documented allergy to methyl salicylate exacerbated by systemic administration of acetylsalicylic acid after patch tests to acetylsalicylic acid were negative.

Shelley [26] reported the case of a 6-year-old boy who was admitted to hospital with generalized pustular psoriasis due to an exquisite hypersensitivity to salicylates of tree, shrub, and medical origin. Sweet birch (*Betula lenta*) pollen was incriminated as the antigenic agent since the tree produces large quantities of methyl salicylate, and the boy's outbreaks occurred after he hiked in the Pennsylvania woods and chewed birch leaves and twigs as well as wintergreen leaves. The boy's mother and aunt were also allergic to acetylsalicylic acid. Speer [6] reported the case of a 16-year-old who developed recurrent attacks of urticaria and angioedema after exposure to candy, two different brands of toothpaste, and two different liniments, all containing oil of wintergreen. The amount of methyl salicylate contained in the toothpaste was 0.4% and 0.2% while that in the liniments was 15% and 18.3%. Although the patient developed urticaria after exposure to methyl salicylate and acetylsalicylic acid, Speer concluded that the lack of previous reports of the two agents causing urticarial reactions in the same patient indicated that he was dealing with coincidence rather than cross-sensitivity.

Central Nervous System Reactions

Central nervous system symptoms of mild chronic salicylate toxicity include headache, dizziness, tinnitus, difficulty in hearing, dimness of vision, mental confusion, lassitude, and drowsiness. A more severe degree of salicylate intoxication is characterized by CNS disturbances that may include seizures and coma. Fever is usually prominent especially in children [7]. Severe acute salicylism includes a variety of neurological signs and symptoms such as disorientation, irritability, hallucinations, lethargy, stupor, coma, and seizures [18].

Dermatological Reactions

As indicated in the section on allergic reactions, the ingestion of oil of wintergreen has been reported to precipitate urticaria in at least one patient [6].

Gastrointestinal Reactions

Gastrointestinal irritation caused by salicylates may produce nausea and vomiting, hyperventilation, and increased GI losses which combine to produce mild dehydration [18,27]. Dehydration is also enhanced by decreased intake of fluid [27]. Hypokalemia may result from increased GI and renal losses and systemic alkalosis [18,27].

Renal Reactions

Heng et al. [28] reported on a patient who experienced persistent interstitial nephritis as well as full-thickness skin and muscle necrosis as a result of topical application of methyl salicylate and menthol followed by use of a heating pad, despite the manufacturer's warning against the use of heating pads with the preparation.

Fertility, Pregnancy, and Lactation

Data on the ingestion of oil of wintergreen preparations during pregnancy and lactation were not retrieved from the literature. However, methyl salicylate's pharmacological actions are closely related to those of other salicylates, and safe use of salicylates during pregnancy has not been established. Salicylates have been shown to be teratogenic and embryocidal in various species of animals [29,30]. In humans, studies of the teratogenic effects of salicylates have been mixed. In some studies, chronic maternal salicylate ingestion has been associated with decreased fetal birthweight; an increased incidence of stillbirth, neonatal mortality, antepartum and postpartum maternal hemorrhage, complicated deliveries, prolongation of gestation, and spontaneous labor [29–33]. Because of its potential toxicity and since salicylates are distributed into breast milk, oil of wintergreen should be avoided by pregnant and nursing women [30].

Mutagenicity and Carcinogenicity

Data on the mutagenic and/or carcinogenic potential of *Gaultheria procumbens* have not been retrieved from the literature. Petierno et al. [34] studied the ability of acetylsalicylic acid to induce cytotoxicity, mutation to ouabain resistance, and morphological transformation in cultured C3H/10T1/2 clone 8 (10T1/2) mouse embryo cells. The compounds was cytotoxic from 0.5 mg/ml to 2 mg/ml concentrations as evidenced by decreased plating efficiency. It induced neither detectable base substitution mutations to ouabain resistance, even at cytotoxic concentrations, nor morphological transformation. One study using the Ames *Salmonella* strains [35] and one study using 6 strains of *Salmonella typhimurium* [36] found no evidence of mutagenic activity for acetylsalicylic acid. Although no evidence of mutagenic and/or carcinogenic activities for *Gaultheria procumbens* were retrieved, its use should be minimized and/or avoided whenever possible.

References

1. Tyler VE, Brady LR, Robbers JE (eds) (1976) Pharmacognosy. 7th ed. Philadelphia: Lea & Febiger
2. Millspaugh CF (1974) American medicinal plants. 1st ed. New York: Dover Publications, Inc
3. Trease GE, Evans WC (eds) (1983) Pharmacognosy. 12th ed. London: Bailliere Tindall
4. Wade A, Reynolds JEF (eds) (1977) Martindale: the extra pharmacopoeia. 27th ed. London: The Pharmaceutical Press
5. Duke JA (1985) CRC handbook of medicinal herbs. 1st ed. Boca Raton: CRC Press
6. Speer F (1979) Allergy to methyl salicylate. Ann Allergy 43:36–37
7. Flowers RJ, Moncada S, Vane JR (1985) Analgesic-antipyretic and anti-inflammatory agents: drugs employed in the treatment of gout. In: Gilman AG, Goodman LS, Rall TW, Murad F (eds) The pharmacological basis for therapeutics. New York: Macmillan Publishing Co, pp 674–715
8. Anonymous (1984) USP XII The United States pharmacopeia the national formulary NF XVI. Easton: Mack Publishing Co.
9. Lewis HL, Elvin-Lewis MPF (eds) (1977) Medical botany: plants affecting man's health. 1st ed. New York: John Wiley & Sons
10. Kastrup EK, Olin BR, Connell SI (eds) (1988) Drug facts and comparisons. 1988 ed. St Louis: JB Lippincott Co
11. Anonymous (1989) Salicylates. In: Rumack BH (ed) Poisindex. 61st ed. Englewood: Microdex Inc
12. Levine B, Caplan YH (1984) Liquid chromatographic determination of salicylate and methyl salicylate in blood and application to a postmorten case. J Anal Toxicol 8:239–241
13. Davison C, Zimmerman EF, Smith PK (1961) On the metabolism and toxicity of methyl salicylate. J Pharmacol Exp Ther 132:207–211
14. Danon A, Ben-Shimon S, Ben-Zvi Z (1986) Effect of exercise and heat exposure on percutaneous absorption of methyl salicylate. Eur J Clin Pharmacol 31:49–52
15. Stevenson CS (1937) Oil of wintergreen (methyl salicylate) poisoning: report of three cases, one with autopsy, and a review of the literature. Am J Med Sci 193:772–788
16. Howrie DL, Moriarty R, Breit R (1985) Candy flavoring as a source of salicylate poisoning, Pediatrics 75:869–871
17. Done AK (1978) Aspirin overdose: incidence, diagnosis, and management. Pediatrics 62(suppl):890–897
18. Pribble JP, Elenbaas RM (1988) Poisoning. In: Kimble MA, Young LY (eds) Applied therapeutics: the clinical use of drugs. Vancouver: Applied Therapeutics Inc, pp 1895–1919
19. Gleason MN, Gosselin RE, Hodge HC, Smith RP (eds) (1969) Clinical toxicology of commercial products: acute poisoning. 3rd ed. Baltimore: The Williams & Williams Co
20. Paynter AS, Alexander FW (1979) Salicylate intoxication caused by teething ointment. Lancet 2:1132
21. Johnson PN, Welch DW (1984) Methyl salicylate/aspirin (salicylate) equivalence: who do you trust? Vet Hum Toxicol 26:317–318
22. Maisel GS (1980) Update on child-resistant packaging. Am Pharm NS20:12–13
23. Anonymous (1987) Resolution #4. Can Pharm J 120:439
24. Szczeklik A (1986) Analgesics, allergy and asthma. Drugs 32(Suppl 4):148–163
25. Hindson C (1977) Contact eczema from methyl salicylate reproduced by oral aspirin. Contact Dermatitis 3:348
26. Shelley WB (1964) Birch pollen and aspirin psoriasis: a study in salicylate hypersensitivity. JAMA 189:985–988
27. Temple AR (1978) Pathophysiology of aspirin overdose toxicity, with implications for management. Pediatrics 62(suppl):873–876
28. Heng ML (1987) Local necrosis and interstitial nephritis due to topical methyl salicylate and menthol. Cutis 39:442–444
29. Anonymous (1989) Analgesics and antipyretics. In: McEvoy GK (ed) AHFS drug information 89. Bethesda: American Society of Hospital Pharmacists, Inc
30. Hart LL, Mowers MM (1986) DIAS rounds. Drug Intel Clin Pharm 208:50–51

31. Lewis RB, Schulman JD (1973) Influence of acetylsalicylic acid an inhibitor of prostaglandin synthesis on the duration of human gestation and labor. Lancet 2:1159–1161
32. Collins E, Turner G (1975) Maternal effects of regular salicylate ingestion in pregnancy. Lancet 2:335–338
33. Turner G, Collins E (1975) Fetal effects of regular salicylate ingestion in pregnancy. Lancet 2:338–339
34. Patierno SR, Lehman NL, Henderson BE, Landolph JR (1989) Study of the ability of phenacetin, acetaminophen, and aspirin to induce cytotoxicity, mutation, and morphological transformation in C3H/10T1/2 clone 8 mouse embryo cells. Cancer Res 49:1038–1044
35. Oldham JW, Preston RF, Paulson JD (1986) Mutagenicity testing of selected analgesics in Ames Salmonella strains. J Appl Toxicol 6:237–243
36. Jasiewicz ML, Richardson JC (1987) Absence of mutagenic activity of benorylate, paracetamol, and aspirin in the Salmonella/mammalian microsome test. Mutat Res 190:95–100

Hedeoma pulegioides and Mentha pulegium

E.L. Boyd

Botany

Pennyroyal oil is the volatile oil obtained from the leaves of *Hedeoma pulegioides* L. or *Mentha pulegium* L. Both are members of the Labiatae (mint) family. The former is frequently referred to as American pennyroyal and the latter as European or Old World pennyroyal [1]. Vernacular names for pennyroyal include mock pennyroyal, tick-weed, squawmint, and stinking balm [2].

Chemistry

Both American and European pennyroyal contain pulegone and small amounts of several other ketones such as 1-menthone, d-isomenthone, and piperitone as well as various terpene hydrocarbons [1,3,4]. Sleckman et al. [5] used thin-layer chromatography and densitometry to determine the pulegone contents of *Hedeoma pulegioides* and found its storage was localized in the foliage and stem of the plant. They found that the pulegone concentration was highest (55 mg/g foliage and 3.8 mg/g stem) in the spring.

Pharmacology and Uses

Pennyroyal oil has been used by natural health advocates as an emmenagogue and abortifacient. The leaves of pennyroyal have been used for flavoring, for making tea, and as a spice. They have also been mixed with honey and pepper and used to flavor pork puddings. Decoctions of the whole plant have been used for uterine tumors, uterine fibroids, and indurations of the uterus. The root ground with vinegar has been used as a tumor remedy. Infusions of the leaves have been used for cramps, spasms, and colds. It has also been used for fainting, flatulence, gall bladder ailments, gout, hepatitis, and nervous disorders. Pennyroyal tea has been used for coughs, colds, and menstrual disorders [6]. The tea has been recommended as a stimulant, carminative, diaphoretic, and emmenagogue [7]. The oil has been recommended for topical use to repel gnats, ticks, fleas, and mosquitoes [7].

Adverse Reaction Profile

General Animal Data

Thorup et al. [8] studied the short-term toxic effects of pulegone and menthol on rats. They administered pulegone by gavage for 28 days at 0, 20, 80, and 160 mg/kg bw per day. At the two highest doses pulegone induced atonia, decreased blood creatinine content, lowered terminal body weight, and caused histopathological changes in the liver and the white matter of the cerebellum. The histopathological changes included dose-related vacuolization of hepatocytes in the zone around the central vein.

General Human Data

The use of pennyroyal oil in man has long been associated with toxicity and death [9,10]. Three recent cases of pennyroyal oil poisoning have been reported [11-13]. One woman who ingested up to 30 ml (estimated 24 g) of the oil experienced abdominal cramps, nausea, vomiting, and alternating lethargy and agitation. She later developed kidney failure, massive hepatic necrosis, and evidence of disseminated intravascular coagulation and died seven days after ingestion of the oil [11]. Another woman ingested 15 ml of the oil and within 2 h vomited twice and passed out. She was treated in the hospital and released 96 h after admission. A physical examination two weeks later was normal [12]. Another woman ingested 10 ml of the oil and experienced rash, dizziness, vomiting, and abdominal pain [11].

Although serious toxicity with the tea has not been reported, some women have switched to the more toxic oil when the tea did not induce menses [11,12].

Central Nervous System Reactions

Central nervous system symptoms have been reported in several patients who have ingested pennyroyal-containing preparations. The symptoms include lethargy, agitation, and dizziness [11]. Early [14] reported a case of pennyroyal ingestion that resulted in generalized seizures and auditory and visual hallucinations. Five days after the onset of her illness the patient was clear cognitively. Braithwaite [15] reported a case of pennyroyal essence ingestion (0.5 oz — approximately 15 ml — of 1 in 10 or 1 in 20 of the essential oil) that resulted in the patient losing consciousness. When aroused, her chief symptom was a marked feeling of numbness and tingling in her hands. On the day of ingestion the patient talked strangely and at random, and the day after ingestion the patient was able to get out of bed but still was dizzy and lightheaded.

Dermatological Reactions

There are at least two reports in the literature of patients experiencing dermatological reactions after ingestion of pennyroyal-containing preparations [9,11]. Sullivan et al. [11] reported the symptoms of one of their patients who came to the emergency room after ingestion of two 0.5-oz bottles of pennyroyal oil 2 h earlier to abort a suspected pregnancy. The patient presented with a generalized urticarial rash that spontaneously resolved while she was in the emergency department. Vallance [9] described a fatal case of pennyroyal poisoning in a patient who was admitted to a general medicine ward with a widespread rash and pyrexia after taking codeine tablets for general malaise and two bottles of a pennyroyal mixture to terminate a 3-month pregnancy. He was not able to ascertain how much pennyroyal the patient had actually taken.

Gastrointestinal Reactions

Adverse gastrointestinal effects including nausea, vomiting (sometimes containing blood), burning in the throat, abdominal pain, and diarrhea are frequent findings in many of the reported cases of toxicity associated with ingestion of pennyroyal-containing preparations [9–12].

Hepatic Reactions

Reports indicate that hepatotoxicity (massive centrilobular hepatic necrosis and hepatomegaly) may occur after pennyroyal oil ingestion. It was postulated that pulegone and/or its metabolite(s) may be responsible for the hepatotoxic effects seen [9,11]. Gordon et al. [16] found that formation of a hepatotoxic metabolite after pulegone administration to mice is apparently mediated by the cytochromes P-450 system, and Buechel et al. [12] used early administration of acetylcysteine after pennyroyal oil ingestion to prevent hepatic toxicity.

Several animal studies [8,17–19] have been conducted to determine the adverse effects of pennyroyal oil and pulegone on hepatic tissue. Gordon et al. [19] conducted studies to determine which terpenes of pennyroyal oil were most likely responsible for the hepatotoxic effects caused by its ingestion, and what structural features of the terpenes were important determinants for the hepatotoxic response. In addition, they also investigated the possible role of glutathione in altering the threshold dose for toxicity. The researchers found that pennyroyal oil in doses of 400 mg/kg i.p. and higher in male mice caused acute hepatic and lung damage. Cellular necrosis was localized to the centrilobular regions of the liver and bronchiolar epithelial cells of the lungs. Capillary gas chromatographic analysis of samples of pennyroyal oil obtained from health food stores showed the presence of several monoterpene constituents. Pulegone was the major terpene and constituted more than 80% of the terpenes in the oils examined. Pulegone and two other terpenes, isopulegone and menthofuran, were found to be both hepatotoxic and lung toxic. Based on results of histological scoring of necrosis, plasma GPT elevations, and hepatic glutathione depletion the researchers concluded that pulegone is the terpene primarily responsible for tissue necrosis.

In a subsequent study Gordon et al. [16] found that pulegone is metabolized by hepatic microsomal mono-oxygenases of the mouse to a hepatotoxin. The formation of a toxic metabolite is apparently mediated by cytochromes P-450 of the phenobarbital class. The researchers found that phenobarbital pretreatment of mice increases, and β-naphthoflavone pretreatment decreases the extent of hepatic necrosis caused by pulegone. Inhibitors of cytochrome P-450, e.g. cobalt chloride and piperonyl butoxide, blocked the hepatotoxicity of pulegone [16].

An analogue of pulegone that was labeled with deuterium in the allylic methyl groups was found to be significantly less hepatotoxic than the parent compound, and these results indicate that oxidation of an allylic methyl group is required for generation of a hepatotoxic metabolite. Menthofuran has been identified as a proximate toxic metabolite of pulegone, and investigations with pulegone-d_6 and $^{18}O_2$ strongly indicate that menthofuran is formed by a sequence of reactions that involve: (a) oxidation of an allylic methyl group, (b) intramolecular cyclization to form a hemiketal, and (c) dehydration to form the furan [16]. Whether or not menthofuran is the only metabolite of pulegone involved in the pathogenesis of hepatotoxicity is not known. Inactivation of cytochrome P-450 that catalyzes the oxidation of pulegone to menthofuran would be expected to protect against hepatotoxicity if the direct damage to the cytochromes does not cause hepatotoxic effects, however, since approximately 90% of hepatic cytochromes can be irreversibly inactivated without causing hepatotoxicity, it is unlikely that direct inactivation of cytochrome P-450 by pulegone plays a major role in hepatotoxicity [16].

Madyastha et al. [18] found that once daily in vivo administration of pulegone at doses of 400 mg/kg bw to male rats decreased the level of microsomal cytochromes P-450 to the extent of 32% and 76% at the end of 24 and 96 h, respectively. They also found that in vitro incubation (15 min) of liver microsomes from phenobarbital-treated rats with pulegone (10 mM), aerobically or anaerobically resulted in the loss (approximately 60%) of cytochromes P-450 in the presence or absence of NADPH. The loss of cytochromes P-450 was accompanied by a concomitant loss in microsomal heme. The destructive process was found to be irreversible, time dependent, linear up to a substrate concentration of 10 mM and followed first-order kinetics.

Mizutani et al. [17] conducted experiments to determine whether pulegone requires oxidation biotransformation in order to be toxic for mouse liver. They used intraperitoneal injections of pulegone that caused extensive liver injury as characterized by an increase in serum glutamic pyruvic transaminase (GPT) activity and centrilobular necrosis of hepatocytes. Treatments of mice with the cytochrome P-450 enzyme inhibitors SKF-525A, metyrapone, piperonyl butoxide, and carbon disulfide prevented or markedly alleviated the hepatotoxicity of pulegone. Induction of the cytochromes P-450 enzymes with phenobarbital or 3-methylcholanthrene did not enhance the hepatotoxic action of pulegone. The results of the study are compatible with the view that some metabolite of pulegone is responsible for the liver injury in mice.

In summary, most studies support the view that some metabolite of pulegone is responsible for the liver injuries that occur after its administration. However, Madyastha et al. [18] did find that pulegone decreased the levels of cytochromes P-450. The balance between the inactivation of cytochromes P-450 by pulegone and the metabolism of pulegone by cytochromes P-450 to toxic metabolites is one of the issues that requires further investigation in order to elucidate mechanisms of toxicity caused by monoterpenes [16].

Respiratory Reactions

As indicated in the section on hepatic reactions, Gordon et al. [19] found that pennyroyal oil in doses of 400 mg/kg i.p. and higher in male mice caused cellular necrosis that was localized to the bronchiolar epithelial cells of the lungs.

Fertility, Pregnancy, and Lactation

It is likely that pennyroyal oil's abortive effects are due to irritation of the uterus with subsequent uterine contractions [13]. Data on the teratogenic effects of pennyroyal containing preparations were not retrieved from the literature nor was any information regarding its effect on fertility and lactation found.

Mutagenicity and Carcinogenicity

Anderson et al. [20] investigated the mutagenic potential of peppermint oil, menthol, menthone and pulegone in the Salmonella/mammalian-microsome test. They found that concentrations of 800, 160, 32 and 6.4 µg per plate of pulegone did not demonstrate any mutagenic properties on the Salmonella tester strains TA1537, TA98, TA1535, and TA100. Data on the carcinogenic potential of pennyroyal containing preparations have not been recovered from the literature.

References

1. Tyler VE (1988) The new honest herbal: a sensible guide to the use of herbs and related remedies. 2nd ed. Philadelphia: George F Stickley
2. Millspaugh CF (1974) American medicinal plants. 1st ed. New York: Dover Publications
3. Wade A, Reynolds JEF (eds) (1977) Martindale: the extra pharmacopoeia. 27th ed. London: The Pharmaceutical Press
4. Tyler VE, Brady LR, Robbers JE (eds) (1976) Pharmacognosy, 7th ed. Philadelphia: Lea & Febiger
5. Sleckman BP, Sherma J, Mineo LC (1983) Determination of pulegone in *Hedeoma pulegioides* and peppermint oil by thin layer chromatography with densitometry. J Liq Chromatogr 6:1175–1182
6. Duke JA (1985) CRC handbook of medicinal herbs. 1st ed. Boca Raton: CRC Press
7. Coon N (1979) Using plants for healing. 2nd ed. Emmaus: Rodale Press
8. Thorup I, Wurtzen G, Carstensen J, Olsen P (1983) Short term toxicity study in rats dosed with pulegone and menthol. Toxicol Lett 19:207–210
9. Vallance WB (1955) Pennyroyal poisoning: a fatal case. Lancet 2:850–851
10. Allen WT (1897) Note on a case of supposed poisoning by pennyroyal. Lancet 1:1022–1023
11. Sullivan JB Jr, Rumack BH, Thomas H Jr, Peterson RG, Bryson P (1979) Pennyroyal oil poisoning and hepatotoxicity. JAMA 242:2873–2874
12. Buechel DW, Haverlah VC, Gardner ME (1983) Pennyroyal oil ingestion: report of a case. J Am Osteopath Ass, pp 793–794
13. Anonymous (1986) Pennyroyal. Lawrence review of natural products: Jan 1986
14. Early DF (1961) Pennyroyal: a rare case of epilepsy. Lancet 2:580–581
15. Braithwaite PF (1906) A case of poisoning by pennyroyal. Brit Med J ii:865
16. Gordon WP, Huitric AC, Seth CL, McClanahan RH, Nelson SD (1987) The metabolism of the abortifacient terpene, (R)-(+)-pulegone, to a proximate toxin, menthofuran. Drug Metab Dispos 15:589–594
17. Mizutani T, Nomura H, Nakanishi K, Fujita S (1987) Effects of drug metabolism modifiers on pulegone-induced hepatotoxicity in mice. Res Commun Chem Pathol Pharmacol 58:75–83
18. Madyastha P, Moorthy B, Vaidyanathan CS, Madyastha KM (1985) In vivo and in vitro destruction of rat liver cytochrome P-450 by monoterpene ketone, pulegone. Biochem Biophys Res Commun 128:921–927
19. Gordon WP, Forte AJ, McMurtry RJ, Gal J, Nelson SD (1982) Hepatotoxicity and pulmonary toxicity of pennyroyal oil and its constituent terpenes in the mouse. Toxicol Appl Pharmacol 65:413–424
20. Andersen PH, Jensen NJ (1984) Mutagenic investigation of peppermint oil in the Salmonella/mammalian-microsome test. Mutat Res 138:17–20

Marsdenia cundurango

D. Frohne

Botany

Marsdenia cundurango Reichb. fil. belongs to the Asclepiadaceae (Asclepia-doideae, Marsdenieae). Vernacular names are condor plant and eagle vine. The plant grows on the west slopes of the Andes in Colombia, Peru, and Ecuador. The part of the plant used as drug is the bark of younger as well as older branches: condurango bark or eagle vine bark.

Chemistry

Marsdenia cundurango bark contains $1-2\%$ of a composition known as condu-ranging consisting of various glycoside esters with a C 21-based steroid structure as aglycone (pregnane derivatives). The substances are named condurangins A, A_0, A_1, B, B_0, C, C_0, C_1, D_0, E_{01}, E_{02}. The acidic components have been shown to be acetic acid and/or cinnamic acid. Some of the glycoside-bound sugars have an unusual structure, e.g., 6-desoxy-3-O-methylallose, oleandrose, or cymarose [1–5]. Condurangins can be considered as bitter principles with saponin properties; surprisingly, they are less soluble in hot than in cold water. Therefore a decoction should be filtered only when cooled down to room temperature.

Other components of the bark are the so-called condurangamines, nicotinic acid esters, hydroxylated pregnane derivatives [6], conduritol, and other cyclitols, chlorogenic and caffeic acid, and in trace amounts, flavonoids, coumarin de-rivatives, and vanillin [7–9].

According to the Swiss and German pharmacopoeias the bark contains a minimum condurangin glycoside content of 1.8%, analyzed as condurangin glycoside A. Spectral photometry was used to determine the content according to the recommendations of Kock and Steinegger [10] and of Steinegger and Brunner [11].

Pharmacology and Uses

Due to the bitter taste of condurangin, condurango bark is a bitter [12]. However, it is only a moderately strong one. The drug is generally used as a liquid preparation — decoction, fluid extract, tincture, or condurango wine — for stimulation of gastric juice secretion in cases of loss of appetite. Its significance as a stomachic agent in modern medicinal practice, however, is negligible.

Recent research by a Japanese research team demonstrated antitumor activity of some isolated condurangins (condurangin glycosides) towards Ehrlich carcinoma cells and sarcoma 180 in mice [13,14]. However, there is no definitive confirmation of the reputed anticancer effect of the drug or crude preparations.

Adverse Reaction Profile

General Animal Data

Toxic effects have not been attributed to the drug itself or to liquid preparations [15,16]. However, a closely related species found in Greece, *Marsdenia erecta*, has been described as the cause of severe poisoning in grazing animals [17,18]. The ester glycoside composition of condurangin, equally present in both species, is held responsible for the toxic effects [19].

In animal experiments, clear signs of poisoning were observed after i.v., s.c., or p.o. administration of the isolated raw mixture of condurangin [19]: salivation and vomiting, hyperactivity with loss of coordination, acceleration of pulse and respiration, and finally, convulsions and death through respiratory paralysis. Similar details on the toxicity of condurangin were already described 100 years ago in a dissertation [20] and were also found in a comprehensive review by Jodelbauer [12]. A certain similarity can be noted with signs of poisoning obtained by parenteral administration of saponins. Depending on the route of administration of condurangin, the LD for cats and dogs was 20 mg/kg body weight (i.v.), 30 mg/kg (s.c.), and 40–45 mg/kg (p. o.). In further experiments in mice, a condurangin mixture from *Marsdenia erecta* was administered by intraperitoneal injection; the LD was 300 mg/kg [17].

During their research on the antitumor activity of isolated condurango glycosides, Hayashi et al. [13,14] also determined LD_{50} values (without further specification):

Condurango glycoside	A_0 :	75 mg/kg
Condurango glycoside	B_0 :	615 mg/kg
Condurango glycoside	C_0 :	375 mg/kg
Condurango glycoside	D_0 :	630 mg/kg

The values for two further D_0 derivatives were 603 and 642 mg/kg [14].

General Human Data

Up to now, apparently no striking side effects have been observed during therapeutic use of the above-mentioned liquid preparations of the drug and, to my knowledge, no recent research has been done on the toxicity of the drug or its isolated compounds. According to the present state of knowledge, there are no objections to the therapeutic use of this drug and its liquid preparations in usual concentrations and quantities.

Fertility, Pregnancy, and Lactation

No data have been recovered from the literature.

Mutagenicity and Carcinogenicity

Condurango cortex — in the form of an aqueous or methanolic extract — produced no mutagenic effects in *Salmonella typhimurium* strains TA 98 and TA 100 [21]. No data on carcinogenicity have been recovered from the literature.

References

1. Berger S, Junior P, Kopanski L (1988) Structural revision of pregnane ester glycosides from Condurango cortex and new compounds. Phytochemistry 27:1451–1458
2. Korte F, Weitkamp H (1956) Zur Konstitution des Kondurangins. Chem Ber 89:2669–2675
3. Takase M, Terada S, Yamamoto H et al. (1982) Studies on the constituents of Asclepiadaceae plants. XLIX. Confirmation of the structures of antitumor-active glycosides in condurango cortex. Chemical transformations of the aglycone moiety. Chem Pharm Bull 30:2429–2432
4. Tschesche R, Welzel P, Snatzke G (1965) Die Konstitution von Kondurangogenin A, dem Aglykon eines Esterglykosids der Kondurangorinde. Tetrahedron 21:1777–1795
5. Tschesche R, Kohl H (1968) Die Struktur der Kondurangoglykoside A, A$_1$ und C, C$_1$. Tetrahedron 24:4359–4371
6. Pailer M, Ganzinger D (1975) Alkaloide aus Cortex Condurango. Marsdenia cundurango Reichb. fil. Monatsh Chem 106:37–54
7. Frohne D (1989) Condurangorinde. In: Wichtl M (ed) Teedrogen. 2nd ed. Stuttgart: Wissenschaftliche Verlagsgesellschaft, pp 133–134
8. Koch-Heitzmann I (1987) Marsdenia cundurango, Portrait einer Arzneipflanze. Z Phytother 8:38–41
9. Koch H, Steinegger E (1981) Zur Kenntnis der Inhaltsstoffe von Condurango Cortex. Pharm Act Helv 56:244–248
10. Koch H, Steinegger E (1978) Spektrophotometrische Bestimmung von Kondurangin. Pharm Act Helv 53:56–58
11. Steinegger E, Brunner P (1977) Konduranginbestimmung in Cortex Condurango und deren Zubereitungen. Pharm Act Helv 52:139–142
12. Jodlbauer A (1924) Bittermittel, in: Hdb Exp Pharmakol, Vol II, Berlin: Springer Verlag, pp 1563–1585
13. Hayashi K, Wada K, Mitsuhashi H et al. (1980) Antitumor active glycosides from Condurango cortex. Chem Pharm Bull 28:1954–1958

14. Hayashi K, Wada K, Mitsuhashi H et al. (1981) Further investigation of antitumor conduran-goglycosides with C-18 oxygenated aglycone. Chem Pharm Bull 29:2725–2730
15. Kobert R (1893) Lehrbuch der Intoxikationen. Stuttgart, Verlag F Enke, p 661
16. Zechner L. Zölss G (1956) Zur Konduranginbestimmung. Sci Pharm 24:107–127
17. Frohne D, Zerlentis C (1962) Über Wirkstoffe der Condurangin-Gruppe in Marsdenia erecta R. Br. Planta Med 10:107–117
18. Zerlentis C (1962) Marsdenia erecta R. Br., eine in den östlichen Mittelmeerländern heimische keimungshemmende Giftpflanze der Asclepiadaceen. Naturwissenschaften 49:21
19. Saner A, Zerlentis C, Stoecklin W, Reichstein T (1970) Die Glykoside von Marsdenia erecta R.Br. I. Isolierungen Glykoside und Aglykone. Helv Chim Act 53:221–245
20. Jukna G (1888) Über Condurangin. Dissertation, Dorpat
21. Yamomoto H, Mizutani T, Nomura H (1982) Studies on the mutagenicity of crude drug extracts. I Yakugaku Zasshi 102:596–601

Medicago sativa

P.A.G.M. De Smet

Botany

Medicago sativa L. belongs to the Fabaceae (= Leguminosae). Vernacular names include alfalfa and lucerne [1,2]. Alfalfa is an ambiguous vernacular term, as it may refer not only to the leguminous herb *Medicago sativa* but also to a grass species. German textbooks list alfalfa grass as a common name of *Phleum pratense* L. [3,4]. Illustrating this ambiguity is the claim by Polk [5] that the alfalfa products that are marketed in the United States as nonorthodox remedies come from a member of the grass family. This statement was rightly challenged by Brandenburg [6,7] who pointed out that in the United States alfalfa is generally associated with *Medicago sativa*, whereas *Phleum pratense* goes by the name of timothy. When asked for comment, Polk [8] conceded that not the grass but the leguminous herb is the most likely source of the alfalfa products commercially available in the United States. He added that, unfortunately, manufacturers merely provide vernacular terms such as alfalfa or alfalfa leaf to identify the ingredient of such products [8,9].

Chemistry

Alfalfa contains the nonprotein amino acid L-canavanine. Bell [10] reported in 1960 that alfalfa seeds contain 5–14 mg/g, and that these concentrations fall rapidly during germination of the seeds. This latter statement was reexamined by Kasai and Sakamura [11] who found that the amount of L-canavanine does not decrease but increases a little during germination of alfalfa seeds in the dark or in the light. According to calculations based on their crude data, they detected approximately 0.06 mg/g in etiolated sprouts and 0.09 mg/g in green sprouts. Natelson, alone [12] and with Bratton [13], analyzed different varieties of alfalfa and recovered concentrations of 8–15 mg/g in the seeds, 0.9–1.2 mg/g in the leaves, and 0.6–0.9 mg/g in the stems. In sharp contrast, Malinow et al. [14] reported a content of only 8 mg/kg in raw alfalfa seeds. This surprisingly low level decreased with autoclavation until L-canavanine was undetectable in seeds autoclaved for 2 h.

Saponins can be present at levels of 3 mg/g in alfalfa seeds [15] and 5–20 mg/g in the green herb [16]. Livingston et al. [17] analyzed the saponin contents of alfalfa sprouts grown from different varieties of alfalfa seeds. The initial levels of 1.1–1.4 mg/g on day 0 increased rapidly during germination to 31–72 mg/g on day 8. Other alfalfa constituents include phenolic compounds, the predominant one being coumestrol [18]. This constituent occurs in amounts of 10–184 mg/kg in alfalfa haylage [19] and 5 mg/kg in fresh sprouts [20]. It is said that alfalfa seeds contain the alkaloids stachydrine and 1-homostachydrine [16,21].

Since alfalfa seeds may be used to grow sprouts for human food consumption, Archer and Gauer [22] investigated whether application of pesticides to alfalfa seed crops may lead to contamination of alfalfa seeds and of the sprouts grown from these seeds. After field application of five different pesticides at two or three times the normal usage rate, the seeds yielded mean residual levels of 0.06 mg/kg aldicarb, < 0.01 mg/kg chlorothalonil, < 0.02 mg/kg chlopyrifos, 0.23 mg/kg methamidophos, and 2.30 mg/kg propargite. The sprouts were found to contain 0.07 mg/kg propargite, but the residual levels of the other four pesticides did not exceed the detection limit.

Pharmacology and Uses

Dietary alfalfa seeds were found to decrease hypercholesterolemia and to reduce atherosclerosis in cholesterol-fed rabbits [15], and a diet rich in ground alfalfa hay prevented hypercholesterolemia and atherosclerosis in cholesterol-fed monkeys [23]. Partially hydrolyzed alfalfa hay saponins may also produce these responses when fed alone [15,24]. Moreover, the reducing effect of alfalfa meal on cholesterol absorption in the rat was lost by extraction of saponins, and it was restored again by the addition of the saponin fraction to the extracted material [25]. Yet it is unlikely that the hypocholesterolemic effects of alfalfa products can be attributed solely to the presence of saponins [26].

Alfalfa seeds were shown to reduce plasma cholesterol levels in a short-term study involving three human normolipidemic subjects who took a high daily dose of 80–160 g [27]. Effects in patients with hyperlipoproteinemia (HLP) were recently reported by Mölgaard et al. [28] who openly gave 40 g of heat-treated alfalfa seeds 3x per day at mealtimes for eight weeks to eight type IIA patients, three type IIB patients, and four type IV patients. While the number of type IV patients was too small for statistical evaluation, it was found that the patients with type II HLP responded with significant decreases in total serum cholesterol, LDL cholesterol, and apolipoprotein B. LDL cholesterol decreased less than 5% in two of the eleven patients, however, which suggests that there may be responders and nonresponders to alfalfa treatment.

In the United States, alfalfa teas, tablets, and capsules are advocated for a variety of ailments, such as arthritic conditions and diabetes, but the therapeutic usefulness of such commercial preparations remains to be proven [2,29]. Alfalfa sprouts are also used as a tasteful ingredient of salads [2].

L-canavanine has cytotoxic and antimetabolic properties, and its potential usefulness as an antitumor agent is under investigation [30–32].

Adverse Reaction Profile

General Animal Data

Diets with 1.0–1.2% of partially hydrolyzed alfalfa hay saponins have not been found to be toxic in monkeys during protracted periods of ingestion [33].

L-canavanine is a structural analogue of L-arginine and may interfere with the binding of this amino acid to enzymes and with its incorporation into proteins [12,31]. Furthermore, hydrolytic cleavage by arginase yields L-canaline, an analogue of ornithine, and L-canaline may inhibit pyridoxal phosphate and enzymes that require the B_6 cofactor [34]. L-canavanine has well-established toxicity in mice [35], rats [31,32], and lower organisms [30], and it has been reported to induce and worsen autoimmunity in monkeys and mice (see the section on autoimmune reactions below).

General Human Data

Alfalfa use in humans has been associated with systemic lupus erythematosus (SLE)-like manifestations, skin reactions, gastrointestinal disturbances, and raised serum urate levels (see the different sections below). In addition, a fatal case of listeriosis was recently traced to the consumption of alfalfa tablets contaminated with *Listeria monocytogenes* [36].

Data on the toxicity of pure L-canavanine in humans have not been recovered from the literature.

Allergic Reactions

Alfalfa was claimed to pose a potential hazard to persons sensitive to grass pollen, because exposure to it might exacerbate allergic symptoms. This statement was apparently based on the assumption that alfalfa is a grass species and may thus cause similar problems as wheat and other grains have been reported to do [5]. As discussed in the botanical section, however, the identification of alfalfa as a grass species is untenable, and it seems unlikely that persons allergic to grass pollen would suffer from cross-sensitization to the leguminous alfalfa herb [7].

Autoimmune Reactions

Alfalfa preparations can induce and reactivate SLE-like manifestations in monkeys [34,37] and in man [38–40]. SLE is an autoimmune disease, which is multisystemic and fluctuating in nature so that SLE patients may present with a variety of signs and symptoms. This has led to the development of criteria by the American Rheumatism Association for the identification of SLE-patients (Table 1).

Monkeys developed a condition similar to SLE when fed a diet containing 45% of raw alfalfa seeds or 40% of alfalfa sprouts for two months or more. Not all animals were susceptible, so that the possibility of a genetically mediated mechanism should be entertained. Characteristic hematological and serological abnormalities were Coombs' positive hemolytic anemia, elevated titer of antinuclear antibodies (ANA), high binding of double-stranded DNA (ds-DNA), and lowered serum complement. Immune complex induced glomerulonephritis and granular deposition of immunoglobulin G and complement at the dermal-epidermal junction were also observed as well as lethargy, alopecia, anorexia, rash, and edema. The syndrome could be reactivated after a recovery period by a second challenge with raw alfalfa seeds [34,37]. Exacerbation of SLE-like signs did not occur, however, when susceptible monkeys were rechallenged with a diet containing 45% of roasted alfalfa seeds that had been autoclaved for 3 h at 15 lb pressure and 120°C [14].

Malinow et al. [38] observed pancytopenia and splenomegaly in a 59-year-old man who had ingested 80–160 g of ground alfalfa seeds daily on eight occasions for periods up to six weeks during five months. The patient had a positive Coombs' test, speckled ANA, slightly increased antibodies to ds-DNA, and reduced total hemolytic component. Following discontinuation of the alfalfa ingestion, the spleen decreased to a normal size, serological and complement studies reverted to negative, and the hematological abnormalities returned slowly toward normal values.

Roberts and Hayashi [39] reported the reactivation of quiescent SLE in two patients following the use of commercial alfalfa tablets (Shaklee, San Francisco). Aside from serological signs, one patient developed proteinuria, malaise, lethargy, depression, and arthralgias after the daily ingestion of 15 tablets for nine months, whereas the other patient showed diffuse proliferative glomerulonephritis after a 2.5-year-long use of 8 tablets per day.

Prete [40] stated that four previously well patients developed a reversible SLE-like syndrome after taking 12–24 alfalfa tablets (Shaklee) per day for 3 weeks to 7 months. Symptoms and signs included arthralgias, myalgias, and mild rash, with positive antinuclear antibodies (solid pattern), and antibodies to ds-DNA in one patient.

Since these latter two reports list arthralgias as adverse effects, it is disturbing that alfalfa preparations are promoted for the treatment of arthritis (see the section on pharmacology and uses).

Table 1. Criteria proposed by the American Rheumatism Association for identifying patients with systemic lupus erythematosus; at least 4 of these 11 manifestations should be present, serially or simultaneously, during any interval of observation [41]

Criterion	Description
1. Malar rash	Fixed erythema, flat or raised, over the malar eminences, tending to spare the nasolabial folds
2. Discoid rash	Erythematous raised patches with adherent keratotic scaling and follicular plugging; atrophic scarring may occur in older lesions
3. Photosensitivity	Skin rash as a result of unusual reaction to sunlight, by patient history or physician observation
4. Oral ulcers	Oral or nasopharyngeal ulceration, usually painless, observed by a physician
5. Arthritis	Nonerosive arthritis involving two or more peripheral joints, characterized by tenderness, swelling, or effusion
6. Serositis	Pleuritis — convincing history of pleuritic pain or rub heard by a physician or evidence of pleural effusion; or Pericarditis — deocumented by ECG or rub or evidence of pericardial effusion
7. Renal disorder	Persistent proteinuria > 0.5 g/day or $> 3+$ if quantitation not performed; or Cellular casts — may be red cell, hemoglobin, granular, tubular, or mixed
8. Neurological disorder	Seizures — in the absence of offending drugs or known metabolic derangements (e.g., uremia, ketoacidosis, or electrolyte imbalance); or Psychosis — in the absence of offending drugs or known metabolic derangements (e.g., uremia, ketoacidosis, or electrolyte imbalance)
9. Hematological disorder	Hemolytic anemia — with reticulosis; or Leukopenia — $< 4000/mm^3$ total on two or more occasions; or Lymphopenia — $< 1500/mm^2$ on two or more occasions; or Thrombocytopenia — $< 100\,000/mm^3$ in the absence of offending drugs
10. Immunological disorder	Positive LE cell preparation; Anti-DNA (antibody to native DNA in abnormal titer); or Anti-samarium (presence of antibody to samarium nuclear antigen); or False positive serological test for syphilis known to be positive for at least six months and confirmed by *Treponema pallidum* immobilization or fluorescent treponemal antibody absorption test
11. Antinuclear antibody (ANA)	An abnormal titer of antinuclear antibody by immunofluorescence or an equivalent assay at any point in time and in the absence of drugs known to be associated with drug-induced lupus syndrome

Alfalfa saponins are unlikely to be responsible, because they are heat stable [14], and their dietary administration to monkeys did not result in SLE-like abnormalities [33,37]. It has been proposed that the effects of alfalfa may be due to the presence of L-canavanine [42]. This constituent is destroyed by auto-clavation of alfalfa seeds [14], and a challenge of susceptible monkeys with a diet containing 1% of L-canavanine sulfate resulted in reactivation of the SLE-like syndrome [34]. L-canavanine was also found to induce and worsen autoim-munity in mice when given in amounts to approximate a 20% alfalfa sprout diet [43].

As L-canavanine occurs in the seeds, sprouts, stems, and leaves of the alfalfa plant (see the section on chemistry), it would seem prudent to caution SLE patients against the use of any alfalfa preparation. It is still uncertain, however, that the SLE-like effects of alfalfa are caused by L-canavanine. Weissberger and Armstrong [44] analyzed commercial alfalfa tablets of the same origin (Shaklee) as the tablets that were actually associated with SLE-like reactions in doses of 8–24 tablets per day (see the case reports above). They found L-canavanine levels of 17 ± 1 μg/tablet, which implies that the patients who experienced SLE-like adverse reactions from the tablets were exposed to 0.14–0.41 mg L-canavanine per day. Whether such low levels of human exposure are indeed sufficient for the induction of SLE-like effects warrants investigation.

Another aspect that still needs further exploration is the exact mechanism of the SLE-like reactions to alfalfa and L-canavanine [39,45–47].

Dermatological Reactions

According to text books, *Medicago sativa* has been associated with photosensi-tivity reactions in animals [1,48]. A diet containing *Medicago sativa* was reported to induce photosensitization from porphyrins in albino rats, the photosensitivity being related to the pheophorbide *a* and the chlorophyllide *a* content of the plant material [49]. Concrete references about alfalfa-induced photosensitivity in man are not available. It should not be forgotten, however, that alfalfa products have been reported to induce SLE-like effects in humans (see the section on autoim-mune reactions) and that photosensitivity is one of the various manifestations of SLE (Table 1).

Kaufman [50] reported six cases of patchy, pruritic, erythematous, and edematous skin reactions following the use of alfalfa seeds in capsule form or as a herbal tea. Two of these cases were described in detail. They involved elderly females with arthritis who had been taking for two months four to six cups daily of an infusion prepared by boiling 2–4 tablespoons of alfalfa seeds in 1 pt (473 ml) of water. In one patient, the eruption spread from the hands to the arms and the face. The other patient developed patches only on the lateral aspects of both thighs, which makes a photosensitive reaction unlikely. The pruritic nature of the eruptions argues against the possibility of an SLE-like erythematous rash.

Endocrine Reactions

The alfalfa constituent coumestrol has weak estrogenic properties. As measured by a mouse uterine weight bioassay, it is some 200 times less potent than estron and almost 3000 times less potent than diethylstilbestrol [51]. In spite of this apparently low level of potency, cattle fed alfalfa haylage containing as little as 37 mg/kg coumestrol as their major feed may show deleterious estrogenic effects [19].

Elakovich and Hampton [51] were unable to detect coumestrol in a brand of alfalfa seed tablets but found coumestrol concentrations of 20–194 mg/kg in three brands of commercial alfalfa tablets. The brand with the highest level would provide slightly more than 1.1 mg coumestrol when taken in the maximum label-recommended dosage of 9 tablets daily. As this amount is well below the 37 mg/kg tested in alfalfa haylage feeding experiments with cattle, it is unclear whether it might represent any health hazard.

Gastrointestinal Reactions

Ingestion of large amounts of alfalfa seeds (e.g., 120 g per day) can be associated with flatulence, abdominal discomfort, loose stools, diarrhea, and loss of appetite [27,28].

Metabolic Reactions

In the study that Mölgaard et al. [28] performed in hyperlipoproteinemic patients (see the section on pharmacology and uses), the mean serum urate was raised significantly from 296 to 336 μmol/l by 120 g of heat-treated alfalfa seeds per day. This effect was attributed to the presence of purines in the seeds. It would thus be prudent to avoid treatment with alfalfa seeds in patients with gout.

Fertility, Pregnancy, and Lactation

Medicago sativa and *Trifolium* species (clovers) are used widely for the supplemental feeding of live-stock. In view of the extensive field observations and experimental work on these plants, Keeler [52] does not consider it likely that teratogenic effects would have been overlooked. He recalls, however, that the phytoestrogens in these plants may produce signs as difficult labor, infertility, and full-term fetal death or abortion.

Whether such animal data may have any relevance for humans is unclear, especially since the reported amounts of coumestrol in commercial alfalfa products would seem to be much lower than the levels to which livestock is exposed (see the section on endocrine reactions).

Human data on the ingestion of alfalfa preparations during pregnancy or lactation were not retrieved from the literature.

Mutagenicity and Carcinogenicity

Data on the mutagenic and/or carcinogenic potential of *Medicago sativa* have not been recovered from the literature.

References

1. Kingsbury JM (1964) Poisonous plants of the United States and Canada. Englewood Cliffs: Prentice-Hall, Inc
2. Tyler VE (1987) The new honest herbal. A sensible guide to herbs and related remedies. 2nd edn. Philadelphia: George F Stickley Company, pp 18–20
3. Hoppe HA (1975) Drogenkunde. Vol 1. Angiospermen. 8th edn. Berlin: Walter de Gruyter
4. List PH, Hörhammer L (1977) Hagers Handbuch der pharmazeutischen Praxis. 4th edn. Vol 6. Chemikalien und Drogen, Teil A: N-Q. Berlin: Springer-Verlag
5. Polk IJ (1982) Alfalfa pill treatment of allergy may be hazardous. JAMA 247:1493
6. Brandenburg DM (1982) Alfalfa grass and legume. JAMA 248:2836
7. Brandenburg DM (1983) Alfalfa of the family Leguminosae. JAMA 249:3303
8. Polk IJ (1982) Personal communication, May 4
9. Polk IJ (1982) Alfalfa grass and legume. JAMA 248:2837
10. Bell EA (1960) Canavanine in the Leguminosae. Biochem J 75:618–620
11. Kasai T, Sakamura S (1986) Reexamination of canavanine disappearance during germination of alfalfa (*Medicago sativa*). J Nutr Sci Vitaminol (Tokyo) 32:77–82
12. Natelson S (1985) Canavanine to arginine in alfalfa (*Medicago sativa*), clover (*Trifolium*), and the jack bean (*Canavalia ensiformis*). J Agric Food Chem 33:413–419
13. Natelson S, Bratton GR (1984) Canavanine assay of some alfalfa cultivars (Medicago sativa) by fluorescence practical procedure of canavanine preparation. Microchem J 29:26–43
14. Malinow MR, McLaughlin P, Bardana EJ Jr, Craig S (1984) Elimination of toxicity from diets containing alfalfa seeds. Food Chem Toxicol 22:583–587
15. Malinow MR, McLaughlin P, Stafford C, Livingston AL, Kohler GO (1980) Alfalfa saponins and alfalfa seeds. Dietary effects in cholesterol-fed rabbits. Atherosclerosis 37:433–438
16. List PH, Hörhammer L (1976) Hagers Handbuch der pharmazeutischen Praxis. 4th edn. Vol 5. Chemikalien und Drogen (H-M). Berlin Springer-Verlag
17. Livingston AL, Knuckles BE, Teuber LR, Hesterman OB, Tsai LS (1984) Minimizing the saponin content of alfalfa sprouts and leaf protein concentrates. Adv Exp Med Biol 177:253–268
18. Bickoff EM, Livingston AL, Witt SC, Knuckles BE, Guggolz J, Spencer RR (1964) Isolation of coumestrol and other phenolics from alfalfa by countercurrent distribution. J Pharm Sci 53:1496–1499
19. Lookhart GL (1980) Analysis of coumestrol, a plant estrogen, in animal feeds by high-performance liquid chromatography. J Agric Food Chem 28:666–667
20. Knuckles BE, deFremery D, Kohler GO (1976) Coumestrol content of fractions obtained during wet processing of alfalfa. J Agric Food Chem 24:1177–1180
21. Der Marderosian A, Liberti LE (1988) Natural product medicine. A scientific guide to foods, drugs, cosmetics. Philadelphia: George F Stickley
22. Archer TE, Gauer WO (1985) Residues of five pesticides in field-treated alfalfa seeds and alfalfa sprouts. J Environ Sci Health [B] 20:445–456
23. Malinow MR, McLaughlin P, Naito HK, Lewis LA, McNulty WP (1978) Effect of alfalfa meal on shrinkage (regression) of atherosclerotic plaques during cholesterol feeding in monkeys. Atherosclerosis 30:27–43

24. Malinow MW, McLaughlin P, Kohler GO, Livingston AL (1977) Prevention of elevated cholesterolemia in monkeys by alfalfa saponins. Steroids 29:105–110
25. Malinow MR, McLaughlin P, Stafford C, Livingston AL, Kohler GO, Cheeke PR (1979) Comparative effects of alfalfa saponins and alfalfa fiber on cholesterol absorption in rats. Am J Clin Nutr 32:1810–1812
26. Story JA, LePage SL, Petro MS, West LG, Cassidy MM, Lightfoot FG, Vahouny GV (1984) Interactions of alfalfa plant and sprout saponins with cholesterol in vitro and in cholesterol-fed rats. Am J Clin Nutr 39:917–929
27. Malinow MR, McLaughlin P, Stafford C (1980) Alfalfa seeds: effects on cholesterol metabolism. Experientia 36:562–563
28. Mölgaard J, Von Schenck H, Olsson AG (1987) Alfalfa seeds lower low density lipoprotein cholesterol and apolipoprotein B concentrations in patients with type II hyperlipoproteinemia. Atherosclerosis 65:173–179
29. Worthington-Roberts B, Breskin M (1983) Fads or facts? A pharmacist's guide to controversial 'nutrition' products. Am Pharm NS23:410–422
30. Rosenthal GA (1977) The biological effects and mode of action of L-canavanine, a structural analogue of L-arginine. Q Rev Biol 52:155–178
31. Thomas DA, Rosenthal GA, Gold DV, Dickey K (1986) Growth inhibition of a rat colon tumor by L-canavanine. Cancer Res 46:2898–2903
32. Thomas DA, Rosenthal GA (1987) Toxicity and pharmacokinetics of the nonprotein amino acid L-canavanine in the rat. Toxicol Appl Pharmacol 91:395–405
33. Malinow MR, McNulty WP, Houghton DC et al. (1982) Lack of toxicity of alfalfa saponins in monkeys. J Med Primat 11:106–118
34. Malinow MR, Bardana EJ Jr, Pirofsky B, Craig S, McLaughlin P (1982) Systemic lupus erythematosus-like syndrome in monkeys fed alfalfa sprouts: role of a nonprotein amino acid. Science 216:415–417
35. Tschiersch B (1962) Zur toxischen Wirkung der Jackbohne. Pharmazie 17:621–623
36. Farber JM, Carter AO, Varughese PV, Ashton FE, Ewan EP (1990) Listeriosis traced to the consumption of alfalfa tablets and soft cheese. New Engl J Med 322:338
37. Bardana EJ Jr, Malinow MR, Houghton DC, McNulty WP, Wuepper KD, Parker F, Pirofsky B (1982) Diet-induced systemic lupus erythematosus (SLE) in primates. Am J Kidney Dis 1:345–352
38. Malinow MR, Bardana EJ Jr, Goodnight SH Jr (1981) Pancytopenia during ingestion of alfalfa seeds. Lancet 1:615
39. Roberts JL, Hayashi JA (1983) Exacerbation of SLE associated with alfalfa ingestion. New Engl J Med 308:1361
40. Prete PE (1985) The mechanism of action of L-canavanine in inducing autoimmune phenomena. Arthritis Rheum 28:1198–1200
41. Tan EM, Cohen AS, Fries JF et al. (1982) The 1982 revised criteria for the classification of systemic lupus erythematosus. Arthritis Rheum 25:1271–1277
42. Corman LC (1985) The role of diet in animal models of systemic lupus erythematosus: possible implications for human lupus. Semin Arthritis Rheum 15:61–69
43. Prete PE (1984) Effects of in vivo L-canavanine on immune function in normal DBA/2 and autoimmune (NZB and NZB × NZW F$_1$) mice. Arthritis Rheum 27(Suppl 4):29
44. Weissberger LE, Armstrong MK (1984) Canavanine analysis of alfalfa extracts by high performance liquid chromatography using pre-column derivatization. J Chromatogr Sci 22:438–440
45. Alcocer-Varela J, Iglesias A, Llorente L, Alarcon-Segovia D (1985) Effects of L-canavanine on T cells may explain the induction of systemic lupus erythematosus by alfalfa. Arthritis Rheum 28:52–57
46. Alcocer-Varela J, Alarcon-Segovia D (1985) The mechanism of action of L-canavanine in inducing autoimmune phenomena. Arthritis Rheum 28:1200
47. Thomas TJ, Messner RP (1986) Effects of lupus-inducing drugs on the B to Z transition of synthetic DNA. Arthr Rheumat 29:638–645
48. Mitchell J, Rook A (1979) Botanical dermatology. Plants and plant products injurious to the skin. Greengrass: Vancouver

49. Towers GHN (1980) Photosensitizers from plants and their photodynamic action. Prog Phyto-chem 6:183–202
50. Kaufman WH (1954) Alfalfa seed dermatitis. JAMA 155:1058–1059
51. Elakovich SD, Hampton JM (1984) Analysis of coumestrol, a phytoestrogen, in alfalfa tablets sold for human consumption. J Agric Food Chem 32:173–175
52. Keeler RF (1972) Known and suspected teratogenic hazards in range plants. Clin Toxicol 5:529–565

Mentha piperita and *Mentha spicata*

I.H. Bowen and I.J. Cubbin

Botany

The genus *Mentha* belongs to the family Labiatae, and several species are used medicinally. *Mentha piperita* L. [1–3], a cross between the two older species *M. spicata* and *M. aquatica*, is commonly called peppermint but may also be referred to as brandy mint, curled mint, or balm mint among other names. It is widely considered to exist in varietal forms; the main two are the black and white peppermints, the best oil being obtained from the white variety [1,2]. According to the BPC the black variety yields more essential oil, but the oil from the white variety has a more delicate aroma [4]. The higher yielding variety is more frequently used pharmaceutically. *Mentha spicata* L., which has formerly been described as *M. crispa* or *M. viridis*, has a large number of vernacular names including spearmint, garden mint, mackerel mint, and yerba buena [1–3]. Occasionally the wild or hairy mint *M. aquatica* or *M. saliva* is collected. The so-called purple mint (*Perilla frutescens*) is a Japanese plant excluded from this contribution. *M. arvensis*, the Japanes mint, is also excluded, but this plant has been used to adulterate *M. piperita* [5]. It is readily distinguishable from the other species, however, by its stunted, feeble growth [6]. It is unlikely that other botanical sources are included, except that high-yielding strains and cultivars of both *M. piperita* and *M. spicata* are almost certainly involved in improving oil production. The aerial parts of both these species and their respective oils form the articles of commerce commonly encountered. The essential oil, which may be present up to 1.5% (although Wichtl [6] reports up to 4%) depending on the varietal form, is of variable quality. The English peppermint oil has historically been regarded [7] as the finest quality, and great care has been taken to exclude *M. arvensis* from the crop since this, with its high proportion of menthol (70–90%) can completely ruin the product.

Chemistry

Tannins represent 6–12% of the fresh weight. In peppermint oil, a pale yellow liquid, menthol is present to 50–60%, crystallizing at low temperatures. Menthone

(15–32%), a number of esters calculated as menthyl acetate (4–14%), and small amounts of cineole and other terpenes are also present [1–5]. Immature plants contain some pulegone (1–3%) and menthofuran giving an inferior oil [3]. The dementholized oil of *M. arvensis* has been used as a substitute for peppermint oil, with menthol occasionally being added to bring the content up to pharmacopeial standards. A simple color test may be used to distinguish these oils [8,9]. Wichtl additionally lists flavonoid and triterpene as components of peppermint leaf [6].

Oil of spearmint contains (−)-carvone (55–70%); (−)-limonene, phellandrine and dihydrocarveol acetate are also present, accompanied by esters of acetic, butyric, and caproic or caprylic acids [1,2].

Pharmacology and Uses

Peppermint and the constituents of the oil have wide application as flavorings in pharmaceutical and dental preparations. Peppermint is also marketed for the treatment of gastrointestinal disorders and figures prominently as a carminative, antispasmodic and antinauseant in mixtures used as stomachics [10–13]. Peppermint oil inhibits smooth muscle and relaxes the lower esophageal sphincter, and in vitro and in vivo experiments in animals and man indicate that peppermint oil and menthol act by calcium channel blockade. The effect is most pronounced on the gut, and it is unlikely that serum concentrations are reached at normal therapeutic doses to have any effect on the heart or nervous system [14–17]. A delayed-release capsule containing peppermint oil [18] has use in the treatment of irritable bowel syndrome, and injection of the oil along the biopsy channel of the colonoscope is reported to give fast relief of colonic spasm during endoscopy [19]. On the other hand, Nash [20] reports that peppermint oil does not relieve the pain of irritable bowel syndrome, and Rogers [21] considers the action of peppermint oil to be more complex than simple inhibition of gastrointestinal smooth muscle. Measurement of pressure activity of the colon following intraluminal administration of peppermint oil in five normal subjects produced unexpected results suggesting stimulation of smooth muscle, and he proposes further studies to define the effect of peppermint oil on alimentary motility. Wichtl [6] lists cholagogue as one of the actions of peppermint oil, and recent work has shown that menthol/ursodeoxycholic acid preparations significantly reduce the size of gallstones by dissolution, and the incidence of stone calcification was also reduced [22]. The effect on bile flow was not reported, however. Externally, menthol is a frequent constituent of liniments and ointments, having a cooling or mild anesthetic action, and also finds use as an inhalation or constituent of lozenges/pastilles to clear congested nasal passages, the menthol increasing the nasal sensation of airflow [23]. Menthol may also be added to cigarettes to utilize this cooling effect. One report records reduced fatigue and increased mental capacity of flight controllers while their working environment was enhanced by volatile plant aromatics, including peppermint [24].

Spearmint is frequently encountered as a flavoring in gum, toothpaste, and mouthwashes, being employed for the latter purpose in local remedies throughout Europe [25].

Pharmacokinetics

Pharmacokinetic studies on the delayed release peppermint oil preparations 'Colpermin' (Tillots Laboratories) and 'Mintec' (S.K. & F. Ltd.) indicated that Colpermin was excreted more slowly than Mintec and concluded that Colpermin seemed to deliver peppermint oil more effectively to the distal small bowel and ascending colon than does Mintec. The pharmacokinetic data may be relevant to choice of preparation for the treatment of altered colonic mobility. Menthol is excreted in the urine as the glucuronide, but this accounts for only 50% of the administered dose, the fate of the remainder being unknown [26,27].

Adverse Reaction Profile

General Animal Data

In a series of toxicity studies on peppermint oil and its major constituents menthol and menthone in rats, Wurtzen and Carstensen [28–30] have demonstrated spaces in the white matter of the cerebellum at various dose levels. No behavioral changes were observed nor any obvious clinical symptoms associated with the encephalopathy. This effect was observed with the oil and with menthone but not with menthol. The no-effect level for peppermint oil for humans was calculated at 10 mg/kg per day, equivalent to consumption of 28 g/day of peppermint lozenges containing 4% peppermint oil.

No toxicity studies of spearmint have been recovered from the literature.

General Human Data

Peppermint teas generally contain only low amounts of menthol and menthone [31], and where adverse effects have been encountered they are mainly associated with a relatively high intake of menthol via confectionery, pharmaceuticals, or other products in which peppermint oil or menthol figure as significant components of the formulation. Normal usage of peppermint teas, even over prolonged periods, rarely leads to adverse effects [6].

Heng [32] reports severe necrosis and interstitial nephritis in an elderly patient after topical application of a preparation containing menthol and methyl salicylate, followed by prolonged use of an electrically heated pad.

The estimated lethal dose for menthol in man may be as low as 2 g [33,34], but there are reports of individuals surviving doses as high as 8–9 g [35].

The product information of an enteric coated capsule containing 0.2 ml peppermint oil lists skin rashes, headache, bradycardia, muscle tremor, and ataxia as rarely reported side effects [36]. Recurrent muscle pains have also been associated with the ingestion of peppermint oil [37].

Allergic Reactions

Allergic reactions to peppermint appear to be rare or of a relatively minor nature.

Burr [38], investigating food-allergic asthma, reported one positive response to peppermint but concluded that the effect was small and probably not a major contributor to the patient's asthma. Eight workers in a penicillin factory gave positive histamine-release reactions on exposure to peppermint [39], a flavor additive, the response probably being pseudo-allergic (nonimmunological mechanism). Fisher [40] in a brief review of menthol reactions reports cases of urticaria, allergic cheilitis, and stomatitis on exposure to a variety of products containing menthol, including pharmaceuticals, toothpaste, and cigarettes and comments that while allergic reactions are rare, they may include shaking chills from use of topical menthol products, particularly in elderly persons. Hausen [41] documents persistent cheilitis due to the carvone content of a spearmint-flavored toothpaste, and Lubow [42] records a single incident of plasma cell gingivitis due to regular use of a peppermint dental preparation. Menthol has been reported to cause hypersensitivity characterized by urticaria [43] or dermatitis [44]. These reactions generally subside within a short time of discontinuation of use of the product.

Auricular Reactions

Schmidt [45] reports the occurrence of otitis externa and damage to the tympanic membrane following use of a group of local anesthetics including Bonain's liquid, which contains phenol, menthol, and cocaine hydrochloride. The contribution, if any, of the menthol to the adverse reaction is not clear.

Cardiovascular Reactions

Bradycardia has been reported in a patient addicted to menthol cigarettes [46], while excessive consumption of peppermint-flavored confectionery has caused fibrillation [47]. In both cases, reduction in the menthol/peppermint intake reversed the condition.

Dermatological Reactions

Relatively mild dermatological reactions to the skin and mucous membranes are described above [40–44], and in a Polish study [48] approximately 1% of patients exhibited a reaction to menthol. More seriously, Parys [49] describes a case of chemical burns to the hand of a worker in a pharmaceutical factory due to spillage of neat peppermint oil and recommends protective measures (gloves) for workers. Isolated incidents due to accidental or inappropriate use of the products suggest caution in the handling and application of the oil or menthol products, particularly the application of neat oil to treat rheumatism [2].

Gastrointestinal Reactions

Although peppermint has many uses in the treatment of GI disorders (see pharmacology and uses), nevertheless there are reports of GI irritation or aggravation of GI complaints due to use of peppermint preparations including confectionery. Reported conditions include stomatitis, severe esophagitis, gastritis, unexplained diarrhea, and pancreatitis. Attention is drawn to the presence of peppermint in antacid formulations which could exacerbate some GI conditions [50]. In the case of delayed release peppermint oil, administration to a patient with concurrent diarrhea led to anal burning due to the excreted peppermint [51]. This did not occur when the diarrhea was controlled, the oil remaining in the GI tract for a longer time and with good patient tolerance and absence of any burning sensation. The product information of an enteric coated capsule with peppermint oil cautions that preexisting heartburn may be exacerbated [36].

Respiratory Reactions

Martindale [33] records the warning that nasal preparations containing menthol may cause spasm of the glottis in young children, and that cases of instant collapse have been reported in infants following local application of menthol (see also the section on allergic reactions).

Fertility, Pregnancy, and Lactation

No data for peppermint or spearmint oils have been recovered from the literature to suggest toxic effects in pregnancy or during lactation. Pulegone, a component of oil of pennyroyal (*Mentha pulegium*) and a known abortifacient [52], is absent from good-quality peppermint oil. Oil from young plants may contain some pulegone [3], and inferior oils may contain traces, but it is highly unlikely that peppermint-flavored products would give cause for concern in this respect in normal use or at therapeutic doses. In a screening of medicinal plants for antifertility activity the related species *Mentha arvensis* was examined but not found to have any significant activity [53], while a more detailed study found weak antiovulatory action but no abortifacient or spermicidal action [54].

Mutagenicity and Carcinogenicity

In studies of mutagenicity [55] menthone has been shown to be mutagenic in the Salmonella/mammalian microsome test, but despite the presence of up to 30% menthone in samples of peppermint oil no mutagenic effects could be detected using the oil or with menthol, the major component of peppermint. Carcinogenic effects of the oil have not been recovered from the literature, but a recent survey [56] of the incidence of esophageal cancer reveals a higher incidence among smokers of menthol cigarettes than in other population groups. The study was, however, relatively small and confined to one ethnic group.

References

1. Trease GE, Evans WC (1983) Pharmacognosy. 12th ed. Eastbourne: Bailliere Tindall, pp 421–424
2. Grieve M (1974) A modern herbal. London: Jonathan Cape, pp 533–543
3. Tyler VE, Brady LR, Robbers JE (1976) Pharmacognosy. 7th ed. Philadelphia: Lea and Febiger, pp 142
4. Anonymous (1968) British pharmaceutical codex. London: Pharmaceutical Press, p 590
5. Clark RJ, Menary RC (1981) Variations in composition of peppermint oil in relation to production areas. Econ Bot 35:59–69
6. Wichtl M (ed) (1984) Teedrogen: Ein Handbuch für Apotheker und Arzt. Stuttgart: Wissenschaftliche Verlagsgesellschaft mbH, pp 255–257
7. LeStrange R (1977) A history of herbal plants. New York: Aris Pub. Co., p 179
8. Hanbury D, Fluckinger FA (1874) Pharmacographia. London: MacMillan and Co., p 436
9. Wallis TE (1967) A Textbook of Pharmacognosy. 5th ed. London: Churchill, pp 338–340
10. Robson NJ (1987) Carminative property of peppermint in magnesium trisilicate mixture B.P. Anaesthesia; 42:776–777
11. Jaffe G, Grimshaw JJ (1982) A comparison between Gastrils and Aludrox in the treatment of gastric hyperacidity in general practice. J Int Med Res 10:437–442
12. Kapila YV, Dodds WJ, Helm JF, Hogan WD (1984) Relationship between swallow rate and salivary flow. Dig Dis Sci 29:528–533
13. DeVault KR, Castell DO (1987) Effects of antireflux therapies on salivary function in normal humans. Dig Dis Sci 32:603–608
14. Anonymous (1988) Hole for the mint [Editorial]. Lancet 2:1144–1145
15. Taylor BA, Duthie HL, Luscombe DK (1985) Calcium antagonist activity of menthol on gastrointestinal smooth muscle. Br J Clin Pharmacol 20:293P–294P
16. Taylor BA, Luscombe DK, Duthie HL (1983) Inhibitory effect of peppermint oil on gastrointestinal smooth muscle. Gut 24:A992
17. Hawthorn M, Ferrante J, Luchoswki E, Rutledge A, Wei XY, Triggle DJ (1988) The actions of peppermint oil and menthol on calcium channel dependent processes in intestinal, neuronal and cardiac preparations. Aliment Pharmacol Therap 2:101–118
18. Dew MJ, Evans BK, Rhodes J (1984) Peppermint oil for the irritable bowel syndrome: a multicentre trial. Brit J Clin Pract 38:394, 398

19. Leicester RJ, Hunt RH (1982) Peppermint oil to reduce colonic spasm during endoscopy. Lancet 2:989
20. Nash P, Gould SR, Barnardo DE (1986) Peppermint oil does not relieve the pain of irritable bowel syndrome. Br J Clin Prac 40:292–293
21. Rogers J, Tay HH, Misiewicz JJ (1988) Peppermint oil. Lancet 2:98
22. Leuschner U, Leuschner J, Lazarovici D, Kurtz W, Hellstern A (1988) Dissolution of gallstones with ursodeoxycholic acid menthol preparation: a controlled perspective double blind trial. Gut 29:428–432
23. Eccles R, Griffiths DH, Newton CG, Tolley NS (1988) The effects of menthol isomers on nasal sensation of airflow. Clin Otolaryngol 13:25–29
24. Leshchinskaya YS, Makarchuk NM, Lebeda AF, Krivenko VV, Sgibnev AK, Bajatskaya TS (1983) Effect of phytonicides on cerebral circulation in flight controllers during their professional activities. Kosm Biol Aviakosm Med 17:80–83
25. Tammaro F, Xepapadakis G (1986) Plants used in phytotherapy, cosmetics and dyeing in the Pramanda district (Epirus, N-W Greece). J Ethnopharmacol 16:167–174
26. White DA, Thompson SP, Wilson CG, Bell GD (1987) A pharmacokinetic comparison of two delayed-release peppermint oil preparations, Colpermin and Mintec, for treatment of the irritable bowel syndrome. Int J Pharm 40:151–155
27. Bell GD (1988) Peppermint oil. Lancet 2:99
28. Thorup I, Wurtzen G, Carstensen J, Olsen P (1983) Short-term toxicity study in rats dosed with peppermint oil. Toxicol Lett 19:211–215
29. Thorup I, Wurtzen G, Carstensen J, Olsen P (1983) Short-term toxicity study in rats dosed with pulegone and menthol. Toxicol Lett 19:207–211
30. Madsen C, Wurtzen G, Carstensen J (1986) Short-term toxicity study in rats dosed with menthone. Toxicol Lett 32:147–152
31. Miething H, Holz W (1988) Menthol und Menthon in Pfefferminztees – Ermittlung der Freisetzungskinetiken. Pharm Ztg 133:16–17
32. Heng MC (1987) Local necrosis and interstitial nephritis due to topical methyl salicylate and menthol. Cutis 39:442–444
33. Wade A (ed) (1982) Martindale: the extra pharmacopoeia. 28th Ed. London: The Pharmaceutical Press, p 352
34. Cooper P (1974) Poisoning by drugs and chemicals, plants and animals – an index of toxic effects and their treatment. London: Alchemist, p 133
35. Schwenkenbecher A (1985) Über Mentholvergiftung des Menchen. Münch Med Wschr 1908; 55:1495–6 [Quoted in Wirth W, Gloxhuber C. Toxikologie für Ärzte, Naturwissenschaftler und Apotheker. Stuttgart, New York: Georg Thieme, p 295]
36. Anonymous (1986) Mintec capsules. Pharm J 237:355
37. Williams B (1972) Palindromic rheumatism. Med J Aust 2:390
38. Burr ML, Fehily AM, Stott NCH, Merrett TG (1985) Food allergic asthma in general practice. Hum Nutr Appl Nutr 39A:349–355
39. Moller NE, Skov PS, Noru S (1984) Allergic and pseudo-allergic reactions caused by penicillins, cocoa and peppermint additives in penicillin factory workers examined by basophil histamine release. Acta Pharmacol Toxicol 55:139–144
40. Fisher AA (1986) Reactions to menthol. Cutis 38:17–18
41. Hausen BM (1984) Tooth-paste allergy. Dtsch Med Wschr 109:300–302
42. Lubow RM, Cooley RL, Hartman KS, McDaniel RK (1984) Plasma-cell gingivitis: report of a case. J Periodontol 55:235–241
43. Papa CM, Shelly WB (1964) Menthol hypersensitivity. JAMA 189:546
44. Rudzki E, Grzywa Z, Bruo W (1976) Sensitivity to 35 essential oils. Contact Dermatitis 2:196
45. Schmidt S-H, Hellstom S (1986) Late effects of local anaesthetics on tympanic membrane structure. Am J Otolaryngol 7:346–352
46. Luke E (1962) Addiction to mentholated cigarettes. Lancet 1:110
47. Thomas JG (1962) Peppermint fibrillation. Lancet 1:222
48. Rudzki E, Kleniewska D (1970) The epidemiology of contact dermatitis in Poland. Br J Derm 83:543–545

49. Parys BT (1983) Chemical burns resulting from contact with peppermint oil. Burns Inc Therm Inj 9:374-375
50. Roberts HJ (1983) Caution regarding peppermint mints. South Med J 10:1331
51. Weston CFM (1987) Anal burning and peppermint oil. Postgrad Med J 63:717
52. Gordon WP, Huitric AC, Seth CL, McClanahan RH, Nelson SD (1978) The metabolism of the abortifacient terpene, (R)-(+)- pulegone, to a proximate toxin, menthofuran. Drug Metab Disp 15:589-594
53. Kholkute SD, Mudgal V, Deshpande PJ (1976) Screening of indigenous medicinal plants for antifertility potentiality. Planta Med 29:151-155
54. Kamboj VP, Dhawan BN (1982) Research on plants for fertility regulation in India. J Ethnopharmacol 6:191-226
55. Andersen PH, Jensen NJ (1984) Mutagenic investigation of peppermint oil in the Salmonella/mammalian-microsome test. Mutat Res 138:17-20
56. Hebert JR, Kabat GC (1988) Menthol cigarettes and oesophageal cancer. Am J Public Health 78:986-987

Panax ginseng

U. Sonnenborn and R. Hänsel

Botany

Panax ginseng C.A. Meyer ("Korean" ginseng) and its congeners belong to the family Araliaceae [1,2]. The same is true for *Eleutherococcus senticosus* Maxim. (syn. *Acanthopanax senticosus*, "Siberian" ginseng) [3]. The natural habitat of *Panax ginseng* is South and North Korea, northeastern China (Manchuria), and parts of the far eastern Soviet Union [4,5]. Other *Panax* species such as *P. notoginseng* Burk. ("San-Chi" ginseng), *P. pseudoginseng*, and *P. japonicus* ("Chikusetsu" ginseng) grow in southwestern China and Vietnam, in the Himalayan region, and in Japan. *P. quinquefolius* ("American" ginseng) and *P. trifolius* ("dwarf" ginseng) are the typical ginseng species of Canada and the USA [4,5]. Wild ginseng plants, which can hardly be found today, originally grew in the shady mixed mountain forests of Southeast Asia and North America. Nowadays, ginseng is cultivated on large plantations in Korea and to a somewhat lesser extent in China, Japan, Canada, and the USA [6].

In contrast to the *Panax* species, *Eleutherococcus* (*Acanthopanax*) *senticosus* is a thorny shrub that even today can be found growing wild in the southeastern part of the Soviet Union, northern China, Korea, and Japan [3]. It is propagated especially in the USSR as a potent substitute for *P. ginseng*, exhibiting similar pharmacological properties [7,8].

Only the roots of *Panax ginseng* are used pharmaceutically [2,9]. The main root is a fleshy tap root, branched into smaller rootlets. At the age of 4 to 6 years, when most of the cultivated plants are harvested, their roots usually are about 2 to 3 cm in diameter and about 10 to 20 cm long [2].

Two kinds of "Korean" ginseng roots are found on the world market: red and white ginseng. Both originate from *Panax ginseng*, but they are processed differently for preservation purposes [2,5]. While after harvesting white ginseng is bleached with SO_2 and then dried, red ginseng is treated with hot water vapor prior to drying. By the latter procedure the roots obtain their characteristically red color [2]. Only minor qualitative and quantitative differences concerning the chemical composition of the main active principles of white or red ginseng roots have been recognized so far [2,4,5,10,11]. In the USA, the roots of *Panax quinquefolius* are also sold as red or white ginseng[11]. Part of the yearly American ginseng harvest is exported to Hong Kong [6], from where it is distributed to various Asian countries and even back to the USA [12]. *Eleutherococcus senticosus* is nearly exclusively harvested and manufactured in the USSR [2].

The root of *Panax ginseng* is an official drug in Korea, China, Japan, USSR, Austria, Switzerland, and Germany. In other countries with high ginseng consumption, especially in the USA, ginseng is recognized only as a food supplement ("health food") [13].

Chemistry

Current knowledge sees the main active principles of *Panax ginseng* as triterpenoidal saponins (ginsenosides) which derive from the tetracyclic dammaran sceleton [2,4,5]. In addition, the roots contain ginsenoside Ro, a triglycoside of oleanolic acid which is widely distributed in the plant kingdom. The aglycones of all other ginsenosides are protopanaxadiol and protopanaxatriol. Ginsenosides Ra, Rb_1, Rb_2, Rc, and Rd belong to the former, ginsenosides Re, Rf, Rg_1, Rg_2, and Rh_1 to the latter group. The quantitatively main ginsenosides of the diol and the triol series in *P. ginseng* are Rb_1 and Rg_1, respectively [4,5]. The total ginsenoside content of the roots depends on the age of the plant and on the part of the root under study [14]. On average the ginsenoside content is between 0.7 and 3.0% in a 6-year-old main root of *P. ginseng* [9,15]. About two- to threefold of this amount may be found in the lateral roots and up to tenfold in the slender rootlets [9]. No significant differences could be detected in the major saponins between wild and cultivated ginseng specimens [16]. Roots obtained from different *Panax* species, however, show large variations with regard to content and spectrum of the ginsenosides [4,5,11,17].

Besides the ginsenosides, the roots of *P. ginseng* contain about 0.05% of essential oil [5]. Ether-soluble substances are beta-elemene and several structurally related polyacetylenes with distinct pharmacological activities, such as panaxynol, panaxatriol, panaxydol, and others [5,18–23].

In addition, peptidoglycanes with hypoglycemic activity (panaxanes) [24–27] and a peptide with insulinomimetic properties [28] have been isolated from Korean ginseng. Han and colleagues [29] found several phenolic substances in *P. ginseng*, such as salicylate and vanillic acid, which showed antioxidant and antifatigue effects in animal experiments.

An extraordinarily high amount of germanium in *P. ginseng* roots has been described [30], but this finding has never been proven by others [31,32]. There is one report [33] which suggests the presence of estrone in ginseng roots. However, Obermeier [34] and Youn [32] could not reproduce this result. Moreover, the *P. ginseng* roots studied by Youn [32] also did not contain estriol or estradiol.

Pharmacology and Uses

For more than two thousand years *Panax ginseng* has been used in traditional oriental medicine as a tonic (supplementing) drug for increasing general strength and removing fatigue [35].

In contrast to a common opinion among Western pharmacologists, numerous reports about the biochemical and pharmacological effects of ginseng have appeared in the past twenty years, especially in Oriental and Russian journals, even to the point that *P. ginseng* belongs to the most intensively studied medicinal herbs today (for reviews see [4,36-39]). However, many studies on the pharmacology of the ginseng drug must be regarded with caution because of the following: (a) route of application (mostly i.p.) is often different from the oral route preferred in human practice; (b) treatment with very high doses is common, which in some examples may well reach toxicological levels; (c) pure ginsenosides (e.g., ginsenoside Rb_1 vs. Rg_1) may exhibit antagonistic effects on the model system tested.

Nevertheless, some pharmacological effects of ginseng have been demonstrated repeatedly in animals by different research groups. These actions may be arranged under two headings: (a) the so-called adaptogenic effect [8], which means mainly an unspecific enhancement of the body's resistance to exogenous stressors or noxes [2,36,38], and (b) an improvement of physical and psychophysical performance [1,37,38]. There are also two studies, however, which could not demonstrate an antifatigue effect in animals [11,40].

A nearly identical pharmacological profile (adaptogenic and antifatigue action) has been described for *E. senticosus*, although other compounds than triterpenoidal saponins are responsible for its effects [3].

The pharmacological actions of *Panax ginseng* have been attributed to the ginsenosides by the majority of researchers [4,36,37,41]. It should be mentioned, however, that Han and colleagues [29] and Kim et al. [22] recently presented some evidence that the effects of *P. ginseng* might also be due to nonginsenoside constituents with antioxidant activity.

In the light of recent knowledge about the adverse effects of free radicals upon a wide range of bodily functions [42-44], antioxidant activity might be of crucial importance for understanding the complex and unspecific mode of action of this drug.

Pharmacokinetics

Pharmacokinetic studies have been performed with different animal species by applying purified ginsenosides from *P. ginseng* [45,46,47] and *P. quinquefolius* [48]. After intravenous injection, it was noted that protopanaxadiol glycosides such as Rb_1 showed a longer elimination half-life, a smaller volume of distribution, and a lower total body clearance than protopanaxatriol glycosides such as Rg_1 [45,48]. This corresponded to their different plasma protein binding, which was over 99% for ginsenosides of the diol series [45,48]. After oral administration, ginsenoside Rg_1 was rapidly absorbed and metabolized [47]. The genuine saponin and its metabolites were also rapidly distributed throughout the body [46,47], with the exception of the brain because the blood-brain barrier was not penetrated [47]. Excretion was via urine and faeces [47]. Chemistry, pharmacology and toxicology of the formed metabolites are unknown.

Adverse Reaction Profile

General Animal Data

Toxicological effects of ginseng have been achieved in animal experiments only by using extremely high doses, not relevant for human practice. Thus, in studies on acute toxicity, LD_{50} values of a crude neutral saponin fraction (containing primarily Rb_1, Rb_2, and Rc) from *P. ginseng* were in the range of 500–910 mg/kg body weight when administered i.p. to mice [49–51]. For i.v. application 367 mg/kg and for p.o. application more than 5000 mg/kg has been determined as LD_{50} of this fraction [49]. For a lipophilic fraction from *P. ginseng* the LD_{50} was between 2000 and 3000 mg/kg, and for a polar fraction (with Rg_1, Rg_2, and Rg_3) an LD_{50} between 500 and 1000 mg/kg was found when injected i.p. into mice [50]. The LD_{50} values for purified ginsenosides administered i.p. to mice were in the range of 305 mg/kg (for Rb_2) to 1340 mg/kg (for Rf) [52].

Subchronic feeding of a crude alcoholic ginseng extract to minipigs for seven days at a dose of 2000 mg/kg per day had no effect on body weight, blood status, or other clinical chemical parameters [53]. Peroral administration of an alcoholic ginseng extract (up to 15 mg/kg per day) to beagle dogs for a period of three months did not affect body weight, eating behavior, general behavior, an blood parameters [54]. On macroscopic and histological examination no effects on organs and tissues were noted. Chronic feeding of ginseng powder (up to 0.25% in the food) to rats for a period of six months could not reveal any effect on body and organ weight, organ histology, or blood parameters [55].

General Human Data

Since about ten years an increasing number of papers has appeared in the international literature which claim adverse effects of ginseng or interactions of ginseng with other remedies (for a recent review see [13]). However, most of these publications are review articles [1,56–64] or comments and letters to the editor [65–70]. They refer to a few original case records [71–78], to a clinical pilot study performed in Australia [79], and to two clinical studies conducted by Siegel in the USA [80–82]. Two case reports presume an interaction between ginseng and the MAO inhibitor phenelzine [74,78].

When one analyzes the original reports, it is striking that in almost all cases (a) incomplete data, e.g., about type of ginseng product, dose, or duration of ingestion are provided, and (b) the communications in general come from Great Britain, North America, or Australia [13]. In these countries preparations containing ginseng are not drugs but belong to the so-called "health foods" which are not liable to legal drug control. This may lead to health hazards for the consumers because falsification of drugs (replacement of *Panax ginseng* by other Araliaceae and more or less related plants) or admixture of other potentially toxic plant material (*Rauwolfia, Mandragora* or *Cola* species) as well as of highly potent chemical substances (phenylbutazone, aminopyrine, procaine, nicotinate, etc.) have been found in some of these products [1,56,65–67,83]. Some preparations labeled as ginseng did not even contain any ginsenosides [1,56,65,83–85]. In addition, Barna [68] recently pointed out that for the "health food supplements" of the American market no dose recommendations are required on the labels, and that ad libitum recommendations are common. The reported adverse effects (see below) may thus have resulted from the uncontrolled use of uncontrolled products.

This problem is illustrated by the report on the so-called ginseng abuse syndrome. This term was coined by Siegel in 1979 [80] in a clinical note about an open study conducted over a period of two years with 133 ginseng users in Los Angeles. This publication was later supplemented with further data [82]. Since the side effects of ginseng use reported here are often cited in reviews and textbooks as evidence for the potential hazard of the ginseng drug, this trial is considered briefly here.

After long-term administration of daily doses up to 15 g ginseng (mean: 3 g/day), 22 out of the 133 patients included in the study experienced adverse effects such as hypertension, often combined with nervousness, sleeplessness, skin eruptions, and morning diarrhea. This complex of symptoms was termed ginseng abuse syndrome (GAS) by Siegel. Doses of 15 g ginseng/day or more resulted in feelings of confusion and depersonalization or depression by an unknown number of patients. The GAS appeared periodically throughout the first 12 months of the trial but was rarely seen after 18 and 24 months. Concomitantly, the patients reported that they had reduced their daily dose to an average of about 1.7 g ginseng.

However, the study showed several methodological flaws: all participants of the study were outpatients, no data about the participants were communicated, a wide variety of ginseng products (e.g., roots, capsules, tablets, teas, extracts) was used, intake was not controlled, no data about the composition of the preparations were supplied, andcomedication was not recorded. Except for the examinations of blood pressure, only subjective statements of the participants were recorded.

In a second study Siegel [81] examined the adverse effects of American ginseng products (teas, capsules, extracts, roots, and cosmetic creams) on two groups of volunteers. Group A contained ten drug addicts, group B eight normal ginseng users. Adverse effects were reported only by the users in group A and corresponded to those seen in the earlier publication [80]. The study shows the same methodological deficiencies as the earlier one, especially with respect to the lack of controls of intake and the wide palette of products allowed. This procedure is hard to understand because Siegel himself in 1977 had already stated that the distribution of mislabeled ginseng products was usual in the USA [83]. During a critical discussion of this paper at a Symposium in Korea in 1980, Siegel had to retract some of his conclusions about the health hazards and abuse potential of the ginseng drug [81]. He finally admitted that these adverse drug reactions would not have occurred if standardized ginseng products had been taken and correct doses used.

The nunfortunate inadequacies in the experimental design of Seigel's studies have also been recognized by others [37,56,66,86–88] The so-called GAS seems to be restricted to the USA and should more likely be attributed to the quality of certain "health foods" and the specific consumer behavior there than to an abuse potential of the ginseng drug.

Cardiovascular Reactions

In a report from Australia [73], a 39-year-old man experienced hypertension, dizziness and inability to concentrate after having ingested a variety of different unknown ginseng preparations for about three years. After cessation of intake blood pressure returned to normal within five days, and the other symptoms also settled. In a letter to the *New Scientist* [71] Brunner claimed that he himself had experienced acute hypertension and pressure headaches after having taken an unspecified ginseng product for eight to ten days.

The occurrence of hypertension after *Panax ginseng* ingestion is in contrast to the results of clinical studies on this topic [101,102,103,104], where rather an opposite effect could be detected. The experiences of Japanese clinicians with several hundred patients who had ingested *P. ginseng* (3–5 g/day) over a period of three to five years (see discussion in [81]) also argues against an increasing effect of *P. ginseng* on blood pressure.

Dermatological Reactions

Skin eruptions were experienced by two volunteers of the Australian pilot study on *Panax ginseng* [79]. They took two capsules daily, each with 500 mg of (presumably) Korean ginseng (Gateway Ginseng Capsules). It is not known, whether the capsules contained root powder or a special extract.

Endocrine Reactions

Mastalgia and Rise of Sexual Responsiveness
A 70-year-old English woman developed symptoms of mastalgia after having ingested a Gin Seng powder regularly for 21 days [76]. After cessation of the Gin Seng administration the symptoms settled. In two further trials with the same prescription the same effects appeared again. Koriech [75] reported about a similar ginseng effect on five women aged 25 to 40 years. All of them developed breast symptoms and felt an increase in "sexual responsiveness." In both reports, exact data are missing, so that it cannot be judged properly whether the observed effects have been really due to the administration of *Panax ginseng*.

Estrogenic Effects
In three case reports from Finland [77] and the USA [72,89] an estrogen-like effect of ginseng was observed in three women after menopause.

In the Finnish paper [77], an estrogenic effect was noted in a vaginal smear from a 62-year-old woman who had ingested an unknown amount of unspecified "Rumanian" ginseng tablets for a period of two weeks. Serum concentrations of estrone, estradiol, and estriol were not affected. Vaginal and cervical epithelia looked normal and no atrophic changes were noticed. Analysis of the tablets proved that they did not contain any estrogenic hormone. On the other hand, it was found that a methanolic extract prepared from the tablets strongly competed with 17-estradiol (type not specified) and R5020 binding sites in human myometrium. This finding, however, is in contrast to the results of Pearce and colleagues [90]. Using the same experimental set-up, the latter authors could not show any affinity of methanolic extracts from *Panax ginseng* to estrogen receptors. This discrepancy was explained by Pearce and coworkers by their finding that the separation of free and bound tracer by charcoal was complicated in the presence of ginseng extract. Since a botanical species named "Rumanian ginseng" does not exist, another possibility for explaining the results of the Finnish case report might be that the "Rumanian" ginseng tablets did not contain *Panax ginseng* but *Eleutherococcus senticosus* ("Siberian" ginseng), used as a *P. ginseng* substitute in eastern Europe. For extracts from this plant an affinity for estrogen receptors has been detected [90].

In the first report from the USA [72], a 72-year-old wan experienced vaginal bleeding after having taken one tablet daily of Geriatric Pharmaton, a Swiss ginseng preparation containing an ethanolic extract from *Panax ginseng* and, in addition, several vitamins and minerals. On the other hand, two controlled clinical trials from Switzerland [91,92] could not reveal any influence of the same standardizef ginseng extract on male or female sexual hormone levels (testosterone, LH, FSH, and estradiol) after up to twelve weeks of treatment. Similar negative results were reported by Fulder and colleagues [93]. In the second report [89], a 44-year-old woman repeatedly used a ginseng face cream (Fang Fang), imported from Shanghai, China. She responded with a drop in follicle-stimulating hormone level and abnormal uterine bleeding whenever she applied the cream. An endometrial biopsy specimen showed a disordered proliferative pattern. After stopping the use of the face cream, FSH level returned to normal, and further bleeding episodes were not observed.

Effects of Adrenal Cortex Function
Corticosteroid hormone output was enhanced in animal experiments by higher amounts of purified ginseng saponins [94–99]. In a controlled study with human volunteers [100] it was noted that red ginseng powder given orally at 7.5 g per day for 10 days promoted the ACTH-induced fall of the eosinophil count, suggesting an effect on the pituitary-adrenocortical system. In another controlled study [91], however, no effects on cortisol levels were observed in young volunteers after ingestion of standardized ginseng extracts with either 4% or 7% ginsenosides (equivalent to about 1–2 g of white root powder).

Gastrointestinal Reactions

Adverse reactions of *Panax ginseng* administration on the gastrointestinal system by 2 out of 25 participants were recognized in a New South Wales trial [79]. Since the drug contains high amounts of saponins with detergent character, the observed adverse drug reaction (diarrhea) can readily be imagined. On the other hand, controlled clinical trials with equivalent or even higher ginseng doses did not reveal such an effect [13]. It is well known that unspecific gastrointestinal side effects are one of the most frequently recognized adverse drug reactions in clinical studies, also seen under placebo.

Muscular Reactions

A WHO report from 1988 cited reservations of the Swedish Department of Drugs about a French trial from 1985 which claimed that ginseng might have improved athletic performance (see [105] and literature cited therein). The Swedish authorities expressed their concern about the finding that postexercise blood concentrations of creatine kinase and SGOT were higher in the ginseng group than in the placebo group. This was interpreted in the way that ginseng may perhaps aggravate the transient muscle damage that is known to result from intensive sustained physical exercise. This interpretation of the French data by the Swedish Authorities is in contrast to the results of other clinical studies on athletic performance and thus awaits further confirmation.

Drug Interactions

A case report from the USA [78] presented a 64-year-old woman who had been treated with the MAO inhibitor phenelzine. When she added Californian "health-food" products which contained ginseng (Natrol High, ginseng tea), she developed insomnia, headache, and tremulousness. She had also used ginseng tea before phenelzine without developing any symptoms. Another case of a possible interaction between ginseng and phenelzine was that of a 42-year-old woman who was treated with phenelzine because of major depressive illness [74]. She was also treated with triazolam and lorazepam. Simultaneously, the patient took an unknown ginseng product as well as an unspecified preparation of bee pollen. The patient soon began to show an improvement in her mood. However, since she now suffered from headaches, irritability, and vague visual hallucinations, she discontinued the phenelzine and subsequently began to show a total depressive relapse. Accordingly, she was restarted on phenelzine but now without any therapeutic effect. Interestingly, this time the patient was no longer taking the above-mentioned unconventional remedies. An interaction between the ginsenosides and the antidepressive phenelzine is imaginable but cannot be proven by these cases.

Fertility, Pregnancy, and Lactation

Human data about ginseng effects during pregnancy could not be retrieved from the literature. Studies on this topic have been performed with experimental animals [53,55,106]. No adverse effects of feeding an ethanolic ginseng extract (15 mg/kg/day) to rats on fertility, lactation, or offspring (F1 and F2 progeny) have been noticed [106]. Hong et al. [55] could not detect any adverse effect on fertility and found no teratogenic potential of *P. ginseng* root powder when administered orally to rats (up to 2.5 g/kg diet). Neither the F1 nor the F2 generation was influenced by the ginseng feeding. Similar results were reported by Soldati [53] for oral ginseng administration to rats [40 mg/kg/day) and to rabbits (20 mg/kg/day). Additionally, Chun and colleagues [107] provided evidence that ginseng root powder (200 mg/day in the diet) and crude saponin fraction (20 mg/kg/day i.p.) prevented the toxic effect of chlorambucil on rat fetal skeletogenesis.

Mutagenicity and Carcinogenicity

No mutagenic or carcinogenic potential of *P. ginseng* [53,108] or *P. quinquefolius* [109] could be detected so far. On the other hand, antitumor and desmutagenic effects of *Panax ginseng* in vitro [110–112] and in vivo [113–115] have been reported by various researchers.

References

1. Phillipson JD, Anderson LA (1984) Ginseng – quality, safety and efficacy? Pharm J 232:161–165
2. Steinegger E, Hänsel R (1988) Lehrbuch der Pharmakognosie und Phytopharmazie. 4th ed. Berlin: Springer-Verlag, pp 615–628
3. Farnsworth NR, Kinghorn AD, Soejarto DD, Waller DP (1985) Siberian ginseng (Eleutherococcus senticosus): current status as an adaptogen. In: Wagner H, Hikino H, Farnsworth NR (eds) Economic and medicinal plant research. vol 1. London: Academic Press, pp 155–215
4. Shibata S, Tanaka O, Shoji J, Saito H (1985) Chemistry and pharmacology of Panax. In: Wagner H, Hikino H, Farnsworth NR (eds) Economic and medicinal plant research. vol 1. London: Academic Press, pp 217–284
5. Shoji J (1985) Recent advances in the chemical studies on ginseng. In: Chang HM, Yeung HW, Tso WW, Koo A (eds) Advances in Chinese medicinal materials research. Singapore: World Scientific Publ Co, pp 455–469
6. Dubick MA (1986) Historical perspectives on the use of herbal preparations to promote health. J Nutr 116:1348–1354
7. Brekhman II, Dardymov IV (1969) Pharmacological investigation of glycosides from ginseng and Eleutherococcus. Lloydia 32:46–51
8. Brekham II, Dardymov IV (1969) New substances of plant origin which increase nonspecific resistance. Ann Rev Pharmacol 9:419–430
9. Sollorz G (1985) Qualitätsbeurteilung von Ginsengwurzeln: quantitative HPLC-Bestimmung der Ginsenoside. Dtsch Apoth Ztg 125:2052–2055
10. Kitagawa I, Taniyama T, Shibuya H et al. (1987) Chemical studies on crude drug processing. V. On the constituents of ginseng radix rubra (2): comparison of the constituents of white ginseng and red ginseng prepared from the same Panax ginseng root. Yakugaku Zasshi 107:495–505
11. Martinez B, Staba EJ (1984) The physiological effects of Aralia, Panax and Eleutherococcus on exercised rats. Japan J Pharmacol 35:79–85
12. Lewis WH (1980) Ginseng revisited. JAMA 243:31
13. Sonnenborn U (1989) Ginseng-Nebenwirkungen: Fakten oder Vermutungen? Med Mschr Pharm 12:46–53
14. Kim MW, Ko SR, Choi KJ, Kim SC (1987) Distribution of saponin in various sections of Panax ginseng root and changes of its contents according to root age. Korean J Ginseng Sci 11:10–16
15. Soldati F, Tanaka O (1984) Panax ginseng: relation between age of plant and content of ginsenosides. Planta Med 50:351–352
16. Yamaguchi H, Matsuura H, Kasai R et al. (1988) Analysis of saponins of wild Panax ginseng. Chem Pharm Bull 36:4177–4181
17. Lui JHC, Staba EJ (1980) Ginsenosides of various ginseng plants and selected products. Lloydia 43:340–346
18. Ahn BZ, Kim SI (1988) Beziehungen zwischen Struktur und cytotoxischer Aktivität von Panaxydol-Analogen gegen L1210 Zellen. Arch Pharm (Weinheim) 321:61–63
19. Ahn BZ, Kim SI (1988) Heptadeca-1,8t-dien-4,6-diin-3,10-diol ein weiteres, gegen L1210-Zellen cytotoxisches Wirkprinzip aus der koreanischen Ginsengwurzel. Planta Med 54:183
20. Hansen L, Boll PM (1986) Polyacetylenes in Araliaceae: their chemistry, biosynthesis and biological significance. Phytochemistry 25:285–293
21. Katano M, Yamamoto H, Matsunaga H (1988) A tumor growth inhibitory substance isolated from Panax ginseng. In: Korea Ginseng and Tobacco Research Institute (ed) Proceedings of the 5th International Ginseng Symposium. Seoul/Korea, pp 33–38
22. Kim H, Lee YH, Kim SI, Jin SH (1988) Effect of polyacetylene compounds from Korean ginseng on lipid peroxidation. In: Korea Ginseng and Tobacco Research Institute (ed) Proceedings of the 5th International Ginseng Symposium. Seoul/Korea, pp 81–86
23. Teng CM, Kuo SC, Ko FN et al. (1989) Antiplatelet actions of panaxynol and ginsenosides isolated from ginseng. Biochim Biophys Acta 990:315–320
24. Konno C, Sugiyama K, Kano M et al. (1984) Isolation and hypoglycaemic activity of panaxanes A, B, C, D and E, glycans of Panax ginseng roots. Planta Med 50:434–438

25. Konno C, Murakami M, Oshima Y, Hikino H (1985) Isolation and hypoglycaemic activity of panaxanes Q, R, S, T and U, glycans of Panax ginseng roots. J Ethnopharmacol 14:69–74
26. Oshima Y, Konno C, Hikino H (1985) Isolation and hypoglycaemic activity of panaxanes I, J, K and L, glycans of Panax ginseng roots. J Ethnopharmacol 14:255–259
27. Tomoda M, Shimada K, Konno C, Hikino H (1984) Structure of panaxan B, a hypoglycaemic glycan of Panax ginseng roots. Phytochemistry 24:2431–2433
28. Ando T, Muraoka T, Yamasaki N, Okuda H (1980) Preparation of antilipolytic substance from Panax ginseng. Planta Med 38:18–23
29. Han BH, Han YN, Park MH (1985) Chemical and biochemical studies on antioxidant components of ginseng. In: Chang HM, Yeung HW, Tso WW, Koo A (eds) Advances in Chinese medicinal materials research. Singapore: World Scientific Publ Co, pp 485–498
30. Asai K (1972) Reports of the Germanium Research Institute, p 1
31. Bernstein M (in preparation) PhD Thesis. Berlin, FRG: Freie Universität Berlin
32. Youn YS (1987) Analytisch vergleichende Untersuchungen von Ginsengwurzeln verschiedener Provenienzen. Berlin, FRG: Freie Universität Berlin, PhD Thesis
33. Anguelakova M, Rovesti P, Colombo C (1971) Communication presenté en III. Congrès International de Dermo-pharmacie. San Remo March 4–7, 1971
34. Obermeier A (1980) Zur Analytik der Ginseng- und Eleutherococcus-droge. Munich, FRG: Ludwig-Maximilians-Universität München, PhD Thesis
35. Hong MW (1978) A history of ginseng. In: Bae HW (ed) Korean ginseng, 2nd ed. Seoul, pp 11–41
36. Fulder SJ (1981) Ginseng and the hypothalamic-pituitary control of stress. Am J Chin Med 9:112–118
37. Owen RT (1981) Ginseng: a pharmacological profile. Drugs of today 17:343–351
38. Sonnenborn U (1987) Ginseng — neuere Untersuchungen immunologischer, pharmakologischer und endokrinologischer Aktivitäten einer alten Arzneipflanze. Dtsch Apoth Ztg 127:433–441
39. Yang ZW (1986) Rhenshen. In: Chang HM, But PPH (eds) Phamacology and applications of Chinese materia medica. Vol 1. Singapore: World Scientific Publishing Co, pp 17–31
40. Lewis WH, Zenger VE, Lynch RG (1983) No adaptogen response of mice to ginseng and Eleutherococcus infusions. J Ethnopharmacol 8:209–214
41. Saito H (1985) Neuropharmacological studies on Panax ginseng. In: Chang HM, Yeung HW, Tso WW, Koo A (eds) Advances in Chinese medicinal materials research. Singapore: World Scientific Publ Co, pp 509–518
42. Armstrong D, Sohal RS, Cutler RG, Slater T (eds) (1984) Free radicals in molecular biology, aging and disease. Aging series. Vol 27. New York: Raven Press
43. Sies H (ed) (1985) Oxidative stress. London: Academic Press
44. Slater TF (1984) Free-radical mechanisms in tissue injury. Biochem J 222:1–15
45. Jenny E, Soldati F (1985) Pharmacokinetics of ginsenosides in the mini pig. In: Chang HM, Yeung HW, Tso WW, Koo A (eds) Advances in Chinese medicinal materials research, Singapore: World Scientific Publ Co, pp 499–506
46. Takino Y, Odani T, Tanizawa H, Hayashi T (1982) Studies on the absorption, distribution, excretion and metabolism of ginseng saponins. I. Quantitative analysis of ginsenoside Rg_1 in rats. Chem Pharm Bull 30:2196–2201
47. Strömbom J, Sandberg F, Dencker L (1985) Studies on absorption and distribution of ginsenoside Rg_1 by whole-body autoradiography and chromatography. Acta Pharm Suecia 22:113–122
48. Chen SE, Sawchuk RJ, Staba EJ (1980) American ginseng. III. Pharmacokinet of ginsenosides in the rabbit. Eur J Drug Metab Pharmacokinetics 5:161–168
49. Nabata H, Saito H, Takagi K (1973) Pharmacological studies of neutral saponins (GNS) of Panax ginseng root. Japan J Pharmacol 23:29–41
50. Takagi K, Saito H, Nabata H (1972) Pharmacological studies on Panax ginseng root: estimation of pharmacological actions of Panax ginseng root. Japan J Pharmacol 22:245–259
51. Takagi K, Saito H, Tsuchiya M (1972) Pharmacological studies on Panax ginseng root: pharmacological properties of a crude saponin fraction. Japan J Pharmacol 22:339–346
52. Kaku T, Miyata T, Uruno T et al. (1975) Chemico-pharmacological studies on saponins of Panax ginseng CA Meyer. II. Pharmacological part. Arzneim Forsch 25:539–547

53. Soldati F (1984) Toxicological studies on ginseng. In: Korea Giseng and Tobacco Research Institute (ed) Proceedings of the 4th International Ginseng Symposium. Daejeon, pp 119–126
54. Hess FG Jr, Parent RA, Stevens KR et al. (1983) Effects of subchronic feeding of ginseng extract G115 in beagle dogs. Food Chem Toxicol 21:95–97
55. Hong SK, Lee SJ, Kim YS et al. (1984) Studies on the safety of Korean ginseng ingested as food substance. In: Korea Ginseng and Tobacco Research Institute (ed) Proceedings of the 4th International Ginseng Symposium. Daejeon, pp 199–213
56. Baldwin CA, Anderson LA, Phillipson JD (1986) What pharmacists should know about ginseng. Pharm J 236:583–586
57. Chen KJ (1981) The effect and abuse syndrome of ginseng. J Tradit Chin Med 1:69–72
58. Lisowski F (1983) Herbal and unconventional remedies in the elderly. Can Pharm J 116: 135–137
59. Meere J (1983) Nevenwerkingen van medicinale planten. Farm Tijdschr Belg 60(1):5–10
60. Messerli FH, Fröhlich ED (1979) High blood pressure – a side effect of drugs, poisons and food. Arch Intern Med 139:682–687
61. Penn RG (1983) Adverse reactions to herbal medicines. Adverse Drug React Bull 102:376–379
62. Röder E (1982) Nebenwirkungen von Heilpflanzen. Dtsch Apoth Ztg 122:2081–2092
63. Vaille C (1982) Le ginseng. Concours Med 104:2267–2270
64. Whitworth JA (1982) Drug-induced hypertension. Curr Ther 23(7):55–61
65. Anonymous (1979) "High tea". Med J Aust 2:232
66. Anonymous (1980) Ginseng. Med Lett Drugs Ther 22:72
67. Anonymous (1986) Herbal medicines – safe and effective? Drug Ther Bull 24:97–100
68. Barna P (1985) Food or drug? – The case of ginseng. Lancet 2:548
69. Dixon P (1985) Ginseng on trial. Here's health (Dec):99
70. Dukes MNG (1978) Ginseng and mastalgia. Brit Med J 1:1621
71. Brunner J (1983) Nasty medicine. New Scientist 97:44
72. Greenspan EM (1983) Ginseng and vaginal bleeding. JAMA 249:2018
73. Hammond TG, Whitworth JA (1981) Adverse reactions to ginseng. Med J Aust 1:492
74. Jones BD, Runikis AM (1987) Interaction of ginseng with phenelzine. J Clin Psychopharmacol 7:201–202
75. Koriech OM (1978) Ginseng and mastalgia. Brit Med J 1:1556
76. Palmer BV, Montgomery ACV, Monteiro JCMP (1978) Ginseng and mastalgia. Brit Med J 1:1284
77. Punnonen R, Lukola A (1980) Oestrogen-like effect of ginseng. Brit Med J 281:1110
78. Shader RI, Greenblatt DJ (1985) Phenelzine and the dream machine – ramblings and reflections. J Clin Psychopharmacol 5:65
79. Cartwright L (1982) You and ginseng: recent human trials. Aust J Pharm 63:44–47
80. Siegel RK (1979) Ginseng abuse syndrome – problems with the panacea. JAMA 241:1614–1615
81. Siegel RK (1980) Ginseng use among two groups in the United States. In: Korea Ginseng and Tobacco Research Institute (ed) Proceedings of the 3rd International Ginseng Symposium. Seoul, pp 229–236
82. Siegel RK (1980) Ginseng and high blood pressure. JAMA 243:32
83. Siegel RK (1977) Kola, ginseng and mislabeled herbs. JAMA 237:24–25
84. Liberti LE, Der Marderosian A (1978) Evaluation of commercial ginseng products. J Pharm Sci 67:1487–1489
85. Ziglar W (1979) An analysis of 54 ginseng products. Whole Foods 2:48–53
86. Brieskorn CH (1979) Streit um Ginseng-Nebenwirkungen – eine schlechte Arbeit. Münch Med Wschr 121:991–992
87. Broese R, Connert J (1979) Streit um Ginseng-Nebenwirkungen. Münch Med Wschr 121:991
88. McIntyre M (1984) Exposed: the inaccurate reporting behind the herbal medicine 'scare'. J Alternat Med (Jan):2–3
89. Hopkins MP, Androff L, Benninghoff AS (1988) Ginseng face cream and unexplained vaginal bleeding. Am J Obstet Gynecol 159:1121–1122
90. Pearce PT, Zois I, Wynne KN, Funder JW (1982) Panax ginseng and Eleutherococcus senticosus extracts – in vitro studies on binding to steroid receptors. Endocrinol Japon 29:567–573

91. Forgo I (1983) Wirkung von Pharmaka auf körperliche Leistung und Hormonsystem von Sportlern. Münch Med Wschr 125:822–824

92. Forgo I, Kayasseh L, Staub JJ (1981) Einfluß eines standardisierten Ginseng-Extraktes auf das Allgemeinbefinden, die Reaktionsfähhigkeit, Lungenfunktion und die gonadalen Hormone. Med Welt 32:751–756

93. Fulder S, Hallstrom C, Carruthers M (1980) The effect of ginseng on the performance of nurses on night-duty. In: Ginseng and Tobacco Research Institute (ed) Proceedings of the 3rd International Ginseng Symposium. Seoul, pp 81–85

94. Cheng XJ, Liu YL, Lin GF, Luo XT (1986) Effects of ginseng root saponins on central transmitters and plasma corticosterone in warm stress-rats. Acta Pharmacol Sin 7:6–8

95. Cheng XJ, Liu YL, Deng YS et al. (1987) Effects of ginseng root saponins on central transmitters and plasma corticosterone in cold stress mice and rats. Acta Pharmacol Sin 8:486–489

96. Filaretov AA, Bogdanova TS, Mityushov MI et al. (1986) Effect of adaptogens on activity of the pituitary-adrenocortical system in rats. Bull Exp Biol Med 101:627–629

97. Hiai S, Yokoyama H, Oura H, Yano S (1979) Stimulation of pituitary-adrenocortical system by ginseng saponin. Endocrinol Japon 26:661–665

98. Hiai S, Yokoyama H, Oura H (1979) Features of ginseng saponin-induced corticosterone secretion. Endocrinol Japon 26:737–740

99. Lu G, Yuan WX, Cheng XJ (1988) Effects of ginseng root saponins on serum corticosterone and brain neurotransmitters of mice under hypobaric and hypoxic environment. Acta Pharmacol Sin 9:489–492

100. Chang YS, Noh HI, Kim SI (1981) Effect of ginseng on the adrenal cortex function. J Korean Med Assoc 24:327–331

101. Imamura Y, Kuwashima K (1988) The effects of red ginseng on blood pressure and the quality of life in essential hypertension. In: Korea Ginseng and Tobacco Research Institute (ed) Proceedings of the 5th International Ginseng Symposium. Seoul, pp 87–91

102. Kaneko H, Nakanishi K, Murakami A, Kuwashima K (1984) Effect of red ginseng on hemodynamic changes by physical exercise. In: Korea Ginseng and Tobacco Research Institute (ed) Proceedings of the 4th International Ginseng Symposium. Daejeon, pp 251–256

103. Kuwashima K, Kaneko H, Nakanishi K (1980) Studies on clinical effects of ginseng: 2nd report. Effects of ginseng at acute massive dosage on circulatory function – a study by digital pletysmography. In: Korea Ginseng and Tobacco Research Institute (ed) Proceedings of the 3rd International Ginseng Symposium. Seoul, pp 193–196

104. Sohn SE, Huh BY, Park SC et al. (1980) The effect of ginseng on blood pressure in spontaneously hypertensive rat and essential hypertension. In: Korea Ginseng and Tobacco Research Institute, ed. Proceedings of the 3rd International Ginseng Symposium. Seoul, pp 1–3

105. Anonymous (1988) Ginseng implicated in muscle damage? WHO Drug Information 2:184

106. Hess FG Jr, Parent RA, Cox GE et al. (1982) Reproduction study in rats of ginseng extract G115. Food Chem Toxicol 20:189–192

107. Chun YH, Kim KR, Rha BY (1982) Effect of Korean ginseng on teratogenicity of chlorambucil on developing fetal skeletogenesis in rats. Korean Univ Med J 19:455–463

108. Lee IP, Yun HC, Stammer N, Langenbach R (1984) Safety evaluation of Panax ginseng extracts: a lack of mutagenicity in the Salmonella typhimurium test and Chinese hamster V79 cells. In: Korea Ginseng and Tobacco Research Institute (ed) Proceedings of the 4th International Ginseng Symposium. Daejeon, pp 75–82

109. Chang YS, Pezzuto JM, Fong HHS, Farnsworth NR (1986) Evaluation of the mutagenic potential of American ginseng (Panax quinquefolius). Planta Med 52:338–339

110. Abe H, Arichi S, Hayashi T, Odashima S (1979) Ultrastructural studies of Morris hepatoma cells reversely transformed by ginsenosides. Experientia 35:1647–1649

111. Odashima S, Nakayabu Y, Honjo N et al. (1979) Induction of phenotypic reverse transformation by ginsenosides in cultured Morris hepatoma cells. Eur J Cancer 15:885–892

112. Odashima S, Ohta T, Kohno H et al. (1985) Control of phenotypic expression of cultured B16 melanoma cells by plant gycosides. Cancer Res 45:2781–2784

113. Han MD, Kim JP (1983) An experimental study on the effect of ginseng extract on the development of stomach cancer in Wistar rats induced by N-methyl-N'-nitro-N-nitrosoguanidine. J Korean Med Assoc 26:1126–1140

192   U. Sonnenborn and R. Hänsel: Panax ginseng

114. Kim JP, Park JG, Lee MD et al. (1985) Co-carcinogenic effects of several Korean foods on gastric cancer induced by N-methyl-N'-nitro-N-nitrosoguanidine in rats. Japan J Surg 15:427–437
115. Yun TK, Yun YS, Han IW (1980) An experimental study on tumor inhibitory effect of red ginseng in mice and rats exposed to various chemical carcinogens. In: Korea Ginseng and Tobacco Institute (ed) Proceedings of the 3rd International Ginseng Symposium. Seoul, 87–113

Pyrrolizidine Alkaloids – General Discussion

J. Westendorf

Botany

The chemical class of pyrrolizidine alkaloids (PAs) contains about 200 structurally related compounds present in more than 350 plant species of the plant families: Apocynaceae, Asteraceae (Compositae), Boraginaceae, Celestraceae, Euphorbiaceae, Fabaceae (Leguminosae) Gramineae, Orchidaceae, Ranunculaceae, Rhicophoraceae, Santalaceae, Sapotaceae, and Scrophulariaceae. Among these are a variety of plants used for medicinal purposes, such as asteraceous plants (*Tussilago farfara, Petasites* spp., *Senecio* spp., *Alkanna tinctoria, Eupatorium* spp.), boraginaceous plants (*Symphytum* spp., *Heliotropium* spp., *Cynoglossum officinale, Echium plantagineum*) and fabaceous plants (*Crotalaria* spp.) [1].

Chemistry

The structure of PAs is based on two inclined five-membered rings with a nitrogen in position 4, a hydroxymethyl group in position 9, and a hydroxy group in position 7. This structure is called the 'necine base'. A variant of this structure is the 'otonecine base', which contains additionally a carbonyl function in position 8 and a methyl group in position 4. PAs with saturated necine bases are nontoxic, whereas all toxic PAs contain a double bond between the 1 and 2 position. According to McLean [2] the following conditions are essential for toxic PAs: (a) a double bond between position 1 and 2; (b) an esterification of the hydroxy groups in position 9 and 7; and (c) a branched carbon chain in at least one of the ester side chains. PAs can readily be oxidized to PA-N-oxides, which can be formed during storage of PA-containing plants or drugs but are also present in natural plant material. The N-oxides are much more water soluble than the parent PAs and are therefore better extracted from plant material during preparation of herbal teas.

The PA content of plant and drug material can be analyzed by methanol extraction and chromatographic separation. Suitable methods are TLC, HPLC, or GC. The most sensitive method is capillary GC/MS [3]. Because PAs are often the toxic but not the biologically active principles of many herbal medicines, methods for the elimination of PAs from the crude plant extracts have been developed. Such an elimination is possible by treatment of alcoholic extracts of the medicinal plants with cation exchange resins in the protonated form [4].

As indicated above, two fundamental groups of PAs exist. To the first group belong PAs with a saturated necine base, which are nontoxic. Medicinal plants which contain only such saturated PAs are *Arnica montana* and *Echinacea* spp. A plant which contains mainly saturated PAs is *Senecio nemorensis fuchsii*. The second group of PAs are those with an unsaturated necine base. Most of these compounds are hepatotoxic and genotoxic, and some are also pneumotoxic. A brief overview of the most important plants containing such toxic PAs is given in Table 1. Additional PA plants are comprehensively reviewed in [1,5–7].

Table 1. Some plants containing toxic pyrrolizidine alkaloids

Official name (Vernacular name)	Comments	Ref.
Alkanna tinctoria (Alkanet)		
Anchusa officinalis (Bugloss)		
Borago officinalis (Borage)		
Crotalaria spp.	Human toxicity well documented.	[8–15]
Cynoglossum spp. (e.g., Hound's tongue)	See the specific contribution.	
Echium spp. (e.g. Viper's grass)		
Erechtites hieracifolia (Pilewort)		
Eupatorium cannabinum (Hemp agrimony)		
Heliotropium spp. (e.g., Common heliotrope)	Human toxicity well documented.	[16–25]
Lithospermum officinale (Gromwell)		
Petasites spp. (e.g., Butterbur)	See the specific contribution.	
Pulmonaria spp. (e.g., Lungwort)		
Senecio spp. (e.g., Groundsel, ragwort)	See the specific contribution.	
Symphytum spp. (e.g., Comfrey)	See the specific contribution.	
Tussilago farfara (Coltsfoot)	See the specific contribution.	

Pharmacology and Uses

Although many medicinal plants contain PAs, it is unknown whether these compounds are responsible for the pharmacological actions of these plants. As the pharmacological actions of certain PA-containing plants are due to one or more non-PA constituents, details on pharmacology and uses are only given in contributions on individual PA-containing plants.

Pharmacokinetics

The pharmacokinetic properties of PAs have not been investigated systematically, but data about single compounds which might have a representative character are available. After oral administration of tritiated PAs (senecionine and seneciphylline) to lactating rats, the PAs were rapidly absorbed. Maximum blood levels were reached in less than one hour [26]. Radioactivity was excreted into the milk with concentrations 50% less compared to the blood concentrations. After six hours 83% of the radioactive necine bases remaining in the blood was not dialyzable, which indicates a tight (possibly covalent) binding to macromolecules, such as albumin. Six hours after administration of the PAs the highest concentrations were detected in the liver and lungs of the rats. This finding is in agreement with the organ-specific toxicity of these compounds.

A study performed with lactating mice, using the same PAs but ^{14}C-labeled and injected via i.p. route, showed that 66–75% of the radioactivity was excreted in the urine, 14–18% in feces, 0.04% in the milk of the animals, and 0.2–0.5% was expired as CO_2. The highest concentrations of radioactivity were found in the liver, and a covalent binding to macromolecules could be demonstrated [27]. The PAs of *Symphytum officinale* have been administered orally and dermally to rats [28]. A renal excretion was observed in both experiments. The amounts excreted were 3.4–9.4% after oral administration and only 0.08–0.41% after dermal application. N-Oxides given orally were reduced, whereas a reduction was not observed after dermal administration. This suggests that the reduction was due to the intestinal flora. A small reduction of indicine N-oxide given i.v. to humans was observed [29], but this may also have been the result of an interaction with the intestinal flora after biliary or direct excretion of the compound into the intestinal lumen and reabsorption of indicine.

The metabolism of PAs is well documented in the literature [30–32]. PAs which have been absorbed from the intestine reach the liver via the portal vein, where they are metabolized. Esterases are able to cleave the linkage between the necine base and the necic acids. PA diesters are thus transformed to monoesters and, finally, to the free necine bases. The rate of the hydrolytic cleavage process decreases with the complexity of the acid moieties and is slowest with macrocyclic diesters. These reactions occur with saturated and unsaturated PAs and are not part of the toxification reactions. On the contrary, they lead to a detoxification of toxic (unsaturated) PAs. Liver enzymes are also able to transform PAs to

N-oxides, which are less toxic because of the more rapid excretion due their hydrophilicity.

Of great relevance for the toxicological properties of PAs are oxidative reactions catalyzed by mixed-functional oxidases and cytochromes, leading to pyrrole-like intermediates. These are the ultimate toxic metabolites of the PAs. The pyrrole derivatives are strong electrophiles which after elimination of necic acid moieties are able to react with nucleophilic compounds in their environment. Covalent linkages to proteins, RNA, and DNA are a result of this reactivity. As the pyrrole intermediates are highly reactive, the majority is trapped shortly after its formation in the liver. This mechanism is the reason for the hepatotoxicity of the PAs. According to Mattocks [30], a correlation exists between the ability of PAs to bind to macromolecules of the liver and the hepatotoxicity of these compounds. Most effective in this way are macrocyclic PA diesters, such as senecionine or seneciphylline, which have been shown directly (using radiolabeled compounds) to bind covalently to liver constituents [27].

Adverse Reaction Profile

General Human Data

There is no doubt that pyrrolizidine alkaloids are toxic to man, and many cases have been reported in which single persons as well as hundreds or even thousands of people have been intoxicated by the intake of PAs in the form of herbal remedies or foods (for example the seeds of *Crotalaria* species as a contaminant of grain food) [8–25]. In almost all cases of severe or fatal intoxications, the patients developed liver damage with cirrhosis and ascites. This type of liver damage is called 'seneciosis' or veno-occlusive disease (VOD) and is a key syndrome of intoxication with PAs. The estimated daily intakes of certain PAs leading to fatal intoxications range from 0.5 mg/kg [20,21] to 3.3 mg/kg [22,23].

Central Nervous System Reactions

Poisoning with *Trichodesma incanum*, which occurred in the Samarkand region of Usbekistan, USSR, in 1942–1951 produced a clinical syndrome called 'Ozhalanger encephalitis' [33,34]. The seeds of the plant, which contaminated food grain, contained 1.5–3.1% PAs, mainly trichodesmine and incanine [35]. Over 200 patients were affected who, after a latent period of about 10 days after the exposure, developed headaches, nausea, and vomiting, followed by delirium and loss of consciousness. A total of 44 persons died, mostly due to respiratory depression. At autopsy, relatively nonspecific lesions were detected in several organs, including the central nervous system. This is the only case reported in which PAs led to nervous dysfunction.

Hepatic Reactions

The toxic action of PAs is mainly directed to the liver. Intoxications with PA-containing plants or plant extracts have been reported in numerous cases of humans and animals. In Switzerland, cases of liver cirrhosis in cows could be correlated with the intake of *Senecio alpinus* [36]. In Australia, endemic liver damage of sheep was due to *Heliotropium europaeum*. This plant contains the toxic PAs heliotrine and lasiocarpine [37].

Numerous human cases of VOD, due to pyrrolizidine alkaloids, have also been reported in the literature. In Afghanistan, the contamination of food with the seeds of *Heliotropium* spp. led to endemic cases of liver failure, many of which were fatal [19]. Liver damage in Bantu Negroes of South Africa has been correlated with the use of *Senecio* spp. [38]. Cases of severe liver damage correlated with the use of PA-containing plants for medicinal purposes have also been observed in Central America. The use of so-called 'bush teas' prepared from *Senecio* and *Crotalaria* spp is very popular in Jamaica. These preparations are used for almost every purpose and are often given to little children. This has been the reason for many cases of liver damage in children, which could definitely be correlated with the uptake of toxic PAs present in these remedies [39].

In Europe, a case of VOD in a newborn infant was recently observed which was associated with the maternal use throughout pregnancy of a herbal cough tea containing *Tussilago farfara* [40]. Although it was later reported that the tea also contained the roots of *Petasites hybridus* [41], there seems little doubt that PAs were responsible for the clinical symptoms of liver damage.

Stuart and Bras [42], who have summarized the symptoms of liver damage due to PA-poisoning, differentiate three clinical stages:

Acute Veno-occlusive Syndrome

Typical for this phase is severe abdominal pain accompanied by emesis, vomiting, and diarrhea. The liver is enlarged, and ascites is often present. Generalized edema and sometimes jaundice are observed. In some cases, the disease progresses dramatically, and the patient dies a few weeks after occurrence of the first symptoms. If the patient survives this phase, complete remission may be possible. The disease can also progress, however, to a subacute or chronic phase.

Subacute Veno-occlusive Syndrome

This stage is characterized by an enlargement of the liver and sometimes of the spleen as well. Other clinical symptoms are often absent. The liver function may be normal, but mild to severe ascites is sometimes present. A progressive fibrotic degeneration of the liver is also typical and the disease often passes to a chronic stage.

Chronic Veno-occlusive Syndrome

The key syndrome of this stage is a cirrhosis of the liver, which is different from other forms of liver cirrhosis because portal regions are not involved. A progressive liver failure, detectable by the decrease of serum albumine and affinity of serum cholinesterase occurs, and the general condition of the patient deteriorates more and more. Due to the decrease of serum protein levels, edemas occur, and the patient may develop anorexia. The mortality rate is usually much higher than that in other forms of cirrhotic liver diseases.

Identical symptoms have been observed in animals, such as cattle and sheep consuming PA-containing plants, and they have also been reproduced by feeding PAs to laboratory animals [43]. There can therefore be no doubt that a causal relationship between the ingestion of toxic PAs and the development of the liver damage outlined here exists.

Pulmonary Reactions

Besides liver failure, some cases of pulmonary involvement have been reported [15,44–46]. In one of these cases, a 19-year-old African died from congestive heart failure after the consumption of a herbal tea containing the seeds of *Crotalaria laburnoides*. Vascular changes of severe primary pulmonary hypertension were observed histologically. The same symptoms of pulmonary hypertension with hypertensive vascular changes of the lung together with a right ventricular hypertrophy of the heart could be demonstrated in rats fed with powdered seeds of the plant in their diet. However, no special PA could be made responsible for this effect [44].

Experimental toxicity studies with certain PAs in rats have shown that the alkaloids fulvine and monocrotaline can affect the lungs besides the liver [14,47,48]. Because lung tissue is not able to transform the compounds into the pyrrole-intermediates [49,50], the toxic metabolites apparently originate in the liver and may then be transported with the blood stream to the lung, to allylate lung tissue.

Fertility, Pregnancy, and Lactation

Reports in the literature about teratogenic effects of PAs are limited. A study with heliotrine injected at doses between 15–300 mg/kg body weight to pregnant rats in the second week of gestation produced abnormalities in the litters only at doses which affected the dams as well [51]. Similar results were obtained in another study with heliotrine and its toxic metabolite dehydroheliotridine [52]. The pyrrole metabolite was five times as effective as the corresponding PA. Teratogenic effects of heliotrine have also been demonstrated in *Drosophila* larvae fed with low doses of the PA [53].

Although there is no doubt that many PAs are able to cross the placenta [54], there are conflicting data about their toxicity towards embryonic tissues. On the one hand, fetal livers seem to be more resistant to toxic PAs than maternal ones [51,53]. On the other hand, however, it has been shown that lasiocarpine given at doses of 35 mg/kg to pregnant rats on days 13 and 17 of pregnancy was harmful for the fetal livers without affecting the mother [55]. It has also been demonstrated in vitro that human fetal liver tissue is capable of metabolizing PAs to toxic pyrroles [56].

A case of VOD in a newborn infant of a mother consuming during pregnancy a herbal cough tea containing 0.6 mg/kg senecionine is discussed in the contribution about *Tussilago farfara*, elsewhere in this book. Although this is the only case reported so far, the use of herbal remedies containing PAs during pregnancy can no longer be claimed to be safe, even when only trace levels of hepatotoxic PAs are present.

It has been shown that PAs given orally to lactating rats and mice are excreted into the milk [26,27]. Schoental reported that after administration of the PAs lasiocarpine and retrorsine to lactating rats the livers of the suckling offspring were severely damaged without affecting the mother [57]. The young animals were most sensitive between 3−7 weeks of age. According to Mattocks and White [58] the susceptibility of rat livers to the PA retrorsine increases rapidly after birth. They demonstrated that the susceptibility of rats at various ages was proportional to their capacity to form and retain pyrolle metabolites. The fact that young rats were more sensitive than adult animals may indicate that young children may be at higher risk when treated with PA-containing remedies. In view of all these data, a risk must be considered for suckling infants when humans take PA-containing drugs during lactation.

Mutagenicity and Carcinogenicity

As outlined in the section on pharmacokinetics, PAs are metabolically converted in the liver to pyrrole derivatives, which are reactive electrophiles and are therefore able to react with DNA. The formation of covalent DNA adducts has been demonstrated definitely.

The so-called covalent binding index to DNA (CBI) for senecionine and seneciphylline is stronger than the corresponding value for benzo(a)pyrene, of equal value as that for the hepatocarcinogen acetylaminofluorene but considerably lower than that of aflatoxins [27]. Several authors have demonstrated that PA metabolites act as bifunctional alkylating agents to perform DNA interstrand cross-links [59–62].

A variety of PAs has been demonstrated to be mutagenic in *Salmonella typhimurium* (Ames assay). Among these were the compounds clivorine, petasitenine, heliotrine, lasiocarpine, ligularidine, and senkirkine [63]. However, the PAs lycopsamine, monocrotaline, retronecine, senecionine, and seneciphylline were negative in this assay, even though some of these compounds were demonstrated to be carcinogenic in rodents. This suggests that this assay is not very sensitive for the detection of the genotoxicity of PAs.

In V79 Chinese hamster fibroblasts in culture, the PAs heliotrine, lasiocarpine, petasitenine, and senkirkine induced chromosomal aberrations and mutations on the HGPRT gen locus [64]. The effect was increased after addition of rat liver microsomes. In the same cells, the induction of sister chromatid exchange has been observed. An addition of an exogenous metabolizing system (chicken embryonic liver cells) was essential for the effectiveness of the PAs [65]. Chromosomal aberrations have also been demonstrated for heliotrine in lymphocytes of *Potorous tridactylus* [66] and man [67]. Senkirkine did not induce chromosomal aberrations in human lymphocytes. However, this is possibly due to a lack of metabolic activation by the cells.

In primary rat hepatocytes, which possess an optimal metabolizing system, a variety of PAs was demonstrated to induce DNA repair, which indicates a DNA damaging effect of the compounds [68]. The following PAs were positive in this assay: monocrotaline, senecionine, seneciphylline, epoxyseneciphylline, jacobine, senecicannabine, senkirkine, petasitenine, acetylpetasitenine, syneilesine, clivorine, dihydroclivorine, neoligularidine, ligularidine, and ligularizine. The compounds retronecine and ligularinine were negative in this assay. This finding is in agreement with the hypothesis about the toxicity of PAs. Ligularinine is a saturated PA and is therefore unable to form pyrrole intermediates. Retronecine is unsaturated, but it is missing the activating necic acid moieties. Rat hepatocytes were most sensitive, but DNA repair induction could also be induced by the PAs in liver cells of mice and hamsters.

The toxic PAs retrorsine and monocrotaline as well as the pyrrole intermediate dehydroretronecine have been demonstrated to induce malignant transformation in BHK21/C13 cells in vitro. Rosmarinine, a saturated PA, was negative in this assay [69].

Mutagenic effects of PAs have also been demonstrated in vivo using *Drosophila melanogaster* [70–75]. The investigations showed chromosomal damage such as point mutations, translocations, and chromosomal breakage for a variety of PAs (heliotrine, lasiocarpine, monocrotaline, senecionine, jacobine, fulvine, retrorsine, and isatidine). The existence of a 1,2-unsaturated necine moiety was also essential in this model. The nature of the esterification influenced the effectivity of the mutagenic action, which is in accordance with the hypothesis about the mechanism of action of the PAs [6].

A number of PAs have been investigated for their carcinogenic action in rodents. A summary of the results obtained by different working groups is given in the IARC monographs [76]. Table 2 summarizes the most important experiments. Sufficient evidence of carcinogenicity in rats exists for the PAs heliotrine, monocrotaline, lasiocarpine, senkirkine, clivorine, retrorsine, symphytine, and petasitenine. Tumors were observed mainly in the liver.

Allen et al. [82] injected 20 mg/kg dehydroretronecine, a pyrrole-like metabolite of monocrotaline, s.c. into 75 rats every second week for a total of 4 months, followed by 10 mg/kg for another 8 months. A second group of 75 rats received s.c. doses of 5 mg/kg monocrotaline every second week for a period of 12 months. Fifteen rats were partially hepatectomized 4 months after the start of the experiment for an investigation of the antimitotic activity of the PAs on the liver. All animals were killed after 22 months. 31/60 rats treated with dehydroretro-

Compound	Number of rats	Route of administration	Duration of experiment (days)	Number and type of tumors	Ref.
Senkirkine	20	22mg/kg i.p., 2x/week for 4 weeks, then 1x/week for 52 weeks	650	9 liver cell adenomas	77
Symphytine	20	13mg/kg i.p., 2x/week for 4 weeks, then 1x/week for 52 weeks	650	3 hemangioendothelial sarcomas 1 liver adenoma	77
Retrorsine	14	drinking water (0.03mg/ml), 3x/week	730	4 hepatomas 1 liver adenoma	78
Isatidine	22	drinking water (0.05/0.03mg/ml), 3x/week	600	10 hepatomas 5 hyperplastic nodules of the liver	78
Lasiocarpine	25	7.8 mg/kg, i.p., 2x/week for 4 weeks, then 1x/week for 52 weeks	532	10 hepatocarcinomas 6 skin carcinomas 5 pulmonary adenomas 2 adenocarcinomas of small intestine 1 cholangiocarcinoma 1 adenoma of the ileum	79
Monocrotaline	50	25 mg/kg, p.o., 1x/week for 4 weeks. then 8mg/kg for 52 weeks	504	10 hepatocarcinomas with lung metastases	80
	50	as above with a diet deficient in lipotrope	504	14 hepatocarcinomas with lung metastases	
Petasitenine	11	drinking water (0.01%)	480	5 hemangiosarcomas 5 hepatocellular adenomas	81

necine developed rhabdomyosarcomas at the site of application, and 5 of these animals had metastases. Only 2 rats treated with monocrotaline developed this kind of tumor, but additionally 2 hepatocellular carcinomas, 2 acute myeloic leukemias, and 1 pulmonary adenoma were observed. The mitotic indices of the liver were reduced in the monocrotaline as well as the dehydroretronecine-treated rats. Megalohepatocytoses were only observed in monocrotaline treated animals.

The experiment provided further evidence that the pyrrole metabolites of the PAs are the ultimate carcinogens. The high reactivity of these compounds is evident from the fact that the injection of dehydroretronecine caused tumors at the site of application.

Although the exposure of humans to toxic PAs has occurred many times in the past, no epidemiological studies are available which document a possible carcinogenic risk from these compounds. However, one must also consider that there are no studies to show the absence of such a risk. Because of the positive results in animal carcinogenicity studies together with the in vitro findings about the genotoxicity of unsaturated PAs, the possibility of a carcinogenic effect of PAs on humans must be taken into consideration. There is no absolutely safe dose for genotoxic carcinogens. Extrapolations of dose-response curves from high to low concentrations are questionable, and animal experiments may not be representative for humans. Nevertheless such calculations are made to get crude information about a carcinogenic risk of certain compounds. Studies recently made for the German Federal Health office [83,84] recommend an allowable upper level of toxic PAs in herbal remedies of 0.1–0.2 ppm. The daily intake of such PAs should not exceed 30 ng (senecionine) and 700 ng (symphytine) per day per person. The difference in safety levels originates from differences in the carcinogenic potency of single PAs (see Table 2). It should, however, be noted that such calculations remain questionable.

All in all, if the therapeutic benefit of certain herbal drugs containing carcinogenic PAs cannot be clearly documented, such drugs should no longer be used.[1]

References

1. Robins DJ (1987) The pyrrolizidine alkaloids. In: Daly JW, Ferreira D, Gould StJ (eds) Progress in the chemistry of organic natural products 41:114–202
2. McLean EK (1974) Senecio and other plants as liver poisons. Isr J Med Sci 10:436–440
3. Lüthy J, Zweifel U, Schlatter C, Benn MH (1980) Pyrrolizidinalkaloide in Huflattich (Tussilago farfara L.) verschiedener Herkunft. Mitt Geb Lebensm Hyg 71:73–80
4. Mauz JC (1987) Vorkommen und Genotoxizität von Pyrrolizidinalkaloiden in Petasites hybridus L. und die Entfernung der Alkaloide aus Arzneipflanzenextrakten. Dissertation Eidgenössische Technische Hochschule Zürich No. 8246
5. Smith LW, Culvenor CCJ (1981) Plant sources of hepatotoxic pyrrolizidine alkaloids. J Nat Prod 44:129–152
6. Mattocks AR (1986) Chemistry and toxicology of pyrrolizidine alkaloids. New York: Academic Press

[1]See also the note added in proof on p. 262

7. Anonymous (1988) Pyrrolizidine alkaloids. Environmental health criteria 80. Geneva: World Health Organization
8. Lyford CL, Vergava GG, Moeller DD (1976) Hepatic veno occlusive disease originating in Ecuador. Gastroenterology 70:105-108
9. Tandon BN, Tandon HD, Tandon RK, Narendranathan M, Joshi YK (1976) Epidemic of veno-occlusive disease in central India. Lancet 2:271-272
10. Krishnamachari KAVR, Bhat RV, Krishnamurty D, Krishnaswamy K, Nagarajan (1977) Aetiopathogenesis of endemic ascites in Sarguja district of Madhya Pradesh. Indian J Med Res 65:672-678
11. Siddiqi MA, Suri KA, Suri MP, Atal CK (1978) Novel pyrrolizidine alkaloid from Crotalaria nana. Phytochemistry 17:2143-2144
12. Siddiqi MA, Suri KA, Suri MP, Atal CK (1977) Genus Crotalaria. Part 34. Cronaburmine, a new pyrrolizidine alkaloid from Crotalaria nana Burm. Indian J Chem 16B:1132-1133
13. Bras G, Jelliffe DB, Stuart KL (1954) Veno occlusive disease of the liver with nonportal type of cirrhosis occurring in Jamaica. Arch Pathol 57:285-300
14. Bras G, Berry DM, Gyorgi P (1957) Plants as etiological factor in veno-occlusive disease of liver. Lancet 1:960-962
15. Stuart KL, Bras G (1957) Veno-occlusive disease of the liver. Q J Med 26:291-315
16. Tandon HD, Tandon BN (1975) Epidemic of liver disease — Gulran District Herat Province, Afghanistan. Alexandria: World Health Organization, Regional Office for the Eastern Mediterranean; Assignment Report No. EM/AFG/OCD/001/RB
17. Tandon BN, Tandon HD, Mattocks AR (1978) Study of an epidemic of veno-occlusive disease in Afghanistan. Indian J Med Res 68:84-90
18. Tandon HD, Tandon BN, Mattocks AR (1978) An epidemic of veno-occlusive disease of the liver in Afghanistan. Am J Gastroenterol 72:607-613
19. Mohabbat O, Srivasta RN, Younos MS, Sediq GC, Menzad AA, Aram GN (1976) An outbreak of hepatic veno-occlusive disease in north-western Afghanistan. Lancet 2:269-271
20. Kumana CR, Ng M, Lin HJ, Ko W, Wu PC, Todd D (1985) Herbal tea induced veno-occlusive disease: quantification of toxic alkaloid exposure in adults. Gut 26:101-104
21. Culvenor CCJ, Edgar JA, Smith LW, Kumana CR, Lin HJ (1986) Heliotropium lasiocarpum Fish and Mey identified as cause of veno-occlusive disease due to a herbal tea. Lancet 1:978
22. Datta DV, Khuroo MS, Mattocks AR, Aikat BK, Chhuttani PN (1978) Veno-occlusive disease of liver due to Heliotropium plant used as medicinal herb (report of six cases with review of literature). J Assoc Phys India 26:383-393
23. Datta DV, Khuroo MS, Mattocks AR, Aikat BK, Chhuttani PN (1978) Herbal medicines and veno-occlusive disease in India. Postgrad Med J 54:511-515
24. Dubrovinskii SB (1952) The etiology of toxic hepatitis with ascites. In: Millenkov SM, Kizhaikin Y (ed) Collection of scientific papers on toxic hepatitis with ascites, Tashkent, USSR. Tashkent Publishing house of the University of Central Asia, pp 9-25
25. Mnushkin AS (1952) The clinical features, pathogenesis and treatment of toxic hepatitis with ascites. In: Milenkov SM, Kizhaikin Y (ed) Collection of scientific papers on toxic hepatitis with ascites. Tashkent, Publishing House of the University of Central Asia, pp 91-98
26. Lüthy L, Heim T, Schlatter C (1983) Transfer of (3H)pyrrolizidine alkaloids from Senecio vulgaris and metabolites into rat milk and tissues. Toxicol Lett 17:283-288
27. Eastman DF, Dimenna GP, Segall J (1982) Covalent binding of two pyrrolizidine alkaloids, senecionine and seneciphylline to hepatic macromolecules and their distribution, excretion and transfer into milk of lactating mice. Drug Metabol Dispos 16:236-240
28. Brauchli J, Lüthy HJ, Zweifel U, Schlatter C (1982) Pyrrolizidine alkaloids from Symphytum officinale L. and their percutaneous absorption in rats. Experientia 38:1085-1087
29. Kovach JS, Ames MM, Powis G, Moertel CG, Hahn RG, Creagan ET (1979) Toxicity and pharmacokinetics of a pyrrolizidine alkaloid, indicine N-oxide in humans. Cancer Res 39:4540-4544
30. Mattocks AR (1968) Toxicity of pyrrolizidine alkaloids. Nature (London) 217:723-728
31. Culvenor CC, Downing J, Jago M (1969) Pyrrolizidine alkaloids as alkylating and antimutatic agents. Ann NY Acad Sci 163:837-847
32. Culvenor CC, Edgar J, Jago M, Outteridge A, Peterson J, Smith L (1976) Hepato- and pneumotoxicity of pyrrolizidine alkaloids and derivatives in relation to molecular structure.

Chem Biol Interactions 12:299-324

33. Shtenberg AI, Orlova NV (1955) The question of the etiology of the so-called "Ozhalangar Encephalitis". Vopr Pitan 14:27-31

34. Ismailov NI, Madzhidov NM, Magrupov AI, Makhkamov GM, Mukminova SG (1970) Clinical signs, diagnosis and treatment of Trichodesma toxicosis (alimentary toxic encephalopathy). Tashkent Meditsina, p 85

35. Yunusov SYU, Plekhanova NV (1959) The alkaloids of Trichodesma incanum. The structure of incanine and trichesmine. Zh Obshch Khim 29:677-684

36. Pohlenz J, Lüthy J (1981) Enzootisches Auftreten einer Pyrrolizidin-alkaloid-Zirrhose beim Rind nach Aufnahme von Senecio alpinus (Alpenkreuzkraut). Schweiz Med Wschr 111:908

37. Culvenor CC (1978) Prevention of pyrrolizidine alkaloid poisoning. Animal adaption of plant control. In: Eff Poisonous Plants Livestock Proc Jt US- Australian Symposium Poisonous Plants, pp 189-200

38. Schoental R (1968) Toxicology and carcinogenic action of pyrrolizidine alkaloids. Cancer Res 28:2237-2246

39. Hill U, Rhodes H, Stofford J, Aub R (1951) Liver disease in Jamaican children. West Indian Med J 1:49-63

40. Roulet M, Laurini R, Rivier L, Calame A (1988) Hepatic veno-occlusive disease in newborn infant of a woman drinking herbal tea. J Pediatr 112:433-436

41. Spang R (1989) Toxicity of tea containing pyrrolizidine alkaloids. J Pediatr 115:1025

42. Stuart K, Bras G (1957) Veno-occlusive disease of the liver. Quart J Med 26:291-315

43. Schoental R (1968) Chemical structures and pathological effects of pyrrolizidine alkaloids. Israel J Med Sci 4:1133-1145

44. Heath D, Shaba J, Williams A, Smith P, Kombe A (1975) A pulmonary hypertension-producing plant from Tanzania. Thorax 30:399-404

45. McGee JOD, Patrick RS, Wood CB, Blumgart LH (1976) A case of veno-occlusive disease of the liver in Britain associated with herbal tea consumption. J Clin Pathol 29:788-794

46. Mehta NY, Karmody AM, McKneally MF (1986) Mediastinal veno-occlusive disease associated with herbal tea ingestion. NY State J Med 86:604-605

47. Schoental R, Magee PN (1959) Further observation on the subacute and chronic liver changes in rats after a single dose of various pyrrolizidine (senecio) alkaloids. J Pathol Bacteriol 78:471-482

48. Barnes JM, Magee PN, Schoental R (1964) Lesions in the lungs and livers of rats poisoned with fulvine and its N-oxide. J Pathol Bacteriol 88:521-531

49. Mattocks AR, White INH (1970) Estimation of metabolites of pyrrolizidine alkaloids in animal tissues. Anal Biochem 38:529-535

50. Butler WH, Mattocks AR, Barnes JM (1970) Lesions in the liver and lung of rats given pyrrole derivatives of pyrrolizidine alkaloids. J Pathol 100:169-175

51. Green C, Christie S (1961) Malformations in foetal rats induced by the pyrrolizidine alkaloid heliotrine. Br J Exp Pathol 42:369-378

52. Peterson JE, Jago MV (1980) Comparison of the toxic effects of dehydroheliotridine and heliotrine in pregnant rats and their embryos. J Pathol 131:339-355

53. Brink NG (1982) Somatic and teratogenic effects induced by heliotrine in Drosophila. Mut Res 104:105-111

54. Sundareson AE (1942) An experimental study of placental permeability to cirrhogenic poisons. J Pathol Bacteriol 54:289-298

55. Newberne PM (1968) The influence of a low lipotrope diet on response of maternal and fetal rats to lasiocarpine. Cancer Res 28:2327-2337

56. Armstrong SJ, Zuckerman AJ (1970) Production of pyrroles from pyrrolizidine alkaloids by human embryo tissue. Nature 228:569-570

57. Schoental R (1959) Liver lesions in young rats suckled by mothers treated with the pyrrolizidine (Senecio) alkaloids lasiocarpine and retrorsine. J Pathol Bacteriol 77:485-504

58. Mattocks AR, White INH (1973) Toxic effects and pyrrolic metabolites in the liver of young rats given the pyrrolizidine alkaloid retrorsine. Chem Biol Interact 15:173-184

59. Robertson H, Seymour J, Hsai M, Allen J (1977) Covalent interaction of dehydroretronecine, a carcinogenic metabolite of the pyrrolizidine alkaloid monocrotaline, with cystein and glutathion. Cancer Res 37:3141-3144

60. Petri T, Bowden G, Huxtable R, Sipes I (1984) Characterization of hepatic DNA damage induced in rats by the pyrrolizidine alkaloid monocrotaline. Cancer Res 44:1505–1509
61. Petry T, Bowden G, Bühler D, Sipes K (1986) Genotoxicity of the pyrrolizidine alkaloid jacobine in rats. Toxicol Letters 32:275–281
62. Hincks J, Coulombe R, Stamitz F, Molyneux R (1987) Genotoxicity of pyrrolizidine and larkspur alkaloids detected by alkaline elution. Proc Am Ass Cancer Res 28:33
63. Yamanaka H, Nagao M, Sugimura T (1979) Mutagenicity of pyrrolizidine alkaloids in the Salmonella microsome test. Mut Res 68:211–216
64. Takanashi H, Umeda M, Hirono J (1980) Chromosomal aberrations and mutation in cultured mammalian cells induced by pyrrolizidine alkaloids. Mut Res 78:67–77
65. Bruggeman IM, Van der Hoeven JCM (1985) Induction of SCE's by some pyrrolizidine alkaloids in V79 Chinese hamster cells co-cultured with chick embryo hepatocytes. Mut Res 142:209–212
66. Brick Y, Jackson W (1968) Effects of the pyrrolizidine alkaloid heliotrine on cell division and chromosome breakage in cultures of leucocytes from the marsupial Potorous tridactylus. Austr J Biol Sci 21:469–481
67. Kraus C, Abel G, Schimmer O (1985) Untersuchung einiger Pyrrolizidinalkaloide auf chromosomenschädigende Wirkung in menschlichen Lymphozyten in vitro. Planta Med, pp 89–91
68. Mori H, Sugie S, Yashimi N, Asad Y, Turuya T, Williams G (1985) Genotoxicity of a variety of pyrrolizidine alkaloids in the hepatocyte primary culture- DNA repair test, using rat, mouse and hamster hepatocytes. Cancer Res 45:3125–3129
69. Styles J, Ashby J, Mattocks A (1978) Evaluation in vitro of several pyrrolizidine alkaloid carcinogenes: observation on the essential pyrrolic nucleus. Carcinogenesis 1:161–164
70. Clark A (1959) Mutagenic activity of the alkaloid heliotrine in Drosophila. Nature 183:731–732
71. Clark A (1963) The brood pattern of sensitivity of the Drosophila tests to the mutagenic action of heliotrine. Z Vererb Lehre 94:115–120
72. Clark A (1982) The use of larval stages of Drosophila in screening for some naturally occurring mutagens. Mut Res 103:89–97
73. Brink N (1982) Somatic and teratogenic effects induced by heliotrine in Drosophila. Mut Res 104:105–111
74. Brink N (1966) The mutagenic activity of heliotrine in Drosophila. I. Complete and mosaic sex-linked lethals. Mut Res 3:66–72
75. Cook L, Holt A (1966) Mutagenic activity in Drosophila of two pyrrolizidine alkaloids. J Gen 59:273–274
76. Anonymous (1976 and 1983) IARC Monographs on the evaluation of the carcinogenic risk to humans. 10:265–343 and 31:206–224
77. Hirono I, Mori H, Haga M et al. (1983) Edible plants containing carcinogens in Japan. In: Miller EC et al. (ed) Naturally occurring carcinogens — mutagens and modulators of carcinogenesis. Baltimore, Maryland, University Park Press, pp 79–87
78. Schoental R, Head M, Peacock P (1954) Senecio alkaloids: primary liver tumours as a result of (I) a mixture of alkaloids from S. jacobea Lin. (II) retrorsine; (III) isatidine. Brit J Cancer 8:458–465
79. Svoboda D, Reddy J (1972) Malignant tumours in rats given lasiocarpine. Cancer Res 92:908–912
80. Newberne P, Rogers A (1973) Nutrition, monocrotaline and aflatoxin B1 in liver carcinogenesis. In: Newman PN (ed). Plant food man 1:23–31
81. Hirono I, Mori H, Yamada K, Hirata Y, Haga M, Tatematsu H, Kanie S (1977) Carcinogenic activity of petasitenine, a new pyrrolizidine alkaloid isolated from Petasites japonicus. J Natl Cancer Inst 58:1155–1157
82. Allen Y, Hsu I, Cartens L (1975) Dehydroretronecine-induced rhabdomyosarcomas in rats. Cancer Res 35:997–1002
83. Lüthy J (1988) Toxikologie von Pyrrolizidin Alkaloiden in Arzneipflanzen: Gutachten im Auftrag des Bundesgesundheitsamtes, Berlin
84. Westendorf J (1988) Pyrrolizidinalkaloid-haltige Arzneipflanzen (mögliche human-kanzerogene Wirksamkeit). Gutachten im Auftrag des Bundesgesundheitsamtes, Berlin

Pyrrolizidine Alkaloids – *Cynoglossum officinale*

J. Westendorf

Botany

Cynoglossum officinale L. belongs to the family of the Boraginaceae and is related to *Symphytum* species. Vernacular names are hound's tongue (English) and Hundszunge (German).

Chemistry

Semen and roots of *Cynoglossum officinale* contain the alkaloids cynoglossine, consolidine, and consolicine. The chemical structures of these alkaloids are unknown. Herb and roots contain choline, bitter principles, and tannin. The herb also contains an essential oil which smells like chamomile and large amounts of mucilage [1]. The plant is rich in pyrrolizidine alkaloids (PAs). The dried herb contains up to 1.5% [2]. The PA composition is different from that of *Symphytum* species. The following PAs have been identified in the dried herb of *Cynoglossum officinale*: heliosupine (0.77%), echinatine (0.22%), acetylheliosupine (0.03%), and 7-angelylheliotridine (0.02%) [3]. These PAs belong to the heliosupine-like necine type and are monoesters or open-chain diesters.

Pharmacology and Uses

Cynoglossum preparations were formerly used internally in diarrhea and externally for the treatment of wounds, bone injuries and contusions. Today the plant is used as a remedy against neuralgia, spastic disorders of the skeletal muscles, and as a sedative [1]. It is believed that the alkaloids consolidine and consolicine, which exert a curare-like inhibiting effect on muscle nerve endings, are responsible for the activity of the plant.

Adverse Reaction Profile

A general discussion of the adverse reactions of herbal medicines containing pyrrolizidine alkaloids is presented in a general contribution elsewhere in this book.

General Animal Data

Poisoning of calves [4] and horses [5] by *Cynoglossum officinale* has been reported.

General Human Data

The Federal Committee for Phytotherapy in Germany (the so-called Kommission E) has recently rejected the therapeutic use of *Cynoglossum officinale* because PAs are present, and because the therapeutic usefulness of the herb is insufficiently documented [6].

Fertility, Pregnancy, and Lactation

A general discussion of the effects of herbal medicines containing pyrrolizidine alkaloids when used during pregnancy or lactation is presented in a separate general contribution elsewhere in this volume. It has been shown by Korkhov and Mats [7] that extracts of *Cynoglossum officinale* induce contractions of the rat uterus due to the presence of heliosupine.

Mutagenicity and Carcinogenicity

A general discussion of the mutagenicity and carcinogenicity of herbal medicines containing pyrrolizidine alkaloids is presented in a separate general contribution elsewhere in this book.

References

1. Geßner O, Orzechowski G (1974) Die Gift- und Arzneipflanzen von Mitteleuropa. Heidelberg; Carl Winter Verlag, p 93
2. Petersen E (1975) Pyrrolizidine alkaloids in Danish species of the family of *Boraginaceae*. Arch Pharm Chem Sci 3:55–64
3. Pedersen E (1970) Minor pyrrolizidine alkaloids from *Cynoglossum officinale* L. Danis Tidsvks Farm 44:288–291
4. Baker DC, Smart RA, Ralphs M, Molyneux RJ (1989) Hounds-tongue *Cynoglossum officinale* poisoning in the calf. J Am Vet Med Assoc 194:929–930

5. Knight AP, Kimberling CV, Stermitz FR, Roby MR (1984) A cause of pyrrolizidine alkaloid poisoning in horses. J Am Vet Med Assoc 185:647–650
6. Thesen R, Braun R (1989) Ganz oder teilweise "negativ" bewertete Arzneistoffe. Pharm Ztg 134:2734–2736
7. Korkhov VV, Mats MN (1979) Effect of cynoglossophine-heliosupine from *Cynoglossum officinale* on the contraction activity of the uterus and the gall bladder. Rastit Resur 15:396–399

Pyrrolizidine Alkaloids — *Petasites* Species

J. Westendorf

Botany

The genus *Petasites* belongs to the family of Asteraceae (Compositae). It comprises several species, which are different in botany as well as in chemotaxonomy.

Petasites hybridus (L.) Gaertn., Meyer et Scherb. (= *P. officinalis* Moench) is the most important representative. Vernacular names are butterbur, butterfly dock, coltsfoot (English); Pestwurz, großblättriger Huflattich, Wasserklette (German); pétaside hybride, pétaside vulgaire, pestilence (French); cavallacio, farfaracio, Petasite (Italian). The botanical similarity to *Tussilago farfara*, which is enhanced by the similarity in nomenclature, often leads to confusion in the use of these plants for medicinal purposes.

Other interesting *Petasites* species are *Petasites albus* (L.) Gaertn., *Petasites spurius* (Retz.) Rchb., *Petasites paradoxus* (Retz.) Baumg., and *Petasites japonicus* Maxim Bakk. Fuki.

Chemistry

The leaves of *P. hybridus* contain a similar spectrum of compounds as the leaves of *T. farfara*, i.e., mucilage, proteins, resin, inulin, dextrine, tannic acids, 0.1% of essential oil, and relatively high amounts of manganese [1].

No adequate data about the pyrrolizidine alkaloid (PA) content of butterbur leaves are available in the literature. There is only one report [2] about the PA content of blossoms and stems, in which 40 mg/kg (net weight) of the PAs senecionine, integerrimine, and senkirkine have been detected. Because the leaves of *Petasites hybridus* are often used as an adulterant of *Tussilago farfara*, a more detailed analysis of the PA content is certainly warranted.

The roots of *P. hybridus* contain a variety of sesquiterpene esters of the eremophilan type, which are called petasines. Some of these compounds contain sulfur (s-petasine, s-isopetasine) and are esters of petasol or isopetasol and β-methylmercaptoacrylic acid. The roots also contain the triterpene bauerenol, 0.1% of essential oil, 3.5% of inuline, 1.8% of pectine, choline, resin, lipids, carbohydrates, mucilage, proteins, and β-sitosterine [1].

An analysis of various commercial charges of *Radix petasitidis* yielded PAs in total amounts of 2–350 mg/kg [3]. The main constituents were senecionine, integerrimine, and senkirkine. Minor amounts of saturated nontoxic PAs have also been detected in this drug [2].

There are some remarkable differences in the PA composition of various *Petasites* species. Only senkirkine could be detected in the roots of *Petasites albus* [2], whereas senkirkine, and the otonecine esters petasitenine and neopetasitenine are present in *Petasites japonicus* [4,5].

Pharmacology and Uses

The use of *Petasites* species for medicinal purposes has a long tradition, especially in Europe and Japan. In the middle ages *P. hybridus* was even used as a remedy against plague, which led to the name 'Pestwurz' (German). Its leaves contain mucilage, and they are used, just like coltsfoot, for diseases of the respiratory tract. They are also used as a diaphoretic, diuretic, and anthelminthic remedy. Moreover, fresh leaves are used externally for several skin diseases.

The roots of *P. hybridus* are used mainly as a spasmolytic drug for the treatment of spastic conditions of the gastrointestinal tract. Petasine and other sesquiterpenes which have papaverine-like musculotrope spasmolytic properties have been seen as responsible for the activity of the drug [10]. In contrast to drugs made from the leaves of *Petasites hybridus*, root preparations are generally not used chronically.

Adverse Reaction Profile

A general discussion of the adverse reaction profile of herbal medicines containing pyrrolizidine alkaloids is presented in a general contribution elsewhere in this book.

Allergic Reactions

Although sesquiterpenes are often responsible for allergic reactions to botanicals, no such reactions have yet been reported for *Petasites*.

Fertility, Pregnancy, and Lactation

A general discussion of the effects of herbal medicines containing PAs when used during pregnancy or lactation is presented in a separate general contribution elsewhere in this book.

Maternal use during pregnancy of a herbal cough tea containing roots of *P. hybridus* has been associated with a fatal case of neonatal hepatic veno-occlusive disease (see the contribution on *Tussilago farfara*).

Mutagenicity and Carcinogenicity

A general discussion of the mutagenicity and carcinogenicity of herbal medicines containing PA's is presented in a separate general contribution elsewhere in this book.

There are references in the literature that chronic treatment of laboratory animals with *Petasites japonicus* resulted in the development of malignant tumors of the liver and other organs. Hirono et al. [6] fed the young flower stalks of *Petasites japonicus* to young ACI rats. One group of 27 rats (12 male and 15 female) received the drug at 4% in the diet for 6 months, followed by 8% and 0% on alternate weeks for at least 480 days. The second group of rats (11 male and 8 female) were treated with 4% drug in the diet for 480 days. In the first group 3 animals died of pneumonia. Eleven out of the 24 surviving rats developed tumors of the liver after 15–16 months of feeding. The tumors were liver cell adenomas (6), liver cell carcinomas (2) and haemangiosarcomas (3). In the second group 8/17 surviving rats developed tumors of the liver: 8 hemangiosarcomas, 4 hepatocellular adenomas and 1 liver cell carcinoma.

Fushimi et al. [7] fed 24 male and 21 female ddN mice with 4% of flower stalks of *Petasites japonicus* in the diet for 480 days. They found that 24/39 surviving animals developed lung adenomas and 6/39 lung carcinomas. Additionally, they observed 4/39 liver reticulum cell carcinomas, 1/39 liver cell hemangiosarcoma, 1/39 thymoma and 2/39 cases of leukemia. Except for 1 tumor of the lung, 1 renal hemangioendothelial sarcoma and 1 spleen hemangioma, no tumors were observed in the control group (23 males and 27 females). Of 20 male and 20 female Swiss strain mice, treated with 4% of flower stalks in the diet for 480 days, only 5/26 surviving animals developed lung adenomas. Additional experiments with C57BL/6 mice (20 males and 20 females) and Syrian golden hamsters (13 males and 17 females), which also received 4% of flower stalks of *Petasites japonicus* in the diet for 480 days, did not show significant tumor induction at any site.

The experiments outlined above demonstrate the capacity of *Petasites japonicus* to induce neoplastic diseases in experimental animals. ACI rats and ddN mice were much more sensitive to the carcinogenic action of the drug than C57BL mice and Syrian golden hamsters which did not show tumors after similar treatment. As we do not know how humans correspond to these animals, a carcinogenic action of *Petasites japonicus* must be taken into consideration. No experiments have yet been reported for *Petasites hybridus* or other *Petasites* species.

References

1. List PH, Hörhammer L (1977) Hagers Handbuch der pharmazeutischen Praxis. 4th edn, Vol 6: Chemikalien und Drogen (A: N-Q). Berlin: Springer-Verlag, pp 535–539
2. Lüthy J, Zweifel U, Schmidt P, Schlatter C (1983) Pyrrolizidin-alkaloide in *Petasites hybridus* L. und *Petasites albus* L. Pharm Helv Acta 58:98–100
3. Mauz JC (1987) Vorkommen und Genotoxizität von Pyrrolizidin-Alkaloiden in *Petasites hybridus* L. und die Entfernung der Alkaloide aus Arzneipfianzenextrakten. Zürich: Eidgenössische Technische Hochschule. Dissertation
4. Yamada H, Tatematsu M, Suzuki M, Hirata Y, Haga M, Hirono I (1976) Isolation and the structures of two new alkaloids, petasitenine and neopetasitenine from *Petasites japonicus* Maxim. Chem Lett 1:461
5. Niwa H, Ishiwata H, Yamada K (1983) Separation and determination of macrocyclic pyrrolizidine alkaloids of the otonecine type present in edible plant *Petasites japonicus* by reversed phase high performance liquid chromatography. J Chromat 257:146–150
6. Hirono J, Mori H, Haga M, Fujii M, Yamada K, Hirata Y, Takanashi H, Uschida E, Hosaka S, Keno J, Matsushima T, Umezawa K, Shirai A (1979) Edible plants containing carcinogenic alkaloids in Japan. In: Miller EC (ed) Naturally occurring carcinogens — mutagens and modulators of carcinogenesis. Tokyo, Baltimore; Japan Sci Soc Press, Univ Park Press, pp 79–87
7. Fushimi K, Kato K, Kato T, Matsubara N (1978) Carcinogenicity of flower stalks of *Petasites japonicus* Maxim. in mice and Syrian golden hamsters. Toxicol Lett 1:291–294

Pyrrolizidine Alkaloids — *Senecio* Species

J. Westendorf

Botany

The genus *Senecio* (ragwort, English; Kreuzkraut, German) belongs to the family of Asteraceae (= Compositae) and is subdivided into more than 1200 species. Some *Senecio* species are also known as *Cineraria* species. *Senecio* plants grow all over the world, but only special types occur on different continents. The following *Senecio* spp. are or have been used for medicinal purposes in Europe: *S. vulgaris, S. nemorensis, S. jacobaea,* and *S. aureus.* Of toxicological interest are also *S. longilobus* and *S. alpinus* because poisoning of livestock with these plants has been reported.

Chemistry

Senecio spp. contain pyrrolizidine alkaloids (PAs) in considerable amounts and varieties. The majority of these PAs are unsaturated and thus toxic. The following PAs have been detected in common *Senecio* species:

 S. vulgaris: Senecionine, seneciphylline, retrorsine, riddeline. The total amount of PAs in fresh plant materials is up to 0.16% [1].

 S. jacobaea: Senecionine, seneciphylline, jacobine, jacocine, jacoline, jaconine. Some of these compounds are unique in the class of PAs because they contain chlorine (jaconine) or epoxy moieties (jacocine, jacobine). The total amount of PAs is between 0.1 and 0.2% [1].

 S. nemorensis ssp. *fuchsii:* Fuchsisenecionine, senecionine. Fuchsisenecionine belongs to the saturated, nontoxic PAs, whereas senecionine is one of the most toxic PAs. The PA content of the plant is 0.37% (fuchsisenecionine) and 0.007% (senecionine) [2]. The unsaturated PAs 9-angelylretronecine and retroisogenine together with some other saturated PAs but without senecionine have been detected in the plant by Gottlieb [3].

 S. aureus: Florisenine, otosenine, floridanine. These compounds are unsaturated PAs of the otonecine type with macrocyclic esterstructures. The compounds florisenine and otosenine also contain epoxy structures in the acid moiety of the molecule. The total amount of PAs was reported to be 0.06% [4].

Pharmacology and Uses

A clear pharmacological classification of the different *Senecio* species and of their preparation is not possible. Medicinal uses include dysmenorrhea (*S. nemorensis* ssp. *fuchsii*), diseases of the urinary tract (*S. vulgaris*), spastic conditions of smooth muscles, headache (*S. jacobaea*) etc. No correlation between the pharmacological activity and certain chemical constituents of these plant drugs can be made.

Adverse Reaction Profile

A general discussion of the adverse reactions of herbal medicines containing PAs is presented in a general contribution elsewhere in this volume.

Hepatic Reactions

Several literature reports have described in detail that the use of *Senecio* species can result in hepatic veno-occlusive disease in man. Willmot and Robertson [5] reported as early as 1920 that contamination of wheat with *Senecio ilicifolius* and *Senecio burchelli* had affected whole South African families from time to time. They called this condition 'senecio disease' and noted that its chief symptoms were abdominal pain and vomiting with ascites. They investigated about 11 cases, most of which were in children; the majority of these patients died [5]. Another series of South African poisonings due to contamination with *Senecio* was reported three decades later by Selzer and Parker [6]. More recently, hepatic injury was observed in two American infants, who had been treated with a herbal tea adulterated with *Senecio longilobus*; one of the cases was fatal [7,8]. Furthermore, hepatomegaly and sudden ascites developed in a Portuguese father and his son following the use of a herbal tea prepared from an unspecified *Senecio* plant [9].

Fertility, Pregnancy, and Lactation

A general discussion of the effects of herbal medicines containing PAs, when used during pregnancy or lactation is presented in a separate general contribution elsewhere in this book.

Mutagenicity and Carcinogenicity

A general discussion of the mutagenicity and carcinogenicity of herbal medicines containing PAs is presented in a separate general contribution elsewhere in this book.

Several long-treatment experiments in laboratory animals with preparations made from *Senecio* species have been reported in the literature.

Senecio nemorensis ssp. *fuchsii* [10]: A crude alkaloidal extract of the plant was given in doses of 8 mg and 40 mg/kg p.o. 5 times per week for at least 104 weeks to 20 male and 20 female Sprague-Dawley rats per dose. Of 14 animals treated with 8 mg/kg, 13 developed tumors of the liver. Female rats were much more sensitive than males (11 versus 2 tumors). Only 1/40 animals of the control group developed a liver tumor. At the high concentration 34/40 rats developed liver tumors, 29 of which were observed in the female group. The incidence of tumors in extrahepatic tissues was significantly increased in the female group but not in males.

Senecio longilobus [11]: Continuous feeding of 0.75% or 0.5% of the plant material in the diet of Harlan rats shortened the lifetime of the animals to 131 and 200 days without induction of tumors. When the animals were fed alternately a diet with or without 0.5% *S. longilobus* for 1 week for at least 470 days, 16/47 animals developed liver cell carcinomas and 1/47 angiosarcoma. A dose regimen of feeding 0.5% *S. longilobus* in the diet for 1 month followed by 2 weeks of normal diet for at least 1 year was also effective in inducing liver tumors (4/23 carcinomas).

References

1. Molyneux R, Johnson A, Reitman J, Benson M (1979) Chemistry of toxic range plants: determination of pyrrolizidine alkaloid contents and composition in senecio species by NMR-spectroscopy. J Agric Food Chem 27:494–499
2. Wiedenfeld H, Röder E (1979) Das Pyrrolizidin-Alkaloid Senecionin aus Senecio Fuchsii. Phytochem 18:1083–1084
3. Gottlieb R (1990) Senecio fuchsii: GC-MS-Auswertung der vorhandenen Pyrrolizidin-Alkaloide. Dtsch Apoth Ztg 130:285–288
4. Röder E, Wiedenfeld H, Koenig A (1987) Pyrrolizidin-Alkaloide aus Senecio aureus. Planta Med 1:57–59
5. Willmot FC, Robertson GW (1920) Senecio disease, or cirrhosis of the liver due to senecio poisoning. Lancet 2:848–849
6. Selzer G, Parker RGF (1951) *Senecio* poisoning exhibiting as Chiari's syndrome: a report of 12 cases. Am J Pathol 27:885–907
7. Stillman AE, Huxtable R, Consroe P, Kohnen P, Smith S (1977) Hepatic veno-occlusive disease due to pyrrolizidine (Senecio) poisoning in Arizona. Gastroenterology 73:349–352
8. Fox DW, Hart MC, Bergeson PS, Jarrett PB, Stillman AE, Huxtable RJ (1978) Pyrrolizidine (*Senecio*) intoxication mimicking Reye syndrome. J Pediatr 93:980–982
9. De Peyer R, Schindler AM (1987) Hepatomegalie et ascite soudaines chez un carreleur portugais et son fils. Schweiz Med Wschr 117:767–772
10. Habs H, Habs M, Marquardt H, Röder E, Schmähl D, Wiedenfeld H (1982) Carcinogenic and mutagenic activity of an alkaloidal extract of Senecio nemorensis ssp. fuchsii. Arzneim Forsch 32:144–148
11. Harris P, Chen K (1970) Development of hepatic tumours in rats following ingestion of *Senecio longilobus*. Cancer Res 30:2881–2886

Pyrrolizidine Alkaloids — *Symphytum* Species

J. Westendorf

Botany

The genus *Symphytum* belongs to the family of Boraginaceae and comprises the species *Symphytum officinale* L., *Symphytum asperum* Lepechin, *Symphytum × uplandicum* Nyman — a hybrid derived from *S. officinale* and *S. asperum* — and *S. tuberosum* L. Vernacular names for *S. officinale* are common comfrey (English); gemeiner Beinwell, Komfrey (German); grand consoude (French); and consolida maggiore (Italian). *S. asperum* is known in Germany as rauher Beinwell. *S. × uplandicum* is called Russian comfrey, and *S. tuberosum* is known as tuberous comfrey. The roots of *Symphytum* species are used for medicinal purposes and are known as Radix consolidae (historical) or Symphyti radix.

Chemistry[1]

Symphyti radix contains allantoin (0.6–0.8%), mucilage and tannic acids, as well as minor amounts of the alkaloids symphytocynoglossine, consolidine, and consolicine [1]. The following pyrrolizidine alkaloids (PAs) are present in *Symphytum* species:

S. officinale: Symphytine, lycopsamine, acetyllycopsamine, lasiocarpine, heliosupine, and echinatine [2]. The amount in dry roots varies between 0.3 and 0.4% [3]. A considerable proportion of the PAs may be present as N-oxides. The PA content of the leaves is usually lower than that of the roots [4].

S. × uplandicum Nyman: Echimidine, symphytine, lycopsamine, intermedine, 7-acetyllcopsamine, 7-acetylintermedine, symlandine, uplandine. There are only quantitative data available about the PA content of the leaves (0.01–0.15%) [5]. This content varies with seasons and the age of the plants. A study performed by Mattocks [4] shows that small leaves from *S. × uplandicum* (variety Bocking no. 14) harvested early in the season contained 0.049% PAs, whereas large old leaves contained only 0.003% of PAs. It is probable that the roots contain higher concentrations than the leaves.

---

[1] See also the note added in proof on p. 262

S. asperum: Asperumine, heliosupine, echimidine, 7-acetyllycopsamine, 7-acetylintermedine, echimidine, symphytine, symlandine. The roots contain 0.14–0.37% of total PAs, whereas the leaves contain only 0.01% [6].

S. tuberosum: Symlandine, echimidine. The PA content of dry leaves was reported to be 0.003–0.004% of N-oxides [7]. In view of the data on other *Symphytum* spp., it is not very likely that *S. tuberosum* contains only two different PAs.

Ready-to-use preparations made from comfrey may contain considerable amounts of PAs. It has been reported that comfrey pepsin capsules made from the roots contained 2900 mg/kg of total PAs; brands made from comfrey leaves contained 270 mg/kg PAs [8]. Comsumption of two capsules per meal for six months would lead to the ingestion of 162 mg PAs (leaf preparation) or 1740 mg (root preparation).

Pharmacology and Uses

Tea preparations of dry roots are used internally and externally for the treatment of wounds, bone injuries, contusions, and arthritic disorders. It is believed that the positive influence of *Symphytum* preparations when used externally is based on its content of allantoin [9]. The astringent effect to tannic acids present in drugs made from *Symphytum* is also useful in the treatment of these disorders.

Pharmacokinetics

As *Symphytum* preparations are often used for topic application, it is of interest whether or not the PAs present in these preparations are absorbed through the skin. At the present time there is only one study available about the transdermal absorption of PAs from *Symphytum officinale*. When a crude alcoholic extract of the plant was tested in rats, the percutaneous absorption of the PAs was 20–50 times lower than the absorption following oral administration [10].

Adverse Reaction Profile

A general discussion of the adverse reactions of herbal remedies containing pyrrolizidine alkaloids is presented in a general contribution elsewhere in this book.

General Animal Data

The *Symphytum* alkaloids symphytocynoglossine, consolidine, and consolicine have a curare-like inhibiting effect on muscle nerve endings. Administered to laboratory animals, these compounds cause a paralysis of the skeletal muscles, whereas root extracts from *Symphytum* first enhance the excitability of muscular reflexes, followed by an inhibition and finally anesthesia [11].

General Human Data[1]

Due to the presence of toxic PAs, *Symphytum* preparations have been removed from the nonprescription market in Poland [12]. The Australian National Health and Medical Research Council has recommended that comfrey be available only from pharmacists, medical practitioners, or, in isolated communities, other licensed individuals [13].

Hepatic Reactions

The internal use of *Symphytum* preparations for medicinal purposes may cause severe hepatic damage. A 13-year-old boy with Crohn's disease who had been regularly treated with a tea made from comfrey leaves developed a veno-occlusive disease [14]. The same disorder occurred in a 49-year-old woman who had taken a herbal beverage containing PAs and comfrey pepsin capsules. The daily intake of PAs from the tea was 0.5–1.5 µg/kg body weight per day and 14.1 µg/kg body weight per day from the capsules; the latent period until hospitalization was 4 months [15]. Hepatic veno-occlusive disease was also observed in a 47-year-old woman who had chronically used large amounts of comfrey tea and comfrey pills [16].

Fertility, Pregnancy, and Lactation

A general discussion of the effects of herbal medicines containing pyrrolizidine alkaloids when used during pregnancy or lactation is presented in a separate general contribution elsewhere in this book.

Mutagenicity and Carcinogenicity

A general discussion of the mutagenicity and carcinogenicity of herbal medicines containing pyrrolizidine alkaloids is presented in a separate general contribution elsewhere in this book.

---

[1]See also the note added in proof on p. 263

Hirono et al. [17] have shown that ACI rats which received leaves or roots of *Symphytum officinale* in dietary concentrations between 5% and 33% developed tumors in multiple organs. Liver adenomas were the most prominent tumor type observed. At the same dietary levels, the roots of *Symphytum officinale* were more potent than the leaves. Other tumors induced by *Symphytum officinale* were liver hemangiosarcomas, adrenal cortical adenomas, urinary bladder carcinomas and urinary bladder papillomas. Especially the induction of liver adenomas together with liver hemangiosarcomas is typical for PAs.

References

1. Roth L, Daunderer A, Korman K (1988) Giftpflanzen — Pflanzengifte: Vorkommen, Wirkung, Therapie — allergische und phototoxische Reaktionen. 3rd ed. Landsberg: Ecomed, p 633
2. Petersen E (1975) Pyrrolizidine alkaloids in Danish species of the family of Boraginaceae. Arch Pharm Chem Sci 3:55–64
3. Lüthy J (1987) Vorkommen und Analytik von Pyrrolizidinalkoloiden in Arzneipflanzen und pharmazeutischen Zubereitungen. BGA-Gutachten, Berlin
4. Mattocks AR (1980) Toxic pyrrolizidine alkaloids in comfrey. Lancet 2:1136
5. Culvenor C, Edgar J, Frahn J, Smith L (1980) The alkaloids of *Symphytum* × *uplandicum* (Russian comfrey). Austr J Chem 33:1105–1113
6. Roitman J (1981) Comfrey and liver damage. Lancet 1:944
7. Bhandar P, Gray AI (1985) Pyrrolizidine alkaloid N-oxides from *Symphytum tuberosum*. J Pharm Pharmacol 37:50P
8. Huxtable RJ, Lüthy J, Zweifel U (1986) Toxicity of comfrey-pepsine preparations. N Engl J Med 315:1095
9. Wagner H (1985) Pharmazeutische Biologie: 2. Drogen und ihre Inhaltsstoffe. 3rd ed. Stuttgart: Gustav Fischer Verlag, p 196
10. Brauchli J, Lüthy J, Schlatter C (1982) Pyrrolizidine alkaloids from *Symphytum officinale* L. and their percutaneous absorption in rats. Experientia 38:1085–1087
11. Geßner O, Orzechowski G (1974) Die Gift- und Arzneipflanzen von Mitteleuropa. 3rd ed. Heidelberg: Carl Winter Verlag, p 92
12. Levin LS, Berska F, Fry J (1988) Self-medication in Europe — report on a study of the role of non-prescription medicines. Copenhagen: World Health Organisation Office for Europe 15:251
13. Abbott PJ (1988) Comfrey: assessing the low-dose health risk. Med J Aust 149:678–682
14. Weston CFM, Cooper BT, Davies JD, Levine DF (1987) Veno-occlusive disease of the liver secondary to ingestion of comfrey. Br Med J 295:183
15. Ridker PM, Ohkuma S, McDermott WV, Trey C, Huxtable RJ (1985) Hepatic veno-occlusive disease associated with the consumption of pyrrolizidine-containing dietary supplements. Gastroenterology 88:1050–1054
16. Bach N, Thung SN, Schaffner F (1989) Comfrey herb tea-induced hepatic veno-occlusive disease. Am J Med 87:97–99
17. Hirono I, Mori H, Haga M, Fujii M, Yamada K, Hirata Y, Takanashi H, Uchida E, Kosaka S, Keno J, Matsushima T, Umezawa K, Shirai A (1979) Edible plants containing carcinogenic alkaloids in Japan. In: Miller EC (ed) Naturally occurring carcinogens — mutagens and modulators of carcinogenesis. Tokyo, Baltimore; Japan Sci Soc Press, Univ Park Press, pp 79–87

Pyrrolizidine Alkaloids — *Tussilago farfara*

J. Westendorf

Botany

Tussilago farfara L. belongs to the plant family of Asteraceae (Compositae). Vernacular names are: Huflattich, Brustlattich, Brandlattich, Roßhuf (German), coltsfoot, horsefoot (English), pas d'ane (French), farfaro (Italian). The yellow blossoms (Flores Farfarae, harvested between February and April) and the leaves (Farfarae Folium, harvested between May and June) are used for medicinal purposes [1].

Chemistry

The leaves of coltsfoot contain 6–10% mucilage, which yield upon acid hydrolysis 5% uronic acids, 30% fructose, 24% galactose, 21% arabinose, 15% glucose, and 10% xylose [2]. Another author indicates a carbohydrate content of 67% galacturonic acid with rhamnose [3]. The blossoms of coltsfoot contain essential oils, inulin, flavonoids, organic acids (ascorbic acid, malic acid, tartaric acid, caffeic acid, ferulic acid, p-hydroxybenzoic acid) and tannic acids. Of possible pharmacological and/or toxicological interest are the sesquiterpene lactones, tussilagone, and petasitolid which have been identified in *Tussilago farfara* [4,5]. Among the inorganic constituents are relatively large amounts of potassium nitrate and up to 3% of zinc in the ash of the roots [6].

The following pyrrolizidine alkaloids (PAs) have been detected in *T. farfara*: senkirkine [7], senecionine [8], tussilagine and isotussilagine [9]. Senkirkine and senecionine belong to the PAs with an unsaturated necine moiety which is essential for the toxic properties of these class of chemicals, whereas tussilagine and isotussilagine are saturated and, thus, nontoxic. Rosberger et al. recovered 140 mg/kg senkirkine and 7 mg/kg senecionine from the pre-blooming flowers of North American coltsfoot; mature whole plants yielded 49 mg/kg senkirkine and 1 mg/kg senecionine [10]. *T. farfara* of European origin usually contains much smaller amounts of toxic PAs than plants grown in China [8]. After preparation of a tea from young shoots of *T. farfara* of Chinese origin, up to 80% of the PA senkirkine could be detected in the aqueous phase [8].

Pharmacology and Uses

T. farfara belongs to the pharmacological class of mucilaginous drugs. Its mucilage exerts a protective effect on the mucous membrane of the larynx and the oral cavity by covering the surface. This results in an inhibition of cough reflexes caused by bacteria and necrotic tissue. The astringent effect of tannic acids and a slight antibacterial activity of *T. farfara* preparations [11] due to its content of polyhydroxy cinnamic acids, such as caffeic acid, also positively influences the symptoms of catarrhal disorders. *T. farfara* is used in tea preparations which often contain complex mixtures of different medicinal plants. Among these are additives containing essential oil, such as aniseed and peppermint extracts, which exert secretomotoric and antiseptic activity, and plant extracts with expectorant properties, such as licorice root. As respiratory disorders are often chronical, many patients take *T. farfara* preparations over prolonged time periods.

From the flowers of *Tussilago farfara* of Chinese origin the sesquiterpene lactone tussilagone has been isolated which has been shown to exert stimulating effects on the blood pressure and respiration of rats, cats, and dogs after intravenous injection [5]. The practical impact of this observation, however, remains doubtful, because the effect was very transient and has not yet been demonstrated after oral administration.

Adverse Reaction Profile

A general discussion of the adverse reactions of herbal medicines containing PAs is presented in a general contribution elsewhere in this volume.

Allergic Reactions

It was reported that coltsfoot has only weak allergenic capacity in guinea pig sensitization experiments [12]. Although the components responsible for these effects are unknown, it is most likely that they are attributable to the sesquiterpene lactones present in the plant. Up to now, there is no published evidence that allergic reactions occur during the human use of oral preparations of *T. farfara*.

Fertility, Pregnancy, and Lactation

A general discussion of the effects of herbal medicines containing PA when used during pregnancy or lactation is presented in a separate contribution elsewhere in this volume.

There is one case report in the literature that maternal use of a coltsfoot tea preparation during the entire pregnancy resulted in hepatic veno-occlusive disease of the infant, who died on the 38th day after birth [13]. The incriminated tea was said to contain about 9% of coltsfoot leaves along with a mixture of several other plants. Chemical analysis revealed 0.6 mg/kg senecionine. This would imply a senecionine concentration of the pure unmixed leaves of 6.7 mg/kg, which is compatible with the finding of Rosberger et al. [10] who detected 6 mg/kg of senecionine in the young leaves of *T. farfara*. However, the absence of senkirkine, which normally is present in the plant in concentrations up to 10 times those of senecionine [8], led to the suspicion that *Petasites hybridus* was present in the tea mixture instead of *Tussilago farfara* [14]. Later research showed that the cough tea contained not only *T. farfara*, but also roots of *Petasites hybridus* [15].

Nevertheless, the use of a tea prepared from pure coltsfoot leaves might provide up to 10 times the amount of senecionine that was recovered from the incriminated cough tea. On the basis of this calculation, the use of coltsfoot tea during pregnancy can not be claimed to be safe.

Mutagenicity and Carcinogenicity

A general discussion of the mutagenicity and carcinogenicity of herbal medicines containing PAs is presented in a separate general contribution elsewhere in this volume.

The carcinogenicity of *T. farfara* has been tested in rats [16]. Twelve ACI rats (6 male and 6 female) received 16% of coltsfoot buds of Chinese origin in the diet over a period of 600 days and developed multiple tumors of the liver (8 hemangioendothelial sarcomas, 1 hepatocellular adenoma, 1 hepatocellular carcinoma) and 1 papilloma of the bladder. With 8% of *T. farfara* in the diet, given to 5 male and 5 female rats, only one hemangioendothelial sarcoma of the liver was observed. In view of the type of tumors developed, it is very likely that the PAs present in the plant (senkirkine and senecionine) were responsible for the tumor induction. Because of these experiments, it can not be fully excluded that the chronic use of *T. farfara* preparations for medicinal purposes entails a carcinogenic risk.

References

1. Böhme H, Hartke K (1978) In: Deutsches Arzneibuch. 8th ed. Stuttgart: Govi-Verlag, pp 405–411
2. Franz G (1969) Untersuchungen über die Schleimpolysaccharide von *Tussilago farfara* L., *Symphytum officinale* L., *Borago officinalis* L., and *Viola tricolor* L. Planta Med 17:217–220
3. Haarland E (1972) Studies on pectins from the leaves of *Tussilago farfara* L. Act Chem Scand 26:2322–2328
4. Hausen BM (1980) Allergiepflanzen, Pflanzenallergene: Handbuch und Atlas der allergiein-duzierenden Wild- und Kulturpflanzen; Kontaktallergene. 1st ed. Munich: Ecomed, p 230

5. Li YP, Wang YM (1988) Evaluation of tussilagone: a cardiovascular-respiratory stimulant isolated from Chinese herbal medicine. Gen Pharmac 19:261–263
6. Geßner O, Orzechowski G (1974) Die Gift- und Arzneipflanzen von Mitteleuropa. 3rd ed. Heidelberg: Universitätsverlag, p 403
7. Culvenor C, Edgar J, Smith L, Hirono L (1976) The occurrence of senkirkine in Tussilago farfara. Aust J Chem 29:229–230
8. Lüthy J, Zweifel U, Schlatter Ch, Benn M (1980) Pyrrolizidin-Alkaloide in Huflattich (*Tussilago farfara* L.) verschiedener Herkunft. Mitt Geb Lebensm Hyg 71:73–80
9. Röder E, Wiedenfeld H, Josh E (1981) Tussilagin — ein neues Pyrrolizidinalkaloid aus Tussilago farfara. Planta Med 43:99–102
10. Rosberger D, Resch J, Meinwald J (1981) The occurrence of senecionine in Tussilago farfara. Mitt Geb Lebensm Hyg 72:432–434
11. Didry N, Pinkas M, Torck M, Dubreuil L (1982) Sur la composition chimique et l'activité du Tussilage. Ann Pharm Franc 40:70–80
12. Zeller W, De Gols M, Hausen BM (1985) The sensitizing capacity of Compositae plants. Arch Dermatol Res 277:28–35
13. Roulet M, Laurini R, Rivier L, Calame A (1988) Hepatic veno-occlusive disease in newborn infant of a woman drinking herbal tea. J Pediatr 122:433–436
14. Röder E (1988) Wie gefährlich ist Huflattich als Hustentee? Dtsch Apoth Ztg 128:2321–2322
15. Spang R (1989) Toxicity of tea containing pyrrolizidine alkaloids. J Pediatr 115:1025
16. Hirono I, Mori H, Haga M, Fujii M, Yamada K, Hirata Y, Takanashi H, Uchida E, Kosaka S, Keno J, Matsushima T, Umezawa K, Shirai A (1979) Edible plants containing carcinogenic alkaloids in Japan. In: Miller EC (ed) Naturally occurring carcinogens — mutagens and modulators of carcinogenesis. Tokyo, Baltimore; Japan Sci Soc Press, Univ Park Press, pp 79–87

Sesquiterpene Lactones — General Discussion

B.M. Hausen

Botany

Sesquiterpene lactones (SL) are aromatic compounds widely distributed in certain families of the plant kingdom. Although known since the last century as the bitter principles of various species, most publications related to their isolation, structural elucidation, chemotaxonomy, biosynthesis, and biological effects have been issued during the past three decades [1–3]. While SL have been found only sporadically in the families of Winteraceae, Magnoliaceae, Apiaceae, Illiciaceae, Aristolochiaceae, Acanthaceae, Lauraceae, and Frullaniaceae (lichens), they do most abundantly occur in the Asteraceae (= Compositae). At least 1400 SL have already been isolated and identified from this family [3].

Chemistry

The classification of SL is based on their different sesquiterpenic ring systems. Among the major types of guaianolides, eremophilanolides, eudesmanolides, pseudoguaianolides, and xanthanolides, the germacranolides are considered the largest class [2,3]. While previously SL were mainly studied as chemotaxonomical markers in the plant families and genera, more recently increased attention has been paid to their biological activities [4,5]. Generally in individual species yields only one skeletal type of SL. However, in certain species up to four different SL types may occur. The structural feature of an exocyclic methylene group conjugated to the lactone carbonyl — the rule in a large number of SL — has emerged as functional in plant growth regulation. Such SL are also found as insect repellent constituents in different species [6–12].

Generally the highest concentration of SL is found in the leaves and flowers. Certain species store large amounts in their glandular or capitate glandular hairs (trichomes) [13,14]. When touched, these glands easily release their content of SL which subsequently elicit their various biological or pharmacological activities [15].

Pharmacology and Uses

Anticancer activity of the SL found in Asteraceae and some other plants have received considerable interest in the past two decades [5,16,17]. In structure-activity relationship studies it was shown that all cytotoxic, antileukemic, tumor-inhibiting and immunostimulating SL belong to those types that are equipped with an α,β-unsaturated exocyclic lactone [4,18]. Only a selection can be given by the following references [19–44]. Certain SL also exhibit antibacterial, antifungal, anthelmintic, antihyperlipidemic, and cardiavascular properties [34,40,45–55]. The SL of bitter sneezeweed (*Helenium amarum*) show a potent analgesic effect [56].

Digitalis-like potential has been shown for judaicin found in *Artemisia judaica* L. This SL prolonged the P-R interval in a dose of 0.2 mg/kg by 36.3% after 30 min in the isolated rat heart. After 2 h a prolongation of 90% was reached. These values approximated those of digoxin studied for comparison [20]. An antiburn effect related to some SL is said to exist as well [57].

Some SL show anti-inflammatory activity. Among the compounds studied in an edema-induced carrageenan inflammatory screen (in rats, 2.5 mg/kg) helenalin was the most effective. Similarly, helenalin suppressed delayed hypersensitivity in a methylated bovine albumine and chicken egg system [58,59]. However, neither the mentioned system nor the used animals (rats) are relevant in studying anti-inflammatory effects in delayed hypersensitivity reactions. Whether the claimed anti-inflammatory activity diminishes the known sensitizing capacity of helenalin has not been determined. Aqueous extracts of *Centipeda minima* O Ktze have been demonstrated to possess an antiallergenic activity as well. Two pseudoguaianolides of this species – 6-O-senesiolyx plenolin and arnicolide C – proved to be effective in a passive cutaneous anaphylaxis test carried out by inhibition studies of pigment leakage in rats (oral administration of 50 mg/kg) [60].

Adverse Reaction Profile

General Animal Data

A list of SL-containing species poisonous to sheep and cattle was published in 1976 [5]. Especially *Helenium* species (sneezeweeds) and *Hymenoxys* species (rubberweeds) have a bad reputation. Their principles are highly toxic, killing more than 8000 sheep each year in the United States. The first signs of poisoning seen in animals are dullness and depression. They lie down and feel weak. With standing up they begin to tremble and are unable to keep on their legs. Respiration and pulse become rapid and irregular. In other instances nausea with vomiting is the prominent sign. Postmortem examination shows gastrointestinal irritation and congestion of liver and kidney. The lungs exhibit necrotic areas due to ingesta which entered the trachea during vomiting [61–63]. Among the toxic SL identified as livestock poisons are tenulin in *Helenium amarum* (bitter sneezeweed) [64] and hymenoxon in *Hymenoxys odorata* (bitter rubberweed) [63].

Mammalian toxicity has also been attributed to the SL alantolactone from *Inula helenium* L. (alant, elecampane) [65]. This plant is for example also used in ear-nose-throat medicine to dissolve cerumen. Experimental studies indicate that toxicity of certain SL is due to a degranulation of tissue mast cells [66].

Allergic Reactions

Allergic contact dermatitis due to the presence of SL found in species of the Asteraceae, Lauraceae, Magnoliaceae, and Frullaniaceae has been described frequently in the medical literature [67–83]. More than 80 SL have been proven either in epicutaneous tests or in experimental sensitization to possess allergenic properties. Some of them could also be used in highly pure form in animal experiments to determine their absolute sensitizing capacity [83–85]. All studies performed until now with SL point to the fact that the α-methylene on the lactone combines a remarkable number of different biological activities. Plant constituents with this group are responsible not only for cytotoxic, antifungal, antibacterial, tumor-inhibiting, and immunostimulating activities but also for allergenicity. To confirm the hypothesis that the presence of an α-methylene group exocyclic to the lactone is involved in the induction of contact hypersensitivity binding of SL to amino acids has been performed experimentally. The results gave evidence for the supposition that the SL as haptens are coupled to proteins of the skin [79,86,87]. Based on these findings at least half of the known 1400 SL of the Asteraceae family must be considered as potential contact allergens. Picman et al. [79,81] have tried to make use of this effect by proposing to treat parthenin-sensitive patients (parthenin is a major SL of *Parthenium hysterophorus*) with cysteine in order to reduce the development of allergic contact dermatitis. However, we do not know whether this proposal will function in reality.

Furthermore, SL lacking this requisite (methyl instead of methylene group) but displaying other moieties such as an epoxy group or a cyclopentenone ring may also develop sensitizing properties as demonstrated recently with four sesquiterpene lactones [88].

Based on practical knowledge obtained in clinical routine it is often observed that SL-sensitive individuals tend to develop cross-reactions to related SL when coming into contact with other SL-containing species. Such cross-reactivities have not only been observed in numerous cases but also obtained in experimental sensitization and eliciting studies [68,70,72,75,76,80,82,89,90–96]. They thus should not be underestimated. The experience shows that an individual having acquired a delayed hypersensitivity to one or several SL-containing plants should strictly avoid further contact with any other SL-containing species or extract to prevent relapses of allergic contact dermatitis. Such extracts might often be hidden, e.g., in herbal shampoos, natural cosmetics, and certain medicinal ointments.

SL are low molecular weight plant constituents. They are capable of inducing the delayed type of hypersensitivity only when applied to the skin. Taken orally or administered by another route to the organism they usually produce no allergic effects. The induction of contact sensitivity in an individual depends on the concentration of the SL found in the plant, their sensitizing capacity, frequency, and intensity of application as well as the individual disposition of the human being. In case all these factors come together a plant or its extract must be considered as a risk. However, when a person has already become sensitized, renewed contact with the same plant species and its extracts or a botanically related species containing the SL only in low amounts also becomes a risk. Generally it is observed that the higher the degree of specific hypersensitivity in a patient the lower the dose of the plant or extract being sufficient to elicit a relapse. Table 1 lists those medicinal plants that may induce contact allergy in individuals handling them frequently and/or over longer periods. The number of plus signs indicates whether the SL-containing species has a strong $(+ + +)$, moderate $(+ +)$ or weak $(+)$ sensitizing potency.

Only few species of the Asteraceae and other plant families known for their SL content have been implicated in producing, besides delayed hypersensitivity, also allergic reactions of the immediate type. However it could not be demonstrated in patients that SL play any role in the causation of such reactions. Most likely high molecular weight substances of hitherto unknown character must be held responsible [97].

Dermatological Reactions

Although nontoxic, a number of very powerful skin irritating SL have been found in Apiaceae species. These occur in the genus *Thapsia*, all exhibiting a common hexaoxygenated guaianolide nucleus [98,99]. The known livestock poisons helenalin and hymenovin also function as skin irritants by liberating histamine [66].

Out of the thousands of known SL, 65 have been tested for phototoxic effects on the skin in a *Candida albicans* test. Only one, namely glaucolide G, could be shown to be a photosensitizer. The authors (Towers et al.) believe that their microbial test is indicated to prove phototoxicity of SL in man as well [100].

Fertility, Pregnancy, and Lactation

Since the last century most Asteraceae species are known to contain bitter principles that will give — when eaten by dairy cattle — a bitter taste to the milk. When present at a level as low as 1 ppm the bitterness of certain species is definitely recognized by the individuals. Such plants have received the suffix

Table 1. Plants used medicinally containing sesquiterpene lactones with experimentally determined sensitizing capacity. Besides laurel (Lauraceae) all species belong to the Compositae family

Species	Vernacular name	Sensitizing capacity[a]	Sesquiterpene lactones	References
Arnica montana	Arnica	+ + +	Helenalin, 6-O-acetylhelenalin, helenalin methacrylate, arnicolide-A	88,91,102
Arnica longifolia	Longleaf arnica	+ + +	Carabrone	94,103
Chamomilla recutita	Chamomile	+	Anthecotulide	93
Cichorium intybus	Chicory	+	Lactucin, lactucopicrin	107
Cnicus benedictus	Blessed thistle	+ +	Cnicin	Hausen & Schneider unpublished
Cynara scolymus	Artichoke	+ +	Grossheimin	69
Helianthus annuus	Sunflower	+ +	1,2-anhydrido-4,5-dehydroniveusin-A, 1,2-anhydrido-niveusin-A, argophyllin-B, 15-hydroxy-3-anhydrodeoxy-fruticin, 1-O-methyl-4,5-anhydrido-niveusin-A	104
Inula helenium	Alant, Elecampane	+ + +	Alantolactone, isoalantolactone, dihydroisoalantolactone	89,90,96,105,106
Lactuca sativa, Lactuca virosa	Lettuce	+	Lactucin, lactupicrin	107
Laurus nobilis	Laurel, Bay leaf	+ + +	Deacetyl-laurenobiolide, costunolide, eremanthin	67,89
Saussurea lappa	Costus root	+ + +	Costunolide	96,108
Tanacetum cinerariifolium	Pyrethrum, Dalmatian insect flower	+ + +	Pyrethrosin	69,76
Tanacetum parthenium	Feverfew	+ + +	Parthenolide	91,92,109
Taraxacum officinale	Dandelion	+	Taraxinic acid-1'O-β-D-glucopyranosid	110

[a] + + + = strong; + + = moderate; + = weak

"bitter" in their names, such as "bitter weed" or "bitter sneezeweed." Papers concerning the teratogenic and fetotoxic potential of medicinal SL-containing species have not been recovered from the literature.

Mutagenicity and Carcinogenicity

Some SL are said to possess a mutagenic activity. Among these hymenovin, the major toxic constituent of western bitterweed (*Hymenoxys odorata* DC), shows a remarkable mutagenic effect in the *Salmonella* Ames test strains TA 98, TA 1535 and TA 1537 [42]. Correlations between the structure of certain SL and their mutagenicity are discussed by a few authors [101,102]. However, species containing such SL are not used in medicine.

References

1. Fischer NH, Olivier EJ, Fischer HD (1979) The biogenesis and chemistry of sesquiterpene lactones. Prog Chem Org Prod 38:47–430
2. Heywood VH, Harborne JB (eds) (1977) Biology and chemistry of the Compositae. New York: Academic Press
3. Seaman FC (1982) Sesquiterpene lactones as taxonomic characters in the Asteraceae. Bot Rev 48:121–594
4. Lee KH, Huang ES, Piantadosi C, Pagano JS, Geissman TA (1971) Cytotoxicity of sesquiterpene lactones. Cancer Res 31:1649–1654
5. Rodriguez E, Towers GHN, Mitchell JC (1976) Biological activities of sesquiterpene lactones. Phytochem 15:1573–1580
6. Burnett WC, Jones SB, Mabry TJ (1977) Evolutionary implications of sesquiterpene lactones in *Vernonia* (Compositae) and mammalian herbiviros. Taxon 26:203–207
7. Char MBS, Shankarabhat S (1975) Parthenin: a growth inhibitor behaviour in different organisms. Experientia 31:1164–1165
8. Gross D (1975) Growth regulating substances of plant origin. Phytochem 14:2105–2112
9. Kalsi PS, Vij VK, Singh OS, Wadia MS (1977) Terpenoid lactones as plant growth regulators. Phytochem 16:784–786
10. Kalsi PS, Kaur G, Sharma SS, Talwar KK (1984) Dehydrocostus lactone and plant growth activity of derived guaianolides. Phytochem 23:2855–2856
11. Kalsi PS, Khurana S, Talwar KK (1985) Chemistry of costunolide and biological activity of the derived lactones. Phytochem 24:103–109
12. Rees SB, Harborne JB (1985) The role of sesquiterpene lactones and phenolics in the chemical defense of the chicory plant. Phytochem 24:2225–2231
13. Rodriguez E, Dillon MO, Mabry TJ, Mitchell JC, Towers GHN (1976) Dermatologically active sesquiterpene lactones in the trichomes of *Parthenium hysterophorus*. Experientia 32:236–238
14. Spring O, Bienert U (1987) Capitate glandular hairs from sunflower leaves: development, distribution and sesquiterpene content. J Plant Physiol 130:441–448
15. Blakeman JP, Atkinson P (1979) Anti-microbial properties and possible role in host-pathogen interactions of parthenolide, a sesquiterpene lactone isolated from the glands of *Chrysanthemum parthenium*. Phys Plant Pathol 15:183–192
16. Hartwell JL, Abbott BJ (1969) Antineoplastic principles in plants: recent developments in the field. Adv Pharm Chemother 7:117–209
17. Kupchan SM (1970) Recent advances in the chemistry of tumor inhibitors of plant origin. Trans N Y Acad Sci 32:85–106

18. Kupchan SM, Eakin MA, Thomas AM (1971) Structure-cytotoxicity relationships among sesquiterpene lactones. J Med Chem 14:1147–1152
19. Cassady JM, Ojima N, Chang CJ, McLaughlin JL (1979) Dehydrolanuginolide, a cytotoxic constituent from the fruits of *Michelia doltsopa*. Phytochem 18:1569–1570
20. Galal EE, Kandil A, Abdel Latif M, Khedr T, Khafagy SM (1974) Cardiac pharmacotoxic studies of judaicin, isolated from *Artemisia judaica*. Planta Med 25:88–91
21. Grabarczyk H, Drodz B, Hlaclov B, Wojocicchowska J (1977) Sesquiterpene lactones. XV. New cytotoxic active sesquiterpene lactones from *Anthemis nobilis* L. Pol J Pharmacol Pharm 29:419–423
22. Hall JH, Lee KH, Mar EG, Starnes CO (1977) A proposed mechanism for inhibition of cancer growth by tenulin and helenalin and related cyclopentenones. J Med Chem 20:333–337
23. Herz W, Aota K, Hall AL, Srinivasan A (1974) Antileukemic pseudoguaianolides from *Hymenoxys grandiflora*. J Org Chem 39:2013–2014
24. Jamieson GR, Reid EH, Turner BP, Jamieson AT (1976) Bakkenolide-A, its distribution in *Petasites* species and cytotoxic properties. Phytochem 15:1713–1715
25. Jolad SD, Wiedhopf RM, Cole JR (1974) Tumor-inhibiting agent from *Zaluzania robinsonii* Sharp. J Pharm Sci 63:1321–1322
26. Klimash Walady J (1981) Four new cis,cis-germacranolides from cytotoxic fractions of *Melampodium cinereum*. Phytochem 20:840–842
27. Kupchan SM, Maruyama M, Hemingway JC, Fujita T (1968) Vernolepin, a new elemanolide dilactone tumor inhibitor from *Vernonia hymenolepsis*. J Am Chem Soc 90:3596–3597
28. Kupchan SM, Kelsey JE, Maruyama M, Cassady JM, Hemingway JC, Knox JR (1969) Structural elucidation of tumor-inhibitory sesquiterpene lactones from *Eupatorium rotundifolia*. J Org Chem 34:3876–3883
29. Kupchan SM, Fessler DL, Eakin MA, Gialobbe TJ (1970) Reactions of α-methylene lactone tumor inhibitors with a model biological nucleophils. Science 168:376–378
30. Kupchan SM, Maruyama M, Hemingway RJ, Hemingway JC, Shibuya S, Fujita T (1971) Eupacunin, a novel antileukemic sesquiterpene lactone from *Eupatorium cuneifolium*. J Am Chem Soc 93:4914–4916
31. Kupchan SM, Fujita T, Maruyama M, Britton RW (1973) Isolation and structural elucidation of eupaserin and deacetyleupaserin, new antileukemic sesquiterpene lactones from *Eupatorium semiseratum*. J Org Chem 38:1260–1264
32. Kupchan SM, Kelsey JE, Maruyama M, Cassady JM, Hemingway JC, Knox JR (1973) Structural elucidation of novel tumor-inhibitory sesquiterpene lactones from *Eupatorium cuneifolium*. J Org Chem 38:2189–2196
33. Kupchan SM (1975) Advances in the chemistry of tumor-inhibitory natural products. In: Runeckles VC (ed) Recent advances in phytochemistry. New York: Plenum Press, pp 167–188
34. Lamson PD (1913) On the pharmacological action of helenin, the active principle of *Helenium autumnale*. J Pharm Exp Ther 4:471–489
35. Lee KH, Huang ES, Furukawa H (1972) Angustibalin, a new cytotoxic sesquiterpene lactone from *Balduina angustifolia*. J Pharm Sci 61:626–629
36. Lee KH, Meck R, Piantadosi C, Huang ES (1973) Cytotoxicity and in-vivo activity of helenalin esters and related derivatives. J Med Chem 16:299–301
37. Lee KH, McPhail AT, Onan KD, Geissman TA, Waddell TB (1974) Structure and absolute configuration of plenolin, a cytotoxic sesquiterpene lactone. Tetrahedron Lett No. 14:1149–1152
38. Lee KH, Kozuka M, McPhail AT, Onan KD (1974) Structure and absolute configuration of florilenalin, a new cytotoxic guaianolide from *Helenium autumnale*. Tetrahedron Lett No 26:2287–2290
39. Lee KH, Imakura Y, Sims D (1976) Structure and stereochemistry of microlenin, a novel antitumor dimer sesquiterpene lactone from *Helenium microcephalum*. J Chem Soc Chem Comm, pp 341–342
40. Lee KH, Ibuka T, Wu RY, Geissman TA (1977) Structure-antimicrobial activity relationships among the sesquiterpene lactones and related compounds. Phytochem 16:1177–1181
41. Lee KH, Haruna M, Huang HC, Wu BS, Hall IH (1977) Helenalin, an antitumor principle from *Anaphalis morrisonicola*. J Pharm Sci 66:1194–1195

42. MacGregor JT (1977) Mutagenic activity of hymenovin, a sesquiterpene from western bitter-weed. Food Cosm Toxicol 15:225-227
43. Valdes R, Crdoba F (1975) Effect of zevubrevin A and B, two new sesquiterpene lactones on the immune response in mice. Agents Actions 5:64-68
44. Wiedhopf RM, Young M, Bianchi E, Cole JR (1973) Tumor inhibitory agents from *Magnolia grandiflora*. J Pharm Sci 62:345
45. Cavallito CJ, Bailey JH, Kirchener FK (1945) The antibacterial principle of *Arctium minus*. J Am Chem Soc 67:948-950
46. Hall IH, Lee KH, Sumida Y, Waddell TG, Starnes CO, Muraoka O (1980) Antihyperlipidaemic activity of sesquiterpene lactones and related compounds. J Pharm Sci 69:694-698
47. Konder A, Bayer R, Mannhold R, Noack E, Willuhn G (1984) Studies on the inotropic actions of helenalin. Farm Tijdschr Belg 61e:240
48. List PH, Friebel B (1974)Neue Inhaltsstoffe der Blüten von *Arnica montana* L. Arzneim Forsch 24:148-151
49. Nawrot J, Beoszyk E, Harmatha J, Novotny L (1984) The effect of bisabolangelone, helenalin and bakkenolide-A on development and behaviour of some product beetles. Z Angew Entomol 98:394-398
50. Picman AK, Elliot RH, Towers GHN (1981) Cardiac-inhibiting properties of the sesquiterpene lactone parthenin with the migratory grasshopper *Melanoplus sanguinipes*. Can J Zool 59:285-292
51. Spring O, Albert K, Gradmann W (1981) Annuithrin, a new biologically active germacranolide from *Helianthus annuus*. Phytochem 20:1883-1885
52. Spring O, Albert K, Hager A (1982) Three biologically active heliangoloides from *Helianthus annuus*. Phytochem 21:2551-2553
53. Walther A, Hübel W, Nahrstedt A (1982) Herz- und kreislaufwirksame Drogen im Mittelpunkt. Dtsch Apoth Ztg 122:1547-1551
54. Watanabe K, Ohno N, Yoshioka H, Gershenzon J, Mabry TJ (1985) Structure and fungicidal activity of four pseudoguaianolides isolated from *Helenium quadridentatum* Labin. J Agric Food Chem 33:83-86
55. Willuhn G, Röttger PM (1982) Helenalin und seine Derivate, die herzwirksamen Verbindungen der Arnikablüte. Planta Med 45:131
56. Lucas RA, Rosinski S, Kisiel RJ, Dorfman L, MacPhielny HB (1964) A new sesquiterpene lactone with analgesic activity from *Helenium amarum*. J Org Chem 29:1549-1554
57. Mir-Babaev NF, Safaru SR (1983) Antiburn effect of sesquiterpene lactones. Deposited document VINITI 5401-83, 1983, Inst Fiziol Im Karaeva, Baku, USSR; CA 102 03 017613
58. Hall IH, Lee KH, Starnes CO, Sumida Y, Wu RY, Waddell TG et al. (1979) Anti-inflammatory activity of sesquiterpene lactones and related components. J Pharm Sci 68:537-542
59. Hall IH, Lee KH, Sykes HS (1987) Anti-inflammatory agents. IV. Structure-activity relationships of sesquiterpene lactone esters derived from helenalin. Planta Med 53:153-156
60. Wu JB, Chun YT, Ebizuka Y, Sankawa U (1985) Biologically active constituents of *Centipeda minima*: isolation of a new plenolinester and the anti-allergy activity of sesquiterpene lactones. Chem Pharm Bull 33:4091-4094
61. Kingsbury JM (1964) Poisonous plants of the United States and Canada. Englewood Cliffs, NJ: Prentice-Hall, Inc
62. Herz W (1978) Sesquiterpene lactones from livestock poisons. In: Keeler RF, van Kampen KR, James LR (eds) Effects of poisonous plants on livestock. New York: Academic Press
63. Kim HL, Rowe LD, Camp BJ (1975) Hymenoxon, a poisonous sesquiterpene lactone from *Hymenoxys odorata* (bitterweed). Res Comm Chem Pathol Pharmacol 11:647-650
64. Ivie GW, Witzel DA, Rushing DD (1975) Toxicity and milk bittering properties of tenulin, the major sesquiterpene lactone constituent of *Helenium amarum* (bitter sneezeweed). J Agric Food Chem 23:845-849
65. Witzel DA, Ivie GW, Dollahite JW (1976) Mammalian toxicity of helenalin, the toxic principle of *Helenium microcephalum*. Am J Vet Res 37:859-861
66. Elissalde MH, Drowe L, Elissalde GS (1983) Consideration of the structure of sesquiterpene lactones on biological activity: influence of the α-methylene-γ-butyrolactone moiety on mast cell degranulation. Am J Vet Res 44:1894-1897

67. Cheminat A, Stampf JL, Benezra C (1984) Allergic contact dermatitis to laurel (*Laurus nobilis*). Arch Derm Res 276:178–181
68. Foussereau J, Muller JC, Benezra C (1975) Contact allergy to *Frullania* and *Laurus nobilis*. Cont Derm 1:223–230
69. Hausen BM (1988) Allergiepflanzen-Pflanzenallergene. Vol 1: Kontaktallergene. Landsberg: Ecomed-Verlag
70. Lonkar A, Mitchell JC, Calnan CD (1974) Contact dermatitis from *Parthenium hysterophorus*. Trans St John's Hosp Derm Soc 60:43–53
71. Mitchell JC, Schofield WB, Singh B, Towers GHN (1969) Allergy to *Frullania*. Arch Derm 100:46–49
72. Mitchell JC, Fritig B, Singh B, Towers GHN (1970) Allergic contact dermatitis from Frullania and compositae. J Invest Derm 54:233–239
73. Mitchell JC, Geissman TA, Dupuis G (1971) Allergic contact dermatitis caused by *Artemisia* and *Chrysanthemum* species. J Invest Derm 56:98–101
74. Mitchell JC, Dupuis G (1971) Allergic contact dermatitis from sesquiterpenoids of the Compositae family of plants. Br J Derm 84:139–150
75. Mitchell JC, Dupuis G, Geissman TA (1972) Allergic contact dermatitis from sesquiterpenoids in plants. Br J Derm 87:235–240
76. Mitchell JC, Dupuis G, Towers GHN (1972) Allergic contact dermatitis from pyrethrum (*Chrysanthemum* sp.). Br J Derm 86:568–573
77. Mitchell JC, Epstein WL (1974) Contact hypersensitivity to a perfume material, costus absolute. Arch Derm 110:871–873
78. Mitchell JC (1975) Biochemical basis of geographic ecology. Int J Derm 14:301–321
79. Picman AK, Rodriguez E, Towers GHN (1979) Formation of adducts of parthenin and related sesquiterpene lactones with cysteine and glutathione. Chem Biol Interact 28:83–89
80. Picman AK, Picman J, Towers GHN (1982) Cross-reactivity between sesquiterpene lactones related to parthenin in *Parthenium*-sensitive guinea pigs. Cont Derm 8:294–301
81. Picman J, Picman AK (1985) Treatment of dermatitis from parthenin. Cont Derm 13:9–13
82. Schlewer G, Stampf JL, Benezra C (1980) Synthesis of α-methylene-γ-butyrolactones: a structure-activity relationship study of their allergic power. J Med Chem 23:1031–1038
83. Schulz KH, Hausen BM, Wallhöfer L (1975) Chrysanthemen-Allergie. Arch Derm Forsch 251:234–244
84. Benezra C, Stampf JL, Barbier P, Ducombs G (1985) Enantiospecificity in allergic contact dermatitis. Cont Derm 13:110–114
85. Stampf JL, Benezra C, Klecak G, Geilick H (1982) The sensitizing capacity of helenin and two of its main constituents, the sesquiterpene lactones alantolactone and isoalantolactone. Cont Derm 8:16–24
86. Dupuis G, Mitchell JC, Towers GHN (1974) Reaction of alantolactone, an allergenic sesquiterpene lactone with some amino acids. Can J Biochem 52:575–581
87. Dupuis G, Benezra C, Schlewer G, Stampf JL (1980) Allergic contact dermatitis to α-methylene-γ-butyrolactones. Molec Immunol 17:1045–1050
88. Hausen BM, Schmalle HW (1985) Structure-activity aspects of four allergenic sesquiterpene lactones lacking the exocyclic α-methylene at the lactone ring. Cont Derm 13:329–332
89. Benezra C, Schlewer G, Stampf JL (1979) Lactones allergisantes naturelles et synthétiques. Rev Franc Allergol 18:31–33
90. Bleumink E, Mitchell JC, Geissman TA, Towers GHN (1976) Contact hypersensitivity to sesquiterpene lactones in chrysanthemum dermatitis. Cont Derm 2:81–88
91. Epstein WL, Reynolds GW, Rodriguez E (1980) Sesquiterpene lactone dermatitis. Arch Derm 116:59–60
92. Hausen BM, Osmundsen E (1983) Contact allergy to parthenolide Acta Derm-Venerol 63:308–314
93. Hausen BM, Busker E, Carle R (1984) Über das Sensibilisierungsvermögen von Kompositen-arten. VII. Experimentelle Untersuchungen mit Auszügen und Inhaltsstoffen von *Chamomilla recutita* (L.) Rauschert und *Anthemis cotula* L. Planta Med 50:229–234
94. Hausen BM (1985) Kokardenblumen-Allergie. Derm Beruf Umwelt 33:62–65
95. Mensing H, Kimmig W, Hausen BM (1985) Airborne contact dermatitis. Hautarzt 36:398–402

96. Stampf JL, Schlewer G, Ducombs G, Foussereau J, Benezra C (1978) Allergic contact dermatitis due to sesquiterpene lactones. Br J Derm 99:163–168
97. Senff H, Kalveram KJ, Kuhlwein A, Hausen BM (1989) Asthma bronchiale durch Inhalation von Echter Kamille (*Chamomilla recutita* (L.) Rausch. Allergol 12:51–53
98. Christensen SB, Norup E (1985) Absolute configuration of the histamine-liberating sesquiterpene lactones thapsigargin and trilobolide. Tetrahedron Lett No 26:107–110
99. Christensen SB (1985) Radiolabelling of the histamine-liberating sesquiterpene lactone thapsigargin. J Lab Comp Radiopharm 22:71–77
100. Towers GHN, Wai CK, Graham EA, Bandoni RJ (1977) Ultraviolet-mediated antibiotic activity of species of the Compositae caused by polyacetylenic compounds. Lloydia 40:487–498
101. Ciegler A, Detroy RW, Lillehoj EB (1971) Pathulin, penicillic acid and other carcinogenic lactones. In: Ciegler A, Kadis S, Ajl SJ (eds) Microbial toxins. New York: Academic Press, vol 6:409–434
102. Manners CD, Ivie GW, MacGregor JT (1987) Mutagenic activity of hymenovin in *Salmonella typhimurium*: association with the bishemiacetal functional group. Toxicol Appl Pharmacol 45:629–633
103. Hausen BM, Herrmann HD, Willuhn G (1978) The sensitizing capacity of Compositae plants. Cont Derm 4:3–10
104. Hausen BM, Spring O (1989) Sunflower allergy. On the constituents of the trichomes of *Helianthus annuus* L. Cont Derm 20:326–334
105. Bleumink E, Mitchell JC, Nater JP (1973) Contact dermatitis to chrysanthemums. Arch Derm 108:220–222
106. Calnan CD (1978) Dermatitis from *Helenium*. Cont Derm 4:115
107. Hausen BM, Andersen KE, Helander I, Gensch KH (1986) Lettuce allergy: sensitizing potency of allergens. Cont Derm 15:246–248
108. Cheminat A, Stampf JL, Benezra C, Farrall MJ, Frechet JMJ (1981) Allergic contact dermatitis due to costus. Acta Derm-Venerol 61:525–529
109. Hausen BM (1981) Berufsbedingte Kontaktallergie auf Mutterkraut. Derm Beruf Umwelt 29:18–21
110. Hausen BM (1982) Taraxinsäure-1′-O-β-D-glucopyranosid, das Allergen des Löwenzahns. Derm Beruf Umwelt 30:51–53

Sesquiterpene Lactones – *Arnica montana*

B.M. Hausen

Botany

Arnica montana L. belongs to the family of Asteraceae (= Compositae). Besides arnica other vernacular names are mountain arnica, mountain tobacco, leopard's bane, and celtic nard. As arnica has been exploited extensively for hundreds of years it is now a rare species and therefore protected by law in some countries. At present arnica is in such great demand again that the related species *Arnica chamissonis* Less. ssp. *foliosa* (Nuttal) Maguire has been accepted as a substitute in the pharmacopeias of Germany and the Soviet Union.

Chemistry

Arnica montana contains 0.26–0.35% of essential oil. Furthermore tannins, gallic acid, fat, waxes, chlorophyll, inulin, phytosterin, xanthophyll, coumarins, flavonoids, carbon acids, and cynarin have been found [1–3]. Arnica contains at least 16 different sesquiterpene lactones of which helenalin, helenalin methacrylate, helenalin acetate, helenalin isovalerate, helenalin isobutyrate, dihydrohelenalin, carabrone, xanthalogine and the arnicolides A,B,C, and D are the more important. Their concentration varies from 0.1 to 0.3% [1,4–17]. Besides the sesquiterpene lactones (SL) arnica also contains two polyacetylenes and the pyrrolizidine alkaloid N-ethoxycarbonyl-L-prolinamide [1–3].

Pharmacology and Uses

For hundreds of years arnica has been extensively used as a folk remedy for sprains, bruises, painful swellings, injuries, and wounds. Recent data obtained experimentally confirm that arnica preparations and its constituents have the following pharmacological effects: antiseptic, antiphlogistic, antifungal, antibiotic, antisclerotic, antitumorous, bacteriostatic, cytotoxic, and granulopoietic. A survey of these properties and effects is given in the papers by Hahn et al. [18],

Lamson [19], List et al. [8], Trebitsch [13], and Willuhn [20–23]. The cytotoxic and antitumor activities of helenalin and its different esters were proven in different cell lines from human fibroblasts, laryngeal carcinoma, and human cells transformed with simian virus 40, human epidermoid carcinoma of the larynx as well as against Walker 256 carcinosarcoma in rats and lymphocytic leukemia in the mouse [24–29]. The antiseptic, antibiotic, immunostimulating effects and the inhibition of the function of human platelets are correlated with the occurrence of helenalin and its derivatives [30–32]. Kadans [33] claims arnica to be an aphrodisiac as well. The antihyperlipidemic activity of helenalin, dihydrohelenalin and epoxyhelenalin has been studied in mice. They produced a lowering of serum cholesterol by 30% and of serum triglycerides by 25% [34].

Adverse Reaction Profile

General Animal Data

The alkaloid N-ethoxycarbonyl-L-prolinamide, isolated in 1977 [2], has a pyrrolizidine structure but exhibits no hepatotoxic or carcinogenic effect [3,21]. Helenalin is a toxic SL for mammals. The oral median lethal dose varies from 85 mg/kg in hamster to 150 mg/kg in sheep [29].

General Human Data

Poisoning resulting sometimes even in death has been observed after internal use of tincture of arnica in the past century [35–37]. This is one of the reasons why arnica flowers today are allowed for external use only. Abuse of the tincture or decoction of the flowers as an abortifacient caused strong vomiting, exaggerated pulse, redness of the face, stinging pains, heart and respiratory dysfunction, cerebral symptoms, rigor, and bloody expectoration. Most sufferers recovered completely after a period of 3–5 days, but death caused by circulatory paralysis has been observed [36,38]. Pregnant women have been reported to loose their fruit because of this treatment [36].

Allergic Reactions

Irritant and allergic reactions of the skin following the topical application of arnica are known since 1844 [39]. In most cases tincture of arnica was the source. However, other arnica preparations such as ointments, creams, soaps, lotions and shampoos have also been observed to be responsible in certain cases. A paper reviewing the literature from 1844 to 1980 has been published in 1980 [40]. Another article reviews the literature up to 1986 [41]. Van Ketel and Bruynzeel [42] observed an allergic reaction to Arnica "jelly" while de Leeuw [43] saw a case of contact hypersensitivity due to a jogging cream. We have treated two patients with arnica allergy caused by products of the "natural cosmetic" series containing arnica flower extracts as a major component. Arnica contact allergy has been recognized in 11–75% of the clientele of dermatological clinics. An epidemiologic screening among out-patients demonstrated that arnica hypersensitivity is ranking in the first group of sensitizing agents in patients suffering from hand and face dermatitis, cosmetic allergy and ulcus cruris [41,43–45]. Due to the increased use of arnica extracts by supporters of the 'back-to-nature' movement further cases of hypersensitivity have to be expected.

The responsible contact sensitizers are the SL helenalin, helenalin methacrylate, helenalin acetate, helenalin isovalerate, carabrone, arnicolide A and xanthalongin. Their sensitizing potency and allergenic properties have been proven in animal experiments and epicutaneous tests in arnica-sensitive patients [18,34,41,46,47].

Arnica-sensitive individuals are known to cross-react frequently to extracts of other Asteraceae and Lauraceae species containing similar or chemically related SL [38,49]. Thus these patients have to avoid contact with *all* SL-containing plants to prevent relapses of their allergic contact dermatitis.

A patent has been registered in 1984 to separate the allergens from arnica flowers and other Compositae species by high pressure carbon dioxide extraction [50]. Thin-layer chromatographic examination showed that the SL were indeed removed. However, as most of them are the pharmacologically active constituents such allergen-free preparations are actually ineffective.

Dermatological Reactions

See the section on allergic reactions.

Gastrointestinal Reactions

Arnica tincture or decoctions used in former times as abortifacients caused severe diarrhea, vomiting with bloody expectoration, and abdominal pains. Thus gastrointestinal reactions have been observed and must be expected in the future when arnica tea is used [19,36,38,51].

Fertility, Pregnancy, and Lactation

See the section on general human data.

240   B.M. Hausen

Mutagenicity and Carcinogenicity

In the *Salmonella typhimurium* mutagenesis test strains TA 100, TA 98, TA 1535 and TA 1537 helenalin was inactive [52–54]. An extract of arnica showed no mutagenic effect as well [55]. This appears to be unusual as helenalin contains two functional alkylating groups, the α-methylene-γ-butyrolactone moiety and an α,β-unsaturated lactone group said to be generally necessary for mutagenic activity [53].

References

1. Holub M, Samek Z, Poplawski J, (1975) Loliolode from *Arnica montana*. Phytochem 14:1659
2. Holub M, Poplawski J, Sedmera P, Herout V (1977) N-ethoxycarbonyl-L-prolinamide, a new alkaloid from the leaves of *Arnica montana*. Coll Czech Chem Comm 42:151–154
3. Willuhn G, Kresken J (1983) Zur Frage des Vorkommens von Pyrrolizidinalkaloiden in Arnika. Pharm Ztg 128:517
4. Evstratova RI, Sheichenko VI, Rybalkov VS, Bankowski AI (1969) The structure of arnifolin, a sesquiterpene lactone from *Arnica foliosa* Nutt. and *Arnica montana* L. Chim Farm J 3:39–45
5. Herrmann HD, Willuhn G, Hausen BM (1978) Helenalin methacrylate, a new pseudoguaianolide from the flowers of *Arnica montana* L. and the sensitizing capacity of their sesquiterpene lactones. Planta Med 34:229–304
6. Holub M, Samek Z, Toman J (1972) Carabron from *Arnica foliosa*. Phytochem 11:2627–2628
7. Kresken J, Willuhn G (1983) Ein weiteres Helenalin-Derivat aus *Arnica montana* mit bisher nicht beschriebener Konfiguration. Pharm Ztg 128:1610–1611
8. List H, Friebel B (1974) Neue Inhaltsstoffe der Blüten von *Arnica montana* L. Arzneim Forsch 24:148–151
9. Luley G, Willuhn G (1985) Quantitative und qualitative Variabilität der Sesquiterpenlaktone der Arnika-Blüte. Acta Agron Hung Suppl 34:75
10. Poplawski J, Holub M, Samek Z, Herout V (1971) Arnicolides – sesquiterpene lactones from the leaves of *Arnica montana*. Coll Czech Chem Comm 36:2189–2199
11. Schulte KE, Rücker G (1966) Polyacetylene und einige andere neue Inhaltsstoffe der Arnika-Blüten. Arch Pharm 99:468–480
12. Schulte KE, Rücker G, Reitmeyer K (1969) Einige Inhaltsstoffe von *Arnica chamissonis* und anderen Arnika-Arten. Lloydia 32:360–368
13. Trebitsch F (1978) Antimicrobial action of thymol campher compared with 20 pharmaceutical preparations. Aust Dent J 23:152–155
14. Willuhn G, Herrmann HD (1978) DC-Identifizierung der Arnikablüten und Arnikatinktur (DAB 7) anhand ihrer Sesquiterpenlaktone. Pharm Ztg 123:1803–1808
15. Willuhn G, Röttger PM (1982) Helenalin und seine Derivate, die herzwirksamen Verbindungen der Arnikablüte. Planta Med 45:131
16. Willuhn G, Röttger PM, Matthiesen U (1983) Helenalin und 11,13-dihydrohelenalinester aus Arnikablüten. Planta Med 49:226–232
17. Willuhn G, Kresken J, Merfort I (1983) Arnikablüten: Identitäts- und Reinheitspüfung. Dtsch Apoth Ztg 123:2431–2434
18. Hahn G, Mayer A, Soicke H (1984) Bewährte Wirksubstanzen aus Naturstoffen: Arnika. Notabene Med 14:210–222
19. Lamson PD (1913) On the pharmacological action of helenin, the active principle of *Helenium autumnale*. J Pharm Exp Ther 4:471–489
20. Willuhn G (1973) Die Arnika – ein Beispiel gegenwärtiger pharmakognostischer Forschung. Der Inform Apoth 1:1–19
21. Willuhn G (1981) Neue Ergebnisse der Arnikaforschung. Pharmazie in unserer Zeit 10:1–7

22. Willuhn G, Röttger PM, Quack W (1982) Untersuchungen zur antimikrobiellen Aktivität der Sesquiterpenlaktone der Arnikablüten. Pharm Ztg 127:2183–2185
23. Willuhn G (1987) Sesquiterpenlaktone, potentielle Leitsubstanzen für die Arzneistoffindung. Dtsch Apoth Ztg 127:2511–2517
24. Lee KH, Huang ES, Piantadosi C, Pagano JS, Geissman TA (1971) Cytotoxicity of sesquiterpene lactones. Cancer Res 31:1649–1654
25. Lee KH, Furukawa H (1972) Antitumor agents. III. Synthesis and cytotoxic activity of helenalin amino adducts and related derivatives. J Med Chem 15:609–611
26. Lee KH, Meck R, Piantadosi C, Huang ES (1973) Cytotoxicity and in-vivo activity of helenalin esters and related derivatives. J Med Chem 16:299–301
27. Lee KH, Ikuba T, Mar EC, Hall IH (1978) Antitumor agents. Helenalin symdimethylethylene diamine reaction products and related derivatives. J Med Chem 21:698–701
28. Lee KH, Ikuba T, Sims D, Muraoka O, Hall IH (1981) Antitumor agents. 44. Bis(helenalyl)esters and related derivatives as novel potent antileukemic agents. J Med Chem 24:924–927
29. Williams WL, Chang GS, Hall IH, Lee KH (1984) Indirect inactivation of rabbit reticulocyte initiation factor cIi-2 by helenalin and bis(helenalinyl)malonate. Biochem 23:5637–5644
30. Wagner H, Proksch A, Ries-Maurer I (1984) Immunstimulierend wirksame Polysaccharide (Heteroglykane) aus höheren Pflanzen. Arzneim Forsch 34:659–661
31. Wagner H, Proksch A, Ries-Maurer I (1985) Immunstimulierend wirkende Polysaccharide (Heteroglykane) aus höheren Pflanzen. Arzneim Forsch 35:1069–1075
32. Weil D, Reuter HD (1988) Einfluß von Arnika-Extrakt und Helenalin auf die Funktion der menschlichen Blutplättchen. Ztschr Phytother 9:26–28
33. Kadans JM (1972) Aphrodisiacs. J Am Inst Hypn 13:19–22
34. Hall IH, Lee KH, Sumida Y, Waddell TG, Starnes CO, Muraoka O (1980) Antihyperlipidemic activity of sesquiterpene lactones and related compounds. J Pharm Sci 69:694–698
35. Forst AW (1943) Zur Wirkung der *Arnica montana* auf den Kreislauf. Arch Exp Path Pharmakol 201:242–260
36. Merdinger O (1938) Vergiftung mit 'Arnika-Spiritus'. Münch Med Wschr 85:1469–1470
37. Schelenz C (1938) Geschichtliches über Vergiftung mit Arnika. Münch Med Wschr 85:1791–1792
38. Lewin L (1925) Die Fruchtabtreibung durch Gifte und andere Mittel. 4th edn. Berlin: G Stilke
39. Ochsenheimer J (1844) Erythema gangraenosum in Folge der äußerlichen Anwendung von Tinct. arnicae. Österr Med Wschr, pp 226–227
40. Hausen BM, Herrmann HD, Willuhn G (1978) Occupational contact dermatitis from *Arnica longifolia* Eaton. Cont Derm 4:3–10
41. Willuhn G (1986) Arnika-Kontaktdermatitis und die sie verursachenden Kontaktallergene. Dtsch Apoth Ztg 126:2038–2044
42. Van Ketel WG, Bruynzeel DP (1988) Contactallergie voor plantenextracten bevattende therapeutica. Ned Tijdschr Geneesk 132:609–610
43. De Leeuw J, den Hollander P (1987) A patient with a contact allergy to jogging cream. Cont Derm 17:260–261
44. Eberhartinger C (1984) Beobachtungen zur Häufigkeit von Kontaktallergien. Z Hautkr 59:1283–1289
45. Tronnier H (1973) Zur Anwendung von Tensiden in der Kosmetik und ihrer dermatologischen Bewertung. Goldschmidts Inform 26:13–18
46. Wüthrich B (1980) Bedeutung der epikutanen Sensibilisierung bei chronischvenöser Insuffizienz. Schweiz Rdschau Med 69:1374–1383
47. Hausen BM, Schmalle HW (1985) Structure-activity aspects of four allergenic sesquiterpene lactones lacking the exocyclic α-methylene at the lactone ring. Cont Derm 13:329–332
48. Hausen BM (1987) Identification of the allergens of *Arnica montana*. Cont Derm 4:308
49. Hausen BM (1980) Arnika-Allergie. Hautarzt 31:10–17
50. Pfeiffer H, Goebel G, Welge W. Trennung der Allergene der Arnikablüten durch Hochdruck-Kohlendioxid-Extraktion. Ger Offen Pat. No 3319184 11/29/84
51. Anonymous (1981) Warnung vor Arnikatee innerlich. Pharm Ztg 126:2082
52. MacGregor JT (1977) Mutagenic activity of hymenovin, a sesquiterpene lactone from western bitterweed. Food Cosm Toxicol 15:225–227

53. Manners GD, Ivie GW, MacGregor JT (1978) Mutagenic activity of hymenovin in *Salmonella typhimurium*: association with the bishemiacetal functional group. Toxicol Appl Pharmacol 45:629–633
54. Witzel DA, Ivie GW, Dollahite JW (1976) Mammalian toxicity of helenalin, the toxic principle of *Helenium microcephalum*. Am J Vet Res 37:859–861
55. Göggelmann W, Schimmer O (1986) Mutagenic activity of phytotherapeutical drugs. Prog Clin Biol Res 206:63–72

Sesquiterpene Lactones — *Chamomilla recutita*

B.M. Hausen

Botany

In Europe the dried flower heads of chamomile are one of the oldest and most important drug plants. The source species is *Chamomilla recutita* (L.) Rauschert (= *Matricaria chamomilla* L.; family Asteraceae = Compositae). To distinguish true chamomile (often spelled "camomile" as well) from other species such as *Anthemis cotula* or *Anthemis arvensis* in English-speaking countries, *Chamomilla recutita* is commonly termed "German chamomile." In Spain and Latin America chamomile is usually referred to as manzanilla. Related species belonging to the genus *Anthemis* are also named chamomile and are similarly employed. Thus confusion is common. At present chamomile is cultivated in Europe extensively to serve as a drug. Recently the demand has increased so much that more than 60% of the drug must be imported from foreign countries such as Egypt and Argentina. In the United States chamomile is also so highly regarded nowadays that it is becoming one of the most popular herbal teas. A study of German chamomile covering all aspects of biology, chemistry, chemotypes, pharmacology, uses, and adverse effects was published by Schilcher in 1987 [1].

Chemistry

Chamomile contains a large number of flavonoids, coumarins, and other substances which have been investigated extensively in the past 15 years. Besides azulene, chamazulene, and guaiazulene it contains $(-)$-α-bisabolol, apigenin, quercetin-7-D-glucoside, umbelliferone, herniarin, and matricarin. The volatile oil contains chamazulene, farnesene, α-bisabolol oxides A and B, α-bisabolon oxide A and en-yn-dicycloether [1]. Some polyacetylenes are known to occur as well [2]. The commercial drug is divided into six different chemotypes varying mostly in their contents of α-bisabolol, bisabolol oxides A and B, and matricarin [1]. In such chemical races cultivated for drug uses only, the sesquiterpene lactone (SL) anthecotulide is not detectable. This SL, first isolated from the related species *Anthemis cotula* (stinking dog-fennel) [3], occurs only in wild samples of chamomile [4] and in the drug material imported from foreign countries such as Argentina, Egypt, and Chile [5].

Pharmacology and Uses

Chamomile has been reported to exhibit antiphlogistic [6–10], anticonvulsant [11], antimicrobial [10,12], antiseptic [13–15], anti-inflammatory [16–21], spasmolytic [12,17,22], antifungal [23–25], antiherpetic [26], and sedative [27] properties. Immunostimulation has been reported [28], and inhibition of poliovirus [29] is known as well. Local antiphlogistic activity is especially attributed to the flavonoids apigenin, luteolin, quercetin, apigenin-7-D-glucoside, and bisabolol derivatives [8,16,30]. Two groups of constituents are held responsible for the spasmolytic effects: the flavonoids and the coumarins [1].

Chamomile serves in dermatology, stomatology, pulmology, pediatrics, gynecology, gastroenterology and ear-nose-throat disease treatment as an anthelmintic, antispasmodic, carminative, diuretic, expectorant, sedative, stimulant, and tonic [31]. Externally it is applied as a counterirritant liniment for bruises, hemorrhoids, inflammation, and sores.

Adverse Reaction Profile

General Animal Data

Toxicity experiments using mice, rats, rabbits, dogs, and rhesus monkeys exhibited an acute poisoning effect of $(-)$-α-bisabolol, the *cis*-en-yn-dicycloether, and the chamomile oil when applied in high doses [31,32]. Vomiting in dogs is caused by $(-)$-α-bisabolol when 12.6–15.9 ml/kg are reached. However, a determination of the LD_{50} for dogs was not possible [1,7,14,18,32].

Allergic Reactions[1]

Allergic reactions of the delayed type have been described since 1921. A critical bibliographical review of 50 reports of allergic contact dermatitis [5] revealed that in most of these articles *Anthemis cotula* — the stinking dog-fennel — and related species have been the source of the observed lesions. The reason was that the touched plants were referred to as chamomile without any further identification of the species. In only five papers was there a correct botanical identification of the flowers of *Chamomilla recutita* allowing a direct correlation to the observed skin reactions. As *Anthemis cotula* is known for its commonly high amount of the SL anthecotulide some of the described strong eczematous reactions became explainable. In contrast to stinking dog-fennel true chamomile generally contains only traces of anthecotulide, making severe allergic contact dermatitis improbable. Based on this and the fact that millions of people come into contact with chamomile daily, one must consider allergic reactions to true chamomile to be extremely rare. However, in case a chamomile contact allergy has been acquired resulting in a specific anthecotulide hypersensitivity, cross-reactions to other

[1]See also the note added in proof on p. 263

SL-containing plants is common [5,33,34]. A review of all papers concerning chamomile allergy from 1921 to 1984 is given in [5]. Further cases been seen since then only in the Netherlands [35] and Czechoslovakia [36]. In both articles chamomile has been identified correctly.

Hegyi [36] mentions that he has sometimes seen positive patch test reactions to the coumarin herniarin in chamomile-sensitive patients (5 out of 28). However, it is unknown whether these test results have any clinical relevance. In a study with constituents of chamomile other than anthecotulide it was shown that neither the flavonoids apigenin, apigenin-7-D-glucoside, and luteolin nor matricin, farnesene, *cis*-en-yn-dicycloether, the bisabolols and Kamillosan preparations have any allergenic potency when anthecotulide is not present [5,37].

As a contact allergy is acquired only when the sensitizer enters the organism via the skin, the risk of developing allergic skin reactions in chamomile-sensitive patients drinking chamomile tea is very low. Similarly, delayed hypersensitivity does not develop by drinking chamomile tea, as the contact allergens, e.g., anthecotulide, herniarin (?), are not water soluble, i.e., when they are present in the crude drug, soaking with boiling water will not extract the lipophilic constituents into the herbal tea.

See the section on respiratory reactions for additional information.

Central Nervous System Reactions

Della Loggia et al. [27], studying toxicity of chamomile tubular flowers in mice, found no toxic effect up to 1440 mg/kg but noticed a depressive effect on the central nervous system in a long-time mobility test. This effect appeared already at a dose of 90 mg/kg, reaching a maximum at 360 mg/kg, but lasted for only 15 min.

Dermatological Reactions

See the section on allergic reactions.

Gastrointestinal Reactions

Oral application of chamomile in rats produced no effect up to 5 g/kg [1].

Respiratory Reactions[1]

The most common form of the drug is the chamomile tea. In very few cases symptoms of rhinoconjunctivitis, bronchitis, asthma, anaphylactic reactions, and dyspnea have been observed in individuals drinking the tea, inhaling chamomile

[1]See also the note added in proof on p. 263

vapors or being exposed to the dust of the powdered plant [38–44]. In a 58-year-old tea trader severe asthma occurred by inhalation of chamomile as an aerosol used to cure influenza [45]. In prick tests positive reactions to Kamillosan and Eukamillat solutions were obtained. Laboratory studies gave evidence for antibodies against chamomile in the radio allergo sorbent test. The responsible allergens were of protein character as they were readily bound to bromocyano-activated paper discs. It has also been reported that chronic respiratory symptoms are significantly higher in workers employed in processing different types of tea including chamomile. There also seems to be a nonimmunological mechanism by which unspecific hypersensitivity of the respiratory tract is increased when exposure to dust of tea which includes chamomile is prolonged [42,44].

Fertility, Pregnancy, and Lactation

Oral application of (−)-α-bisabolol (up to 1 ml/kg) did not influence the prenatal development of rats and rabbits nor were malformations observed [32]. Data concerning an influence on lactation have not been reported in the literature.

Mutagenicity and Carcinogenicity

Studies with the crude drug extract of chamomile using *Salmonella typhimurium* TA 98 and TA 100 strains showed a relatively high mutagenic activity [46]. However, it is still unknown whether the observed mutagenicity has any clinical relevance at all. No data on carcinogenic effects of chamomile could be recovered from the literature.

References

1. Schilcher H (1987) Die Kamille. Stuttgart: Wissenschaftliche Verlagsanstalt
2. Achterrath-Tuckermann K, Kunde R, Flaskamp E, Isaac O, Thiemer K (1980) Pharmakologische Untersuchungen von Kamilleninhaltsstoffen. Planta Med 39:38–50
3. Bohlmann F, Zdero C, Grenz M (1969) Über ein neues Sesquiterpen aus *Anthemis cotula* L. Tetrahedron Lett, p 2417
4. Yamazaki H, Miyakado M, Mabry TJ (1982) Isolation of a linear sesquiterpene lactone from *Matricaria chamomilla*. Lloydia 45:508
5. Hausen BM, Busker E, Carle R (1984) Über das Sensibilisierungsvermögen von Compositen-Arten. VII. Experimentelle Untersuchungen mit Auszügen und Inhaltsstoffen von *Chamomilla recutita* (L.) Rauschert und *Anthemis cotula* L. Planta Med 50:229–234
6. Della Loggia R (1985) Lokale antiphlogistische Wirkung der Kamillen-Flavone. Dtsch Apoth Ztg 125; Suppl I:9–11
7. Isaac O (1979) Pharmakologische Untersuchungen von Kamillen-Inhaltsstoffen. I. Pharmakologie des Bisabolols und der Bisabololoxide. Planta Med 35:118–124
8. Jakolev V, Isaac O, Thiemer K, Kunde R (1979) Pharmakologische Untersuchungen von Kamilleninhaltsstoffen. II. Neue Untersuchungen zur antiphlogistischen Wirkung des (−)-α-Bisabolols und der Bisabololoxide. Planta Med 35:125–140

9. Jakolev V, Isaac O, Flaskamp E (1983) Pharmakologische Untersuchungen von Kamilleninhaltsstoffen. Planta Med 49:67–73
10. Stern P, Millin R (1956) Die antiallergische und antiphlogistische Wirkung der Azulene. Arzneim Forsch 6:445–450
11. Abdul-Ghani AS, El-Lati SG, Sacaan AI (1987) Anticonvulsant effects of some Arab medicinal plants. Int J Crude Drug Res 25:39–43
12. Cinco M, Banfi E. Tubaro A, Della Loggia R (1983) A microbiological survey on the activity of a hydroalcoholic extract of camomile. Int J Crude Drug Res 21:145–151
13. Detter A (1981) Keimhemmstoffe als Arzneimittel? Untersuchung des wachstumshemmenden Effekts eines Kamillenblüten- und Schafgarbenblütenauszugs. Pharm Ztg 126:1140–1142
14. Isaac O, Thiemer K (1975) Biochemische Untersuchungen von Kamilleninhaltsstoffen. III. In-vitro-Versuche zur antiphlogistischen Wirkung des (−)-α-Bisabolols. Arzneim Forsch 25:1352–1354
15. Thiemer K, Stadler R, Isaac O (1972) Biochemische Untersuchungen von Kamilleninhaltsstoffen. I. Antiseptische Wirkung von Kamillenextrakten. Arzneim Forsch 22:1086–1087
16. Della Loggia R, Tubaro A, Dri P, Killi C, del Negro P (1986) The role of flavonoids in the antiinflammatory activity of *Chamomilla recutita*. Prog Clin Biol Res 213:481–484
17. Forster HB, Niklas H, Luly S (1980) Antispasmodic effects of some medicinal plants. Planta Med 40:309–319
18. Jakolev V, von Schlichtegroll A (1969) Zur entzündungshemmenden Wirkung von (−)-α-Bisabolol, einem wesentlichen Bestandteil des Kamillenöls. Arzneim Forsch 19:615–616
19. Szelenyi I, Isaac O, Thiemer K (1979) Pharmakologische Untersuchungen von Kamilleninhaltsstoffen. III. Tierexperimentelle Untersuchungen über die ulkusprotektive Wirkung. Planta Med 35:218–227
20. Wagner H, Wierer M, Bauer R (1986) In-vitro-Hemmung der Prostaglandin-Synthese durch ätherische Öle und phenolische Verbindungen. Planta Med 46:184–187
21. Zierz P, Lehmann A, Cramer R (1957) Die Beeinflussung akuter Entzündungsvorgänge durch Azulene. Hautarzt 8:552–556
22. Linde H, Cramer G (1972) (−)-α-Bisabolol und cis-2-(hexadiin)-(2,4)-yliden-1,6-dioxaspiro-(4,4)-nonen-(3) in handelsüblichen Kamillenextrakten. Arzneim Forsch 22:583–585
23. Mariann S, Gizella VP, Ede F (1976) Adatok a *Matricaria chamomilla* L. biologiailag aktiv kompenenseinek antifungalis hatasahoz. Acta Pharm Hung 46:234–247
24. Szalontai M, Verzar-Petri G, Florian E, Gimpel F (1975) Weitere Angaben zur bakteriziden und fungiziden Wirkung biologisch aktiver Stoffe von *Matricaria chamomilla* L. Dtsch Apoth Ztg 115:912–913
25. Szalontai M, Verzar-Petri G, Florian E (1976) Adatok a *Matriacaria chamomilla* L. biologiailag aktiv kompenenseinek antifungalis hatasahoz. Acta Pharm Hung 46:232–234
26. Suganda AG, Amoros M, Fauconnier B, Girre L (1984) Actions antiherpétique et antipoliomyelitique du *Matricaria inordora* L. Planta Med Phytother 18:215–255
27. Della Loggia R, Traversa U, Scarcia V, Tubaro A (1982) Depressive effects of *Chamomilla recutita* (L.) Rauschert, tubular flowers on central nervous system in mice. Pharm Res Comm 14:153–162
28. Wagner H, Proksch A, Ries-Maurer I (1985) Immunstimulierend wirkende Polysaccharide (Heteroglykane) aus höheren Pflanzen. Arzneim Forsch 35:1069–1075
29. Vilaginès P, Delaveau P, Vilaginès D (1985) Inhibition de la réplication du poliovirus par un extrait de *Matricaria chamomilla*. Compt Rend Acad Sci 301(III):289–294
30. Hörhammer L (1961) Über die spasmolytische Wirkung von Arzneipflanzen mit hohem Flavonoidgehalt. Dtsch Apoth Ztg 101:1178–1179
31. Isaac O (1980) Die Kamillentherapie — Erfahrung und Bestätigung. Dtsch Apoth Ztg 120:567–570
32. Habersang S, Leuscher F, Isaac O, Thiemer K (1979) Pharmakologische Untersuchungen von Kamilleninhaltsstoffen. IV. Untersuchungen zur Toxizität des (−)-α-Bisabolols. Planta Med 37:115–123
33. Hausen BM (1988) Allergiepflanzen — Pflanzenallergene. Vol 1: Kontaktallergene. Landsberg: Ecomed-Verlag

34. Krauskopf J, Adamkova D (1975) Tri pripady soucasne kontakni precitlivelosti na hermanek pravy (*Matricaria chamomilla*) a kovanec tamaryskovy. Csl Derm 50:299–300
35. Van Ketel WG (1987) Allergy to *Matricaria chamomilla*. Cnt Derm 16:501
36. Hegyi E, Sarsukova M, Traubnerova K (1986) Experimental study with a view of the possible evidence of sensitizing agent of *Matricaria chamomilla*. Farm Obzor 55:29–36
37. Hausen BM, Schmieder M (1986) The sensitizing capacity of coumarins. Cont Derm 15:157–163
38. Benner MH, Lee HJ (1973) Anaphylactic reaction to chamomile tea. J All 52:307–308
39. Casterline CL (1980) Allergy to chamomile tea. JAMA 244:330–331
40. Jadassohn W, Zaruski M (1927) Idiosynkrasie gegen Kamille. Schweiz Med Wschr 57:868–869
41. Jaeggy E (1931) Crises d'urticaire et d'asthma provoquées par des lavements à la camomille. Schweiz Med Wschr 61:572–574
42. Kowalewski F (1984) Rhinokonjunktivitis allergica, ausgelöst durch verschiedene Teesorten. Allergol 7:355
43. Pevny I (1984) Kamillen- und Zitronenöl-Allergie. Akt Derm 10:56–57
44. Zuskin E, Zkuric Z (1984) Respiratory function in tea workers. Br J Indust Med 41:88–93
45. Senff H, Kuhlwein A, Kalveram KJ, Hausen BM (1989) Asthma bronchiale durch Inhalation mit Echter Kamille (*Chamomilla recutita* (L.) Rauschert). Allergol 12:51–53
46. Yamamoto H, Mizutani T, Nomura H (1982) Studies on the mutagenicity of crude drug extracts. J Pharm Soc Japan 102:596–601

Sesquiterpene Lactones – *Laurus nobilis*

B.M. Hausen

Botany

Laurus nobilis L. belongs to the family of Lauraceae. Besides its common name, laurel, other vernacular terms include true laurel, sweet laurel, sweet bay, Roman laurel, and noble laurel. Laurel is native to the Mediterranean area where it has been in use for thousands of years for different purposes.

Chemistry

Leaves and fruits contain up to 4% of essential oil consisting of 50 to 100 different constituents. Usually 1,8-cineole is the main component in Mediterranean bay leaf oils. In such oils 28–62% of cineole may be found. Further important components are α-pinene, β-pinene, citral, methylcinnamate, terpineol, cinnamic acid, eugenol, 3,4-dimethoxyallyl-benzene, geraniol, α-terpineyl acetate. Furthermore fatty acids, starch, and sugars are known. Ten alkaloids have been isolated from the leaves, stem bark, and roots in low amounts. Four of them are aporphines and five are nor-aporphines. Actinodaphnine is the major alkaloid (ca 0.01%) [1]. Although sesquiterpene lactones (SL) are not characteristic for the Lauraceae, 11 different SL have hitherto been isolated [2–12]. Some of them are identical with certain SL found in Asteraceae species, e.g., costunolide from *Saussurea lappa* Clarke. Costunolide has been isolated by several investigators [5,10,13]. Due to different localizations the other minor SL such as artemorin, verlotorin, and reynosin may vary considerably in their concentration. While Strack et al. [10] found 11 SL by high performance liquid chromatography in the leaves (artecanin, ridentin B, visciludin C, deacetylmatricarin, arbusculin C, rothin B, cumambrin A and B, parthenolide, dihydroparthenolide, costunolide), El-Feraly et al. [5] could only detect four SL (artemorin, verlotorin, santamarin, reynosin) besides costunolide in the leaves of their American samples. In our own studies costunolide, dehydrocostuslactone, and eremanthin were found in the oil prepared from the fruits [13]. Cheminat et al. [4] identified costunolide, dehydrocostuslactone, tulipinolide, and deacetyllaurenobiolide in laurel leaves of French origin. Similar differences in the composition of the laurel

SL have been observed by others. Laurenobiolide was sometimes also found [14–17].

Pharmacology and Uses

Today two different preparations of laurel are commercially available besides the dried leaves:

1. An essential oil obtained by steam distillation from the leaves (laurel essential oil, laurel leaf oil)
2. An oil expressed from the laurel berries which is very fat (Oleum lauri expressum).

While the essential oil is used in perfumery and for flavoring of food products and liqueurs [18,19], the fatty oil from the fruits serves in soap making and veterinary medicine. The essential oil has bactericidal and fungicidal properties [20]. The leaves show a blood glucose lowering effect in animals with experimentally induced diabetes mellitus [21]. 3,4-Dimethoxyallylbenzene causes sedation at low doses and prevents death in mice treated with lethal doses of strychnine [20]. Oleum lauri expressum is reputed to have carminative, emmenagogue, and diuretic properties [22]. It has recently been reintroduced by supporters of the "back-to-nature" movement and has been especially recommended against lipomes and in rheumatism treatment [13]. 1,8-Cineole, known for its antibacterial properties, is used in dentifrices as a softening agent to adapt gutta percha fittings and cones to cavities and root canals in teeth [18]. Bay leaf and its oil are said to repel cockroaches and other insects [23–26].

In folk medicine laurel is used against furuncles, lipomes, abscesses, and rheumatism and in the treatment of skin diseases of men and animals [27]. Dried leaves serve as a flavor for fish, meat, poultry, vegetables, and soups. They are also an ingredient of pickling vinegars and spices. In ancient times heros and victors were decorated with a laurel wreath.

Adverse Reaction Profile

General Animal Data

Given orally to mice, laurel leaf oil may cause a reversible narcosis at doses of 40% and 80% in corn oil. A similar effect is observed in stickleback fish (*Gasteresteus aculeatus*) [20].

Allergic Reactions

Around 1990, Ehrmann [28] and Hoffmann [29] were the first to warn that laurel leaf and berry oil may cause severe lesions of the skin; the oil was being used in middle Europe in the felt hat industry as a glaze to improve luster [30–36]. Allergic contact dermatitis was also observed in cooks, homemakers, grocers, pharmaceutical manufacturers, and dentists handling laurel leaves or the essential oil [37–44]. Hand eczema in housewives occasionally is based on specific hypersensitivity to laurel leaves because of their use as a flavoring agent or in cosmetic preparations [18,22,45,46]. After replacement of laurel oil with a substitute no further cases of felt hat dermatitis have been reported. Supported by the present "back-to-nature" movement Oleum lauri expressum is again praised as a remedy against sprains, bruises, lipomes, rheumatism, and other disorders [30,47]. Recently more than 20 cases of severe allergic contact dermatitis were caused by the external application and use of this oil. Some of the SL known to occur in *Laurus nobilis* such as costunolide, eremanthin, and laurenobiolide were found to be responsible for the observed skin reactions [13,22,40,47]. As the acquired hypersensitivity is directed against the α-methylene moiety of the lactone ring, cross-reactions to a large number of other chemically related SL occurring in different Asteraceae species have been observed. These members of the Asteraceae family are botanically not related but contain the same class of SL constituents [4,13,41,48–51]. 1,8-Cineole plays no role as a skin irritant or contact allergen [52].

Dermatological Reactions

See the section on allergic reactions.

Gastrointestinal Reactions

Excessive doses of the essential oil are irritant to the gastrointestinal tract and may cause diarrhea, nausea, and vomiting [27].

Respiratory Reactions

Oily solutions with 1,8-cineole as a major constituent have been associated with lipoid pneumonia [27]. No further data on respiratory disorders could be recovered from the literature.

Fertility, Pregnancy, and Lactation

Data on adverse effects during pregnancy and lactation have not been recovered from the literature.

Mutagenicity and Carcinogenicity

Mutagenic activity of laurel leaves using the *Salmonella typhimurium* TA 98 and TA 100 strains was not detectable [53]. No data on carcinogenic effects could be recovered from the literature.

References

1. Pech B, Bruneton J (1982) Alcaloides du laurier noble, *Laurus nobilis*. J Nat Prod 45:560–563
2. Asakawa J, Benezra C, Ducombs G, Foussereau J, Muller JC, Ourisson G (1974) Cross-sensitization between *Frullania* and *Laurus nobilis*. Arch Derm 110:957
3. Boelens MH, Sindrell RJ (1986) The chemical composition of laurel leaf oil obtained by steam distillation and hydrodiffusion. Progr Essent Oil Res, 16th Int Symp Essent Oils. Berlin: W de Gruyter, pp 99–110
4. Cheminat A, Stampf JC, Benezra C (1984) Allergic contact dermatitis to laurel. Arch Derm Res 276:178–181
5. El-Feraly S, Benigni DA (1980) Sesquiterpene lactones from *Laurus nobilis* leaves. J Nat Prod 43:527–531
6. Hokwerda H, Bos R, Tattje DHE, Malingre TM (1982) Composition of essential oils of *Laurus nobilis* and *Laurus azorica*. Planta Med 44:116–119
7. Huergo HH, Retamar JA (1978) Aceite essencial de *Laurus nobilis*. Riv Ital Ess Piante Off Aro Sap Cosm Aero 60:635–636
8. Kekelidze NA (1985) Production of laurel essential oil from fresh raw material. Maslo Zhir Prom St 10:28
9. Kekelidze NA, Dzhanikashvili MI, Kutateladze VV (1987) Composition of the water soluble fraction of *Laurus nobilis* oil. Maslo Zhir Prom St 4:24
10. Strack D, Oroksch P, Guelz PG (1980) Analysis of sesquiterpene lactones by HPLC. Ztschr Naturforsch 35 c:915–918
11. Tada H, Takeda K (1976) Sesquiterpenes of Lauraceae plants. IV. Germacranolides from *Laurus nobilis*. Chem Pharm Bull 24:667–671
12. Tada H, Takeda K (1971) Structure of the sesquiterpene lactone laurenobiolide. Chem Comm, pp 1391–1392
13. Hausen BM (1986) Lorbeer-Allergie. Dtsch Med Wschr 110:634–638
14. Anac O (1986) Essential oil contents and chemical composition of Turkish laurel leaves. Perf Flavor 11:73–75
15. Salzer UJ (1977) The analysis of essential oils and extracts from seasonings – a critical review. CRC Crit Rev Food Sci Nutr 9:345–373
16. Skrubis BG (1972) Seven wild aromatic plants growing in Greece and their essential oils. Flav Ind 3:566–568 and 571
17. Zola A, LeVanda JP, Guthbrod F (1977) L'huile essentielle de laurier noble. Plant Med Phytother 11:241–246
18. Fisher AA (1970) Sieben Gewürze aus dermatologischer Sicht. Hautarzt 21:295–297
19. Kochi J, Eguma C, Kanazawa K, Sugihara Y. Deodorant. Japan Kokai Patent No 78 66434 06/06/13/78

20. MacGregor JT, Layton LL, Buttery RG (1974) California bay oil. II. Biological effects of constituents. J Agric Food Chem 22:777–780

21. Ashaeva LA, Anchikova LI, Alkhanova NA, Buzuev VV (1984) The study of sugar-decreasing action of *Laurus nobilis* leaves. Farmatsiya 33:49–51

22. Jelen G, Schlewer G, Chabeau G, Foussereau J (1979) Pflanzenallergene in Medikamenten und Kosmetika. Acta Derm Venerol Suppl 85:91–94

23. Garmon L (1982) Kitchen ecology: cukes, spices, bugs. Sci News (Washgt) 12 Sept

24. Muckensturm B, Duplay D, Mohammadi F, Moradi A, Robert PC, Simonis MT, Kienlen JC (1982) Role of natural phenylpropanoids as antifeeding agents for insects. Colloq INRA 7:131–135

25. Saim N, Meloan CE (1986) Compounds from leaves of bay (*Laurus nobilis*) as repellents for *Tribolium castaneum* when added to wheat flour. J Stored Prod Res 22:141–144

26. Verma M, Meloan CE (1981) A natural cockroach repellent in bay leaves. Am Lab 13:66–69

27. JEF Reynolds, Ed (1982) Martindale: the extra pharmacopoeia. London: Pharm Press, 28th Edition

28. Ehrmann S (1902) Toxische und infektiöse Erytheme chemischen und mikrobiotischen Ursprungs. In: Mracek F (ed) Handbuch der Hautkrankheiten. Vienna: A Hölder, pp 621–676

29. Hoffmann E (1904) Über die Primelkrankheit und andere durch Pflanzen verursachte Hautentzündungen. Münch Med Wschr 78:1966–1968

30. Bandmann HJ, Dohn W (1960) Das Lorbeeröl als nicht seltene Ursache allergischer Kontaktekzeme. Münch Med Wschr 102:680–682

31. Biberstein H (1927) Lorbeerdermatitis. Zbl Haut Geschlechtskrankh 24:586

32. Brunner L (1962) Neue beruflich bedingte Hauterkrankungen. Berufsderm 10:61–68

33. Gronemeyer W (1953) Hutbanddermatitis. Dtsch Med Wschr 78:232–234

34. Schultheiss E (1959) Gummi und Ekzem. Aulendorf: Editio Cantor

35. Spier HW, Sixt I (1953) Lorbeer als Träger eines wenig beobachteten kontaktekzematogenen Allergens. Derm Wschr 128:805–808

36. Straub W (1952) Kontaktdermatitis nach Tragen neuer Hüte. Münch Med Wschr 94:597–600

37. Eisner S (1929) Lorbeeröldermatitis. Zbl Haut Geschlechtskrankh 29:603

38. Foussereau J (1963) L'allergie de contact à l'huile de laurier. Bull Soc franc derm 70:698–701

39. Foussereau J, Benezra C, Ourisson G (1967) Contact dermatitis from laurel. I. Clinical aspects. Trans St John's Hosp Derm Soc 53:141–146

40. Foussereau J, Benezra C, Ourisson G (1967) Contact dermatitis from laurel. II. Chemical aspects. Trans St John's Hosp Derm Soc 53:147–153

41. Foussereau J, Muller JC, Benezra C (1975) Contact allergy to *Frullania* and *Laurus nobilis*. Cont Derm 1:223–230

42. Fuchs E (1954) Allergie gegen Lorbeeröl. Dtsch Med Wschr 78:697

43. Jirasek L, Skach M (1962) Perioralni kontakni ekzem s ekzematozni stomatitidon po bobkoven usta (*Laurus nobilis*). Csl Derm 37:18–21

44. Skach M (1964) Eczematous type of stomatitis. Oral Surg Oral Med 18:455–458

45. Düngemann H (1980) In-vivo-Diagnostik bei berufsbedingten Allergien. Arbeitsmed Sozialmed Präventivmed 8:177–182

46. Ebner H, Stöger H (1973) Das sogenannte Hausfrauenekzem. Wien Klin Wschr 83:901–905

47. Ott A (1984) Kontaktallergie auf Lorbeer-Öl. Ärztl Kosmetol 14:35–38

48. Epstein WL, Reynolds GW, Rodriguez E (1980) Sesquiterpene lactone dermatitis. Arch Derm 116:59–60

49. Goncalo S (1987) Contact sensitivity to lichens and Compositae in Frullania dermatitis. Cont Derm 16:84–86

50. Mitchell JC, Geissman TA, Dupuis G (1971) Allergic contact dermatitis caused by Artemisia and Chrysanthemum species. J Invest Derm 56:98–101

51. Stampf JL, Schlewer G, Ducomes G, Foussereau J, Benezra C (1978) Allergic contact dermatitis due to sesquiterpene lactones. Br J Derm 99:163–168

52. Opdyke DLJ (1975) Eucalyptol. Food Cosm Toxicol 13:105–106

53. Rockwell P, Raw I (1979) A mutagenic screening of various herbs, spices, and food additives. Nutr Canc 1:10–15

Sesquiterpene Lactones — *Tanacetum parthenium*

B.M. Hausen

Botany

Tanacetum parthenium Schulz-Bip. [= *Chrysanthemum parthenium* (L.) Bernh.] belongs to the family of Asteraceae (= Compositae) and is commonly called feverfew. Vernacular names also include featherfew, featherfoil, flirtwort, bachelor's buttons, and midsummer daisy. As feverfew has been in use since the times of Dioscorides (first century A.D.) against fever, its name must be understood as a corruption of "febrifuge" (Latin, febrifuga). It has been known especially as a remedy for female diseases, which led to the German term Mutterkraut.

Chemistry

The herb contains 0.02–0.07% of a yellow to dark-green essential oil including L-camphor, L-borneol, and different terpenes as well as their esters. Besides apigenin-7-glucoside the plant contains at least 11 different sesquiterpene lactones, e.g., artecanin, canin, chrysanthemolide, chrysarthemin A and B, 3-β-hydroxyparthenolide, parthenolide, partholide, santamarine, and secotanaparthenolide A [1–6]. Parthenolide is the major sesquiterpene lactone (SL), while the other SL are minor constituents [7,8]. Considerable differences in the parthenolide content of feverfew have been observed in plants from different geographical localities [9]. We obtained up to 0.9% in samples collected near Hamburg, Germany, in 1988 [10]. Two polyacetylene compounds have also been found in the leaves and roots [11,12].

Pharmacology and Uses

Recent studies indicate that feverfew inhibits interactions of human platelets and polymorphonuclear leukocytes with collagen substrates [13–17]. It has been suggested that its medicinal properties are related to the inhibition of secretory activity [18–20]. Other examinations revealed that relief from headache, arthritis, rheumatism, etc. might be due to an active principle in feverfew which inhibits prostaglandin biosynthesis and histamine release from mast cells [17,21,22,23,24]. Cytotoxicity of parthenolide and santamarine has been determined by Ogura et al. [25] in the Eagle's carcinoma of the nasopharynx cell culture system. Parthenolide has an antimicrobial effect [26] and exhibits a distinct anticancer activity as well [7,25]. However, most attention has been attracted in recent times to the therapeutic usefulness of feverfew in the treatment of migraine [27–36]. In a survey of 300 persons eating fresh feverfew leaves over a longer period Johnson et al. [32,33] could demonstrate that 70% claimed to get relief from their symptoms of migraine. In a double-blind placebo-controlled study the authors confirmed that a daily intake of feverfew prophylactically prevents attacks of migraine [34]. These results were recently confirmed by others [37]. Pattrick et al, did not find an apparent benefit from oral feverfew in rheumatoid arthritis [38].

As commercial preparations of dried feverfew usually contain varying amounts of the active principle [39,40], Johnson has registered a patent describing the preparation of an extract enriched by sesquiterpene lactones, as the SL are said to be the effective constituents [41]. Recently Groenewegen et al. [2] could confirm that all active fractions found in feverfew extracts with an antisecretory activity are compounds with an α-methylene-γ-butyrolactone moiety. Five constituents of the feverfew extract verified in an inhibition of secretory activity test in blood platelets and polymorphonuclear leukocytes were identified as SL [2].

Since ancient times feverfew has been used against fever. Further uses have been against headache, migraine, stomach ache, toothache, insect bites, and in the regulation of menstruation and threatened miscarriage [42].

Adverse Reaction Profile

General Animal Data

The feeding of rats with a daily dose of powdered feverfew 100 times more than taken by man did not result in loss of appetite or unexpected weight differences [33].

General Human Data

In users taking feverfew as a preventive medicine against migraine no chronic toxicity tests have yet been performed. However, Johnson [33] as well as Murphy et al. [37] state that they have noticed no serious side effects in sufferers taking the plant over years. Blood tests in long-term users showed no abnormal values. Up to 18% of the patients studied experienced different kinds of side effects [33,34,37,43]. The most troublesome were ulcerations of the mouth and a sore tongue. In some cases inflammation of the oral mucosa and tongue was seen, occasionally accompanied by swelling of the lips. However, such complaints were also noticed in the placebo group [37]. Few individuals complained of an unpleasant taste. Occasionally a loss of taste was experienced. Urinary problems and headache occurred as well. Diarrhea, flatulence, nausea and vomiting were reasons to stop treatment in a few cases. However, most of the minor side effects not causing the patients to stop eating feverfew were apparent only in the first week.

Allergic Reactions

Cases of allergic contact dermatitis due to contact with feverfew are rare. The flower is not native to middle Europe but has been cultivated for decades in private gardens. From there it spread abundantly to the open country, returning to its wild state. The first case of specific hypersensitivity was described by Maiden in Australia in 1909 [44]. Further reports were published between 1967 and 1983 [10,45,46]. Positive patch tests to feverfew or its main SL parthenolide have been obtained in patients suffering from airborne contact dermatitis [47]. Airborne particles of feverfew bear greater amounts of allergen(s) which on contact with the skin can lead to the development of a dermatitis of those parts of the body unprotected by cloths [48,49]. Risk of acquiring feverfew contact allergy has been increased with the introduction of a new ornamental form of *Tanacetum parthenium* to the flower markets under the misleading name of button chamomile [50]. European members of feverfew including the button chamomile yield parthenolide as the main SL of the plant. Experimentally the high sensitizing potency of parthenolide was established in guinea pigs in 1973 and 1983 using different methods [10,51]. Cross-reactions to other members of the Asteraceae family have often been observed in patients allergic to feverfew or parthenolide [10,50,52–55]. For a patient allergic to one or several SL, cross-reactivity means that all other plants of the family must be avoided that are known to contain similar or related SL in order to prevent further relapses of dermatitis. In view of these documented side effects, individuals with a known hypersensitivity to either feverfew (or parthenolide itself), or to other members of the Asteraceae (= Asteraceae) family should not take feverfew internally.

Central Nervous System Reactions

Chronic feverfew users are said to observe a mild tranquillizing and sedative effect [36]. However, such an effect may also be observed in patients receiving placebo [37], and it may thus perhaps be due to an effective reduction of migraine symptoms making the patient more relaxed.

258   B.M. Hausen

Dermatological Reactions

See the section on allergic reactions.

Gastrointestinal Reactions

Users of feverfew who have chewed the leaves prophylactically for years report abdominal pains and indigestion [33,37,43,56]. See also the section on general human data.

Fertility, Pregnancy, and Lactation

Feverfew is capable of causing abortion in cows [33]. Although a similar effect in human females is not documented, Johnson [33] as well as Heptinstall [31] recommend that pregnant women should take no feverfew until more detailed information on the pharmacological effects of feverfew during pregnancy has been obtained. An influence on lactation has not been recognized [31,33,37].

Mutagenicity and Carcinogenicity

No substantial differences in the frequency of chromosomal aberrations and sister chromatid exchanges in lymphocytes and in mutagenicity of urine in Ames *Salmonella* tests have been observed between migraine patients who had chronically used leaves, tablets, or capsules of feverfew and those who had not. There is no evidence of genotoxic, mutagenic, or carcinogenic effects in other reports [29,33,43,57,58].

References

1. Bohlmann F, Czedro C (1982) Sesquiterpene lactones and other constituents from *Tanacetum parthenium*. Phytochem 21:2543–2549
2. Groenewegen WA, Heptinstall S (1986) Compounds extracted from feverfew that have antisecretory activity contain an α-methylene-butyrolactone unit. J Pharm Pharmacol 38:709–712
3. Herout V, Soucek M, Sorm F (1959) Parthenolide, another sesquiterpene lactone with a few-membered ring. Chem & Ind, pp 1069–1070
4. Romo J, Romo de Vivar A, Trevino R, Joseph-Nathan P, Diaz E (1970) Constituents of Artemisia and Chrysanthemum species. Phytochem 9:1615–1621
5. Romo de Vivar A, Jimenez H (1965) Structure of santamarine, a new sesquiterpene lactone. Tetrahedron 21:1741–1745
6. Soucek M, Herout V, Sorm F (1961) Constitution of parthenolide. Coll Czech Chem Comm 26:803–810
7. Bloszyk E, Drozdz B (1978) Sesquiterpene lactones in species of the genus *Chrysanthemum*. Acta Soc Bot Pol 47:3–13

8. Drozdz B, Bloszyk E (1978) Selective detection of sesquiterpene lactones by thin layer chromatography. Planta Med 33:379–384
9. Awang DVC (1987) Feverfew. Pharm J 239:487
10. Hausen BM, Osmundsen PE (1983) Contact allergy to parthenolide in *Tanacetum parthenium* (L.) Schulz-Bip. (feverfew) and cross-reactions to related sesquiterpene lactone containing Compositae species. Acta Derm Venerol 63:308–314
11. Bohlmann F, Arndt C, Bornowski H, Kleine KM, Herbst P (1964) New acetylene derivatives from *Chrysanthemum* species. Chem Ber 97:1179–1192
12. Bohlmann F, von Kap-Herr W, Fanghänel L, Arndt C (1965) Several new constituents of the Anthemideae family. Chem Ber 98:1411–1415
13. Heptinstall S, Williamson L, White A, Mitchell JRH (1985) Extracts of feverfew inhibit granule secretion in blood platelets and polymorphonuclear leucocytes. Lancet I:1071–1074
14. Heptinstall S, Groenewegen WA, Knight DM, Spangenberg P, Lösche W (1987) Studies on feverfew and its mode of action. In: Rose FC (ed) Current problems in neurology. 4. Advances in headache research. London: John Libbey, pp 129–134
15. Heptinstall S, Groenewegen WA, Spangenberg P, Lösche W (1987) Extracts of feverfew may inhibit platelet behaviour via neutralization of sulphydryl groups. J Pharm Pharmacol 39:459–465
16. Lösche W, Mazurov AV, Heptinstall S, Groenewegen WA, Repin VS, Till U (1987) An extract of feverfew inhibits interactions of human platelets with collagen substrates. Thromb Res 48:5118
17. Makheja AN, Bailey JM (1985) A platelet phospholipase inhibitor from the medicinal herb feverfew (*Tanacetum parthenium*). Prostagland Leucotr Med 8:653–660
18. O'Neill LA, Barrett ML, Lewis GP (1987) Extracts of feverfew inhibit mitogen-induced human peripheral blood mononuclear cell proliferation and cytokine mediated responses. Br J clin Pharmacol 23:81–83
19. Rodriguez E, Towers GHN, Mitchell JC (1976) Biological activities of sesquiterpene lactones. Phytochem 5:1573–1580
20. Williamson LM, Harvey DM, Sheppard KJ, Fletcher J (1988) Effect of feverfew on phagocytosis and killing of *Candida quillermondii* by neutrophils. Inflamm 12:11–14
21. Capasso F (1986) The effect of an aqueous extract of *Tanacetum parthenium* L. on arachidonic acid and metabolism by rat peritoneal leucocytes. J Pharm Pharmacol 38:71–72
22. Collier HOJ, Butt NM, McDonald-Gibson WJ, Saeed SA (1980) Extract of feverfew inhibits prostaglandine biosynthesis. Lancet II:922–923
23. Hayes NA, Foreman JC (1987) The activity of compounds extracted from feverfew on histamine release from rat mast cells. J Pharm Pharmacol 39:466–470
24. Pugh WI, Sambo K (1988) Prostaglandin synthetase inhibitors in feverfew. J Pharm Pharmacol 40:743–745
25. Ogura M, Cordell GA, Farnsworth NF (1978) Anticancer sesquiterpene lactones of *Michalia compressa* (Magnoliaceae). Phytochem 17:957–961
26. Blakeman JP, Atkinson P (1979) Antimicrobial properties and possible role in host-pathogen interactions of parthenolide, a sesquiterpene lactone isolated from glands of *Chrysanthemum parthenium*. Physiol Plant Pathol 15:183–192
27. Anonymous (1985) Feverfew. Ir Pharm J 63:21
28. Anonymous (1985) Feverfew – a new drug or an old wives' remedy? Lancet I:1084
29. Anonymous (1986) Herbal medicine – safe and effective? Drug Ther Bull 24:97–100
30. Berry MI (1984) Feverfew faces the future. Pharm J 232:611–614
31. Heptinstall S (1988) Feverfew – an ancient remedy for modern times. J Royal Soc Med 81:373–374
32. Johnson ES (1983) Patients who chew chrysanthemum leaves. Mims Magazine, pp 32–35
33. Johnson ES (1984) Feverfew. London: Sheldon Press
34. Johnson ES, Kadam NP, Hylands DM, Hylands PJ (1985) Efficacy of feverfew as prophylactic treatment of migraine. Br Med J 291:569–573
35. Waller PC, Ramsay LE, Hylands DM, Johnson ES, Kadam NP, McRae KD (1985) Efficacy of feverfew as prophylactic treatment of migraine. Br Med J 291:1128
36. Warren RG (1986) Anti-migraine activity of feverfew (*Tanacetum parthenium*). Aust J Pharm 67:475–477

260   B.M. Hausen: Sesquiterpene Lactones — *Tanacetum parthenium*

37. Murphy JJ, Heptinstall S, Mitchell IRA (1988) Randomised double-blind placebo-controlled trial of feverfew in migraine prevention. Lancet II:189–192
38. Pattrick M, Heptinstall S, Doherty M (1989) Feverfew in rheumatoid arthritis: a double blind, placebo controlled study. Ann Rheum Dis 48:547–549
39. Groenewegen WA (1986) Amounts of feverfew in commercial preparations of the herb. Lancet I:44–45
40. Mervyn L (1986) Standardised feverfew preparations. Lancet I:209
41. Johnson ES, Hylands PJ, Hylands DM (1984) Pharmaceuticals containing sesquiterpene lactones in extracts from *Tanacetum parthenium*. Eur Pat Appl Patent No 98041, Nov 1st
42. Duke JA (1985) Handbook of medicinal herbs. Boca Raton: CRC Press, p 118
43. Turner P (1985) Adverse reactions to drugs in migraine: some recent reports. Hum Toxicol 4:475–476
44. Maiden JH (1909) On some plants which cause inflammation or irritation of the skin. Agric Gaz New South Wales 20:1073–1082
45. Mitchell JC, Geissman TA, Dupuis G (1971) Allergic contact dermatitis caused by Artemisia and Chrysanthemum species. J Invest Derm 56:98–101
46. Robertson WD, Mitchell JC (1967) Allergic contact and photodermatitis. Can Med Assoc J 97:380–386
47. Guin JD, Skidmore G (1987) Compositae dermatitis in childhood. Arch Derm 123:500–502
48. Mensing H, Kimmig W, Hausen BM (1985) Airborne contact dermatitis. Hautarzt 36:398–402
49. Senff H, Kuhlwein A, Hausen BM (1986) Aerogene Kontaktdermatitis. Akt Derm 12:153–154
50. Hausen BM (1981) Berufsbedingte Kontaktallergie auf Mutterkraut. Derm Beruf Umwelt 29:18–21
51. Schulz KH, Hausen BM, Wallhöfer T, Schmidt P (1975) Chrysanthemen-Allergie. II. Experimentelle Untersuchungen zur Identifizierung der Allergene. Arch Derm Forsch 251:235–244
52. Fernandez de Corres L (1984) Contact dermatitis from Frullania, Compositae and other plants. Cont Derm 11:74–79
53. Hausen BM, Schulz KH (1973) Chrysanthemen-Allergie. Berufsderm 21:199–214
54. Hausen BM (1979) The sensitizing capacity of Compositae plants. V. Cross-reactions in Compositae-sensitive patients. Dermatologia 159:1–11
55. Schmidt RJ, Kingston T (1985) Chrysanthemum dermatitis in South Wales. Cont Derm 13:120–121
56. Baldwin CA, Anderson LA, Phillipson JD (1987) What pharmacists should know about feverfew. Pharm J 239:237–238
57. Anderson D, Jenkinson PC, Dewdney RS, Blowers SD, Johnson ES, Kadam NP (1988) Chromosomal aberration and sister chromatid exchanges in lymphocytes and urine mutagenicity of migraine patients: a comparison of chronic feverfew users and matched non-users. Human Toxicol 7:145–152
58. Johnson ES, Kadam NP, Anderson D, Hylands PJ, Hylands DM (1987) Investigation of possible genotoxic effects of feverfew in migraine patients. Human Toxicol 5:533–534

Notes Added in Proof

P.A.G.M. De Smet

Toxicological Outlook on the Quality Assurance of Herbal Remedies: Toxic Metals in Exotic Remedies (p.43)

In January 1984, a 9-month-old Asian boy died in Florida of severe lead poisoning that resulted from the regular administration of three lead-containing Indian folk remedies since he was 2 months old. The highest lead concentration (16 mg/g) was found in ghasard, a brown powder that had been given once daily as a tonic [1].

Pontifax and Garg [2] observed symptoms and signs of lead poisoning in a 35-year-old Asian male diabetic patient living in Canada. He had been treating himself with a traditional herbal remedy acquired in India for 6 weeks. The medicine contained 8 mg/g lead, and daily use of one teaspoon provided approximately 40 mg lead per day. An association between traditional Indian medicines and lead poisoning in Asian immigrants to Canada has also been documented by Lecours et al. [3].

Mitchell-Heggs et al. [4] described combined lead and arsenic poisoning in a 33-year-old Korean woman. She had taken a Korean herbal medicine with a high content of both metals that had been prescribed to her for hemorrhoids.

McElvaine et al. [5] recently reported lead poisoning in a 41-year-old non-Asian woman residing in the United States. She had been taking several kinds of herbal pills provided to her by an Indian medical practitioner with a degree not recognized in the United States. One kind of pill was found to contain 60 mg/g lead (7.5 mg per pill), and another yielded more than 700 mg/g mercury and significant amounts of arsenic and gold. Analysis of similar folk medicines collected in India showed levels up to 7.5 mg/g lead, 440 mg/g mercury, 430 mg/g arsenic, and 2.6 mg/g cadmium.

Toxicological Outlook on the Quality Assurance of Herbal Remedies: Synthetic Drug Substances (p.47)

Steinigen [6] reported the isolation of prednisolone from an ayurvedic powder called Swasahar (origin not specified).

Giam et al. [7] described the adulteration of herbal tablets called Jamu Indonesia, Toko Air Pancur (Johor Bahru, Malaysia) with phenylbutazone and diazepam. The tablets were associated with erythematous rash and liver dysfunction in two patients and with Stevens-Johnson syndrome in a third patient.

Berberine: General Human Data (p.100)

The German Federal Committee for Phytotherapy (the so-called Kommission E) recently reached the decision that the therapeutic use of the bark, root bark, or root of *Berberis vulgaris* cannot be endorsed since conclusive proof of therapeutic activity is lacking, whereas there are risks to be considered [8].

Cinnamomum species: General Human Data (p.108)

The conditional acceptable daily intake (ADI) of ≤1.25 mg/kg bw that had been previously established for cinnamaldehyde was converted in 1980 by the Joint FAO/WHO Expert Committee on Food Additives into a temporary ADI of ≤0.7 mg/kg bw because of inadequacies in the toxicity data [9]. The Committee extended this temporary ADI in 1984 but refused a further extension in 1990 because the data it had requested in 1984 were not forthcoming [10].

For eugenol, an ADI of ≤2.5 mg/kg bw was established in 1982 [11].

Cinnamomum Species: Mutagenicity and Carcinogenicity (p.111)

The *Cinnamomum* constituent eugenol is not considered to have carcinogenic potential [11].

Eucalyptus Species: Fertility, Pregnancy, and Lactation (p.131)

Pages et al. [12] did not observe embryotoxic or fetotoxic effects following subcutaneous administration of 135 mg/kg bw of the essential oil of *Eucalyptus globulus* to mice on days 6 to 15 of the gestation.

Foeniculum vulgare: General Human Data (p.137)

In 1989 the Joint FAO/WHO Expert Committee on Food Additives reduced its temporary acceptable daily intake (ADI) value for trans-anethole from ≤2.5 mg/kg bw to ≤1.2 mg/kg bw since the available data from a chronic rat study raised the possibility that carcinogenic effects had occurred in the liver of female animals [13]. Detailed reports of this rat study have subsequently appeared. Trans-anethole was given for 117-121 weeks to male and female rats at dietary levels of 0%, 0.25%, 0.5%, and 1% (1% corresponding to 100 times the postulated ·maximum human intake). The incidence of benign and malignant hepatic tumors was slightly higher in females of the 1% group than in controls, but the investigators did not consider this increase as evidence of a significant carcinogenic risk for man [14,15].

Pyrrolizidine Alkaloids — General Discussion: Mutagenicity and Carcinogenicity (p.202)

The German Federal Health Office recently announced that it intends to restrict the availability of botanical medicines containing unsaturated pyrrolizidine alkaloids as follows [16,17]:

— Herbal medicines providing > 1 μg internally or >100 μg externally per day, when used as directed, are no longer permitted.
— A higher limit of 10 μg per day is allowed for leaves of *Tussilago farfara* to be used as a herbal tea, since usually only a small fraction of their pyrrolizidine alkaloids passes into the tea. [However, it should not go unnoted that a herbal tea prepared from the young shoots of Chinese *Tussilago farfara* was reported to contain 80% of the major pyrrolizidine alkaloid, senkirkine (see p.223 of this volume)].
— Herbal medicines providing 0.1-1 μg internally or 10-100 μg externally per day, when used as directed, may be applied only for a maximum of 6 weeks per year, and they should not be used during pregnancy or lactation.

Pyrrolizidine Alkaloids — *Symphytum* Species: Chemistry (p.219)

In the 1960s and 1970s, *Symphytum officinale* was repeatedly reported to contain echimidine [18-20]. However, more recent research has shown that this pyrrolizidine alkaloid does not occur in *Symphytum officinale,* but in *Symphytum asperum* and in *Symphytum* x *uplandicum,* an interspecific hybrid of *S. officinale* and *S. asperum* [19,21,22]. In a recent Canadian study, commercial products specifically labeled as „*Symphytum officinale*" were found to contain echimidine and therefore must have come from another *Symphytum* source [22,23].

Pyrrolizidine Alkaloids – *Symphytum* Species: General Human Data (p.221)

In Canada, the Health Protection Branch of Health and Welfare no longer accepts anything but the leaves of *Symphytum officinale* as an ingredient of comfrey preparations for ingestion [24].

Sesquiterpene Lactones – *Chamomilla recutita:* Allergic/Respiratory Reactions (p.244,245)

An additional case of chamomile-induced anaphylaxis was recently described by Subiza et al. [25]. An atopic boy with a history of hayfever and seasonal asthma developed a severe anaphylactic reaction after ingesting, for the first time, chamomile tea. Immunological testing suggested that he had cross-reacted with the chamomile pollens in the tea following prior sensitization to pollens of *Artemisia vulgaris* (mugwort).

Subiza et al. [26] also reported seven hayfever patients with allergic conjunctivitis caused by eye washing with chamomile tea. Two of these patients also had lid angioedema. Conjunctival provocation was positive in all cases, whereas oral challenges with the chamomile infusion were without effect. A positive response to conjunctival provocation could also be obtained in 2 of 100 controls with hayfever. Chamomile pollens were held responsible for the allergic conjunctival reactions to the tea.

References

1. Anonymous (1984) Lead poisoning-associated death from Asian Indian folk remedies – Florida. MMWR 33:638-645
2. Pontifex AH, Garg AK (1985) Lead poisoning from an Asian Indian folk remedy. Can Med Assoc J 133:1227-1228
3. Lecours S, Osterman J, Lacasse Y, Melnychuk D, Gelinas J (1989) Environmental lead poisoning in three Montreal women of Asian Indian origin. Can Dis Wkly Rep 15:177-179
4. Mitchell-Heggs CA, Conway M, Cassar J (1990) Herbal medicine as a cause of combined lead and arsenic poisoning. Hum Exp Toxicol 9:195-196
5. McElvaine MD, Harder EM, Johnson L, Baer RD, Satzger RD (1990) Lead poisoning from the use of Indian folk medicines. JAMA 264:2212-2213
6. Steinigen M (1983) Tätigkeitsbericht des Deutschen Arzneiprüfungsinstituts für das 1. Halbjahr 1983. Pharm Ztg 128:2254-2255
7. Giam YC, Tham SN, Tan T, Lim A (1986) Drug eruptions from phenylbutazone in Jamu. Ann Acad Med Singapore 15:118-121
8. Thesen R, Braun R (1990) Ganz oder teilweise „negativ" bewertete Arzneistoffe. Pharm Ztg 135:580-581
9. Anonymous (1980) Evaluation of certain food additives and contaminants. 23rd Report of the Joint FAO/WHO Expert Committee on Food Additives. Technical Report Series 648. Geneva: World Health Organization
10. Anonymous (1990) Evaluation of certain food additives and contaminants. 35th Report of the Joint FAO/WHO Expert Committee on Food Additives. Technical Report Series 789. Geneva: World Health Organization
11. Anonymous (1982) Evaluation of certain food additives and contaminants. 26th Report of the Joint FAO/WHO Expert Committee on Food Additives. Technical Report Series 683. Geneva: World Health Organization.

12. Pages N, Fournier G, Le Luyer F, Marques M-C (1990) Les huiles essentielles et leurs propriétés tératogènes potentielles: exemple de l'huile essentielle d'Eucalyptus globulus – étude préliminaire chez la souris. Plant Med Phytother 24:21-26

13. Anonymous (1989) Evaluation of certain food additives and contaminants. 33rd Report of the Joint FAO/WHO Expert Committee on Food Additives. Technical Report Series 776. Geneva: World Health Organization

14. Truhaut R, Le Bourhis B, Attia M, Glomot R, Newman J, Caldwell J (1989) Chronic toxicity/carcinogenicity study of trans-anethole in rats. Food Chem Toxicol 27:11-20

15. Newberne PM, Carlton WW, Brown WR (1989) Histopathological evaluation of proliferative liver lesions in rats fed trans-anethole in chronic studies. Food Chem Toxicol 27:21-26

16. Anonymous (1990) Vorinformation: Pyrrolizidinalkaloidhaltige Humanarzneimittel. Pharm Ztg 135:2532-2533 and 2623-2624

17. Anonymous (1990) Aufbereitungsmonographien Kommission E. Pharm Ztg 135:2081-2082

18. Smith LW, Culvenor CCJ (1981) Plant sources of hepatotoxic pyrrolizidine alkaloids. J Nat Prod 44:129-152

19. Huizing HJ (1985) Phytochemistry, systematics and biogenesis of pyrrolizidine alkaloids of *Symphytum* taxa. Ph.D. Thesis. Groningen: State University

20. Awang DVC (1987) Comfrey. Can Pharm J 120:101-104

21. Röder E, Neuberger V (1988) Pyrrolizidinalkaloide in Symphytum-Arten. Ein Beitrag zum qualitativen und quantitativen Nachweis. Dtsch Apoth Ztg 128:1991-1994

22. Awang DVC (1989) Herb report: Comfrey. Am Herb Assoc Newsletter 6 (4):6-7

23. Huxtable RJ, Awang DVC (1990) Pyrrolizidine poisoning. Am J Med 89:547-548

24. Chandler RF (1991) College of Pharmacy Dalhousie University, Halifax. Personal communication

25. Subiza J, Subiza JL, Hinojosa M, Garcia R, Jerez M, Valdivieso R, Subiza E (1989) Anaphylactic reaction after the ingestion of chamomile tea: a study of cross-reactivity with other composite pollens. J Allergy Clin Immunol 84:353-358

26. Subiza J, Subiza JL, Alonso M, Hinojosa M, Garcia R, Jerez M, Subiza E (1990) Allergic conjunctivitis to chamomile tea. Ann Allergy 65:127-132

Subject Index

D. R. Krishna, Kakatiya University, Warangal, India;
U. Klotz, Stuttgart, FRG

Clinical
Pharmacokinetics

A Short Introduction

1990. VI, 149 pp. 26 figs. 18 tabs. Softcover DM 56,–
ISBN 3-540-52458-4

This basic introduction to pharmacokinetics is designed specifically for the young medical doctor. The text keeps the role of
mathematical derivations to a minimum and brings the clinical
importance of pharmacokinetics upstage.
The first section of the book presents the basic principles of drug
disposition, from absorption and distribution to elimination.
Model problems and their solutions are presented in every
chapter, and pathophysiological factors are also taken into
consideration. The second section shows
clinical applications, and how drug treatment and evaluation can be made more
effective. The third section touches upon
international nomenclature and includes
numerous tables which can serve as
quick and useful guidelines in clinical
practice.

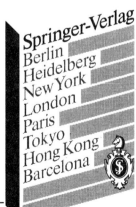

Springer-Verlag
Berlin
Heidelberg
New York
London
Paris
Tokyo
Hong Kong
Barcelona

K.-H. Beyer, Berlin

Biotransformation der Arzneimittel

2., völlig neubearb. Aufl. 1990. XV, 565 S. 5 Abb. 632 Formeln.
Geb. DM 178,– ISBN 3-540-50696-9

Biotransformation ist die biochemische Veränderung von
Arzneimitteln im Organismus. In dem Buch zum Thema
werden 330 Arzneistoffe in alphabetischer Reihenfolge der INN
(International Non-proprietary Names) in Monographie-Form
abgehandelt. Den INN-Namen folgen die chemische Bezeich-
nung nach der IUPAC-Nomenklatur, die CAS-Nr., ein Stichwort
zur Anwendung, die Strukturformel und die Summenformel.
Im anschließenden Monographietext werden die Biotransformation und die Pharmakokinetik beschrieben.
Das Buch schließt eine Lücke, als in medizinischen Lehr- und
Taschenbüchern wohl Angaben über den Indikationsbereich,
die Wirkungsweise und die Dosierung
von Arzneimitteln gemacht werden,
sich jedoch keine Angaben über
das biochemische Verhalten und
den Verbleib im Organismus finden.

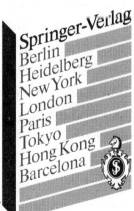

Springer-Verlag
Berlin
Heidelberg
New York
London
Paris
Tokyo
Hong Kong
Barcelona

Preisänderungen vorbehalten.